# THE COMPLETE BOOK OF

# Symptoms AND What They Can Mean

## Lawrence Galton

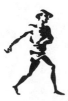

*Simon and Schuster* / *New York*

Designed by Irving Perkins
Manufactured in the United States of America
1  2  3  4  5  6  7  8  9  10

Library of Congress Cataloging in Publication Data

Galton, Lawrence.
  The complete book of symptoms and what they
can mean.

  1. Semiology.  2. Drugs—Side effects.
I. Title.
RC69.G28        616.07'2        77-26684
ISBN 0-671-22691-6

# ACKNOWLEDGMENTS

If this book serves its purpose well, it will be because of invaluable help I have had from many sources. They include medical texts on diseases and their diagnosis and treatment made available by the New York Academy of Medicine. A particularly valuable source has been the *Merck Manual of Diagnosis and Therapy*.

I have also made use of recent research and clinical reports appearing in many medical journals such as the *New England Journal of Medicine*, the *Journal of the American Medical Association, Pediatrics, Obstetrics and Gynecology, Neurology, Cancer, Annals of Surgery, Lancet*, the *British Medical Journal*, and others both of general medicine and the specialties.

Hardly least of all, I am grateful to the many physicians in research and clinical practice—those with whom I have collaborated in the past and others who have generously spent much time with me in interviews, correspondence, and checking of my work. I cannot begin to list them all for lack of space, but I must acknowledge the very special help of Drs. Benjamin F. Miller, Lawrence W. Friedmann, Broda O. Barnes, Daniel Brunner, W. Hugh Missildine, William Likoff, Bernard Segal, Paul Dudley White, Denis Burkitt, Hugh Trowell, Surgeon-Captain T. L. Cleave, Dudley Johnson, Frank A. Finnerty, Jr., and Theodore Cooper.

Finally, my appreciation to Philip James for his superb copy editing.

*To my editor, Peter Schwed,*
*for his encouragement*
*and valuable suggestions*

# Contents

# Introduction

This is a unique book in that it provides a complete guide to more than 350 symptoms and the more than 440 diseases with which they may be associated—and, as well, to the more than 250 symptoms, often confusing, that can be caused by modern drugs. In addition, it lists and describes more than three dozen often-missed diagnoses.

Certainly, the purpose is not to supplant the physician. Self diagnosis and self-treatment are playing with fire. On the other hand, more and more people today are demanding to be informed about matters of health and disease. And more and more physicians are recognizing that the better informed the patient, the better able the doctor to serve.

All of us, when ill, face a series of questions: What is wrong? Something simple, fleeting, of no consequence? Or something serious, urgently requiring medical attention? Patients, not physicians, make the decisions about when to seek help—and if this book serves well, it should help you make wise decisions.

## ABOUT THE SYMPTOMS AND DISEASES SECTIONS

Sections One and Two of this book interrelate symptoms and diseases, presenting each in alphabetical order for quick, convenient reference.

You may use the two sections in several ways.

Suppose, for example, that you have symptoms that lead you to suspect you may have a particular disease. You can immediately refer to that disease in Section Two and determine whether your suspicion is justified.

If your suspicion is wrong, or if you start out with no clear idea of what your symptoms may indicate, you can turn first to Section One.

Say that the symptom of major concern is breathing difficulty. In Section One, you find the heading BREATHING DIFFICULTY (in large capital letters) under which are listed various other symptoms with which it may be associated in different disease states. Is the breathing difficulty accompanied, for example, by such other symptoms as sharp chest pain, cough, pinkish sputum, fever following a shaking chill? That syndrome, or set of symptoms, you discover, suggests pneumonia, and that is so indicated by PNEUMONIA (in small capital letters). You can then turn to the listing for PNEUMONIA in Section Two for more information.

For added convenience, in many instances there are subdivisions under a symptom so that, for example, you find BREATHING DIFFICULTY with such subheadings as "In childhood infections," "In other infections," "In malignancies," "In congenital heart defects," etc.

## ABOUT THE SECTION ON MISSED DIAGNOSES

For one reason or another, some diagnoses are medically missed. And with the cause of one's symptoms not accurately pinned down so treatment may properly be directed at that cause, treatment instead is for symptoms, which is much less than desirable and often much less than helpful.

Section Three presents more than three dozen such conditions. Some are relatively uncommon but others affect, according to authoritative estimates, millions of people.

If you or someone you know is a sufferer from a problem that until now has seemed unfathomable despite numerous medical consultations, it is possible that you may find in this section the clue that can lead to definitive treatment for cause.

## ABOUT THE SECTION ON SYMPTOMS FROM DRUGS

Today, in addition to symptoms stemming from illness, we often face another kind: those produced by modern drugs which, simply because they are potent and effective, almost necessarily have side effects for some people.

Therefore, no book of symptoms can be complete without giving attention to drug-induced symptoms. These may be fully as bothersome and some as serious as, or even more serious than, those of illness unless they are recognized for what they are and suitable measures are taken to counteract them.

In Section Four, the symptoms that may be produced by more than 150 of the most commonly prescribed medications are presented. And, for convenience, they are presented in two ways. One listing shows individual drugs, their trade names and generic names, the purposes for which they are used, and the symptoms to which each may give rise; the second shows individual symptoms and the various drugs capable of producing each.

THE COMPLETE BOOK OF

# Symptoms AND What They Can Mean

# SECTION ONE Symptoms

## Abdomen

*The abdomen, the part of the body lying between chest and hip region, contains the stomach, large and small intestines, appendix, liver, spleen, pancreas, kidneys, gallbladder, urinary bladder.*

## ABDOMINAL DISTENTION

With one or more of the following symptoms: nausea, heartburn, upper abdominal pain, flatulence, belching, feeling of fullness during or after a meal: INDIGESTION.

With abdominal discomfort, nausea, vomiting, diarrhea, scarlet-colored tongue and mouth membranes, and skin and nervous system disturbances: VITAMIN DEFICIENCY (niacin).

With malodorous stools, vomiting attacks, muscle wasting and weakness, failure to thrive, developing in a child after age 6 months but sometimes not until adulthood, and occurring after eating cereals: CELIAC DISEASE.

With intermittent, cramplike pain, vomiting that may become fecal in nature, inability to pass gas or feces or, alternatively, diarrhea, constipation, or diarrhea alternating with constipation: INTESTINAL OBSTRUCTION.

With severe, profuse, watery, sometimes bloody diarrhea, high fever, prostration: ENTEROCOLITIS, PSEUDOMEMBRANOUS.

With abrupt fever, jaundice, fluid accumulation in the abdomen and elsewhere: HEPATITIS, ALCOHOLIC.

With abdominal fluid accumulation, jaundice, and often a tender, rapidly enlarging liver: CANCER OF THE LIVER.

21

With severe upper right abdominal quadrant pain extending into the right shoulder, remaining steadily severe for hours, sometimes with fever, chills, nausea, jaundice: CHOLECYSTITIS, ACUTE.

In a child, accompanied by chronic cough, rapid breathing, barrel-like chest, blueness, chronic respiratory infection, large, frequent, foul-smelling stools: CYSTIC FIBROSIS.

## ABDOMINAL MASS

With abdominal pain, fever, vomiting, diarrhea or constipation, emaciation: ACTINOMYCOSIS.

With pain in the flank (the side of the body between ribs and hip), blood in urine, fever: CANCER OF THE KIDNEY.

In a child, with the mass followed by pain, blood in urine, fever, appetite loss, nausea, vomiting: CANCER OF THE KIDNEY (Wilms' tumor).

Firm mass, but usually not tender, with fever, weight loss, sometimes respiratory distress and urinary obstruction: NEUROBLASTOMA.

## ABDOMINAL PAIN

Pain in the abdomen is a symptom common to many disorders, some within the abdomen itself, some elsewhere, often of relatively minor nature, but sometimes serious. It may accompany many infections and parasitic infestations, malignancies, deficiency states, and a variety of other disorders.

### In common infections

Sudden pain, with nausea, vomiting, gas sounds in the intestines, diarrhea, malaise, appetite loss, sometimes with fever, prostration: GASTROENTERITIS, ACUTE.

Sudden pain, with headache, chills, fever, nausea, vomiting, diarrhea: GASTROENTERITIS, FOOD INFECTION or STAPHYLOCOCCUS TOXIN.

With vague flulike symptoms of malaise, fatigue, headache, fever, chilliness, plus other symptoms that may include sore throat, gland swelling, severe weakness and occasionally nausea, jaundice, faintly red skin eruptions, eyelid swelling: MONONUCLEOSIS, INFECTIOUS.

Centered in lower abdomen in women, with or without a burning sensation during urination or a whitish discharge from the vagina: GONORRHEA.

In lower abdomen in men, accompanied by mild pain on urination, watery, whitish discharge from penis which may be so slight it is not noticed: URETHRITIS, NONGONOCOCCAL.

## In less common infections

With ulcers of mouth, tongue, nose or throat, sometimes of anus, appetite loss, diarrhea: TUBERCULOSIS OF THE ALIMENTARY TRACT.

With fever, chills, headache, pain behind eyes, joint and muscle pain, intolerance of light, nausea, vomiting, sore throat: ROCKY MOUNTAIN SPOTTED FEVER.

With fever, drowsiness or irritability, painful straining at stool, pus and mucus in stools, with stools increasing to 20 or more a day, severe weight loss, in children: BACILLARY DYSENTERY.

Griping pain and urgency to defecate, and pain relief following bowel movement, with such episodes increasing in frequency and development of severe diarrhea, in adults: BACILLARY DYSENTERY.

With chills, fever, severe headache, malaise, occasionally diarrhea, sometimes with backache, weakness, mental depression: BRUCELLOSIS.

With fever, lumpiness of the jaw, diarrhea or constipation, vomiting, emaciation: ACTINOMYCOSIS.

Pain throughout abdomen or localized to one area (most often the lower right quadrant), with one or more other symptoms: diarrhea, constipation, fatigue, slight fever, vague body aches and pains, sometimes painful passage of bloody mucoid stools: AMEBIASIS.

With mucous diarrhea, weight loss, particularly in children: GIARDIASIS.

## In parasitic infestations

Colicky pain, with diarrhea: ROUNDWORM, GIANT INTESTINAL.

In pit of stomach, radiating, with diarrhea: THREADWORM.

With diarrhea, dizziness, exhaustion: TAPEWORM, DWARF.

Abdominal discomfort that may become appendicitislike: TAPEWORM, PORK OR BEEF.

## In malignancies

Pain over the stomach area, usually intensified soon after eating, with one or more other symptoms: vomiting, appetite loss, unexplained weight loss, anemia: CANCER OF THE STOMACH.

Variable, often extending to the back, possibly relieved by sitting up or bending forward, often with appetite and weight loss, jaundice, nausea, vomiting (sometimes with blood in vomitus), constipation or diarrhea (sometimes with stools darkened by blood pigments): CANCER OF THE PANCREAS.

In upper abdomen, vague distress or heaviness, with weakness, fatigue, appetite or weight loss, breastbone tenderness: LEUKEMIA, CHRONIC (myelocytic).

In lower abdomen, vague, with mild digestive complaints, much later with abdominal swelling, pelvic pain, anemia, emaciation: CANCER OF THE OVARY.

In lower abdomen, intermittent, with one or more other symptoms: change in size, form, or number of stools (from few to many or many to few), blood or mucus in stools, unexplained anemia: CANCER OF THE COLON.

In the midabdominal area, crampy, intermittent, with stools darkened by blood pigments, anemia: CANCER OF THE SMALL INTESTINE.

### In deficiency states

With fatigue, appetite loss, lack of energy, aches and pains, often with irritability, poor memory, sleep disturbances, chest pain, constipation: VITAMIN DEFICIENCY (thiamine).

With abdominal distention, nausea, vomiting, diarrhea, scarlet-colored tongue and mouth membranes, skin disturbances, nervous system disturbances: VITAMIN DEFICIENCY (niacin).

### In anemias

With soreness of tongue, burning or tingling sensations of hands and feet, weakness, shortness of breath, palpitation, appetite loss, nausea, vomiting, diarrhea: ANEMIA, PERNICIOUS.

Episodes of severe abdominal pain with vomiting, jaundice, episodes of joint pain with fever: ANEMIA, SICKLE CELL.

Episodes of aching pain in abdomen, back and legs, malaise, chills, fever, with jaundice, spleen enlargement: ANEMIA, HEMOLYTIC.

### In other disorders

Pain and cramps, mild to severe, either about the umbilicus (navel) or generalized to start, then localizing in the right lower abdominal quadrant, later becoming more constant but less intense, aggravated by coughing, sneezing and movement, accompanied by nausea, vomiting, appetite loss, either constipation or diarrhea, with tenderness over the appendix area when pressed: APPENDICITIS.

Diffuse pain, severe, constant, prostrating, so intensified by movement that breathing may become shallow, often with nausea, vomiting, chills, fever, sometimes diarrhea: PERITONITIS.

In the stomach area, extending to back and chest, severe, steady, boring, often partially relieved by sitting up, accompanied by nausea, vomiting, fever: PANCREATITIS.

With intermittent fever, chills, jaundice: CHOLANGITIS, ASCENDING.

In upper right quadrant, extending into right shoulder, severe, remaining steadily severe for hours, sometimes with fever, chills, nausea, abdominal distention, jaundice: CHOLECYSTITIS, ACUTE.

With recurrent diarrhea and flushing of the skin precipitated by eating, alcohol, and emotion: CARCINOID SYNDROME.

Severe, intermittent, cramplike, in the area about the navel, followed by vomiting which may first occur simultaneously with the pain and later independently, becoming fecal in nature, with inability to pass gas or stool: INTESTINAL OBSTRUCTION, MECHANICAL (complete, of the small intestine).

Excruciating, boring pain in abdomen or back, with throbbing: ANEURYSM, ABDOMINAL AORTIC.

Pain in upper abdomen, with one or more of the following: nausea, heartburn, flatulence, belching, feeling of fullness and distention after a meal: INDIGESTION.

On either left or right side, pain may be sharp and knifelike or deep and dull, often relieved by passage of gas or stool, with constipation (small, hard or long, ribbonlike stools) or diarrhea (frequent, semisolid stools), or constipation alternating with diarrhea: COLON, IRRITABLE.

Over the stomach area, typically occurring from one to three hours after a meal, usually relieved by food or an antacid, with nausea and vomiting sometimes following a severe bout of pain: PEPTIC ULCER.

In the upper abdomen, with bloating, belching, intolerance of fried foods: GALLSTONES.

On the left side, usually low, with distention, nausea, vomiting, colic, unyielding constipation or diarrhea, or one alternating with the other, malaise, sometimes with chills, fever: DIVERTICULITIS.

With one or more of the following: nausea, vomiting with blood in vomitus, vertigo, headache, appetite loss, sensation of fullness, malaise: GASTRITIS, ACUTE.

Beginning in the stomach area and sometimes radiating to left shoulder and back, constant or intermittent, mild or severe, often with fever, jaundice: PANCREATITIS, CHRONIC.

Crampy, with nausea, vomiting, diarrhea: GASTROINTESTINAL ALLERGY.

With red skin spots that turn purple, itching, fever, malaise, sometimes joint pain: PURPURA, ALLERGIC.

With one or more of the following symptoms: nausea, vomiting, tearing of eyes, dilation or contraction of pupils, diarrhea, thirst, vertigo, confusion, throat constriction, blood-streaked stools and vomitus, cramps in extremities, collapse: FOOD POISONING, NONBACTERIAL.

Mild, with nausea, heartburn, fullness after eating, chronic or chronic relapsing diarrhea, the stools loose but free of pus or blood and sometimes containing undigested food residue: DIARRHEA, CHRONIC NONINFLAMMATORY.

With chronic diarrhea (several loose, nonbloody stools daily), fever, weight loss, often with abdominal mass, sometimes with colic on top of the abdominal pain: REGIONAL ENTERITIS.

With episodic kidney pain, blood in the urine: POLYCYSTIC KIDNEY DISEASE.

With difficulty in breathing, loss of energy, ankle swelling: CONGESTIVE HEART FAILURE.

With weight loss, diarrhea: BOWEL ARTERY ATHEROSCLEROSIS.

With chest pain, diarrhea, appetite and weight loss, anemia, weakness, fever, nonproductive cough, joint pains and arthritis of knees, wrist, back: WHIPPLE'S DISEASE.

With mild, intermittent diarrhea, nausea, vomiting, massive edema (waterlogging of tissues), especially in a child or young adult: LYMPHANGIECTASIA, INTESTINAL.

Over the stomach with sensation of fullness, persistent vomiting or regurgitation of large amounts of bile-stained fluid, severe thirst, breathing difficulty: GASTRIC DILATION, ACUTE.

With weakness, headache, malaise, sometimes nausea, vomiting: METABOLIC ACIDOSIS.

With distention of abdomen, muscular weakness, sometimes paralysis, breathing difficulty: HYPOKALEMIA.

Colicky, in paroxysms, with abdominal distention, vomiting, diarrhea or constipation, sometimes with muscle pain, convulsive seizures, psychiatric disturbances: PORPHYRIA, ACUTE INTERMITTENT.

Colicky, with sensitivity to light, excessive hair growth and skin pigmentation: PORPHYRIA CUTANEA TARDA.

With flulike symptoms of lassitude, weakness, appetite loss, nausea, drowsiness, fever, headache, sometimes jaundice: HEPATITIS.

With nasal bleeding and other bleeding tendencies, appetite loss, nausea, vomiting, weight loss, malaise, weakness, loss of libido and, in women, absence of menstruation: CIRRHOSIS OF THE LIVER.

In right upper quadrant, dull, aching, occurring in patients with congestive heart failure: CHRONIC PASSIVE CONGESTION.

With pinkish-yellow skin deposits of fat, and the abdominal pain and deposits intensified by increased fat in the diet: HYPERLIPOPRO-TEINEMIA, TYPE 1.

With nervousness, weakness, heat sensitivity, sweating, overactivity, restlessness, weight loss despite increased appetite, tremor, palpitation, stare, abnormal eye protrusion, sometimes with headache, nausea, diarrhea: HYPERTHYROIDISM.

Over stomach area, with pallor, palpitation, headache, sweating, nausea, apprehension, high blood pressure: PHEOCHROMOCYTOMA.

With weakness, appetite loss, nausea, constipation, thirst, excessive urination, calcium stones in urinary tract: HYPERPARATHYROID-ISM.

With fever, weight loss, and one or more of the following: diffuse muscle pain, joint pains, bloody diarrhea, wheezing, pneumonia, hives, reddening of the skin: POLYARTERITIS.

With tiredness, vague limb pain, nosebleeds, followed by joint swellings and pain, sometimes spasmodic twitching movements, body rash, nodules at elbows, knees, wrists: RHEUMATIC FEVER.

In lower abdomen, cramping, with diarrhea, blood and mucus in stools: POLYPS.

Excruciating intermittent pain starting in kidney area and radiating across abdomen into genital area and inner aspects of the thigh, sometimes with nausea, vomiting, chills, fever, urinary frequency: URINARY CALCULI.

## ACHING, GENERALIZED

With one or more of the following: headache, toothache, nasal and postnasal discharge, fever, puffiness about the eyes: SINUSITIS.

Most pronounced in back and legs, with headache, mild distress below the breastbone, chills, fever, weakness, appetite loss, sore throat, unproductive cough, sometimes nasal discharge: INFLUENZA.

With fatigue, appetite loss, lack of energy, and often with irritability, poor memory, sleep disturbances, chest pain, abdominal discomfort, constipation: VITAMIN DEFICIENCY (thiamine).

## AGITATION

With headache, vision blurring, and sometimes confusion, depression, other mental disturbance: CRYPTOCOCCOSIS.

With palpitation, flushing, itching, ear throbbing, coughing, sneezing, breathing difficulty: ANAPHYLAXIS.

With pallor, moist and cool skin, racing pulse: SHOCK.

With tingling or burning sensations, lightheadedness, fainting: RESPIRATORY ALKALOSIS.

## ANEMIA

Anemia (see also Section Two) is a condition in which red cells in the blood either are deficient in number or contain inadequate amounts of hemoglobin (the red pigment that transports oxygen to body tissues).

In mild anemia, symptoms may be limited to diminished energy and a tendency to become fatigued easily. In more severe anemia, they may include weakness, vertigo, headache, ringing of the ears, spots before the eyes, drowsiness, irritability, euphoria, psychotic behavior, failure of menses, loss of libido, low-grade fever, gastrointestinal complaints, jaundice, congestive heart failure.

Massive bleeding from a wound or chronic slow loss of blood such as from a bleeding ulcer or excessive menstrual flow may lead to anemia. Pernicious anemia results from lack of intrinsic factor, a material in the stomach required for absorption of vitamin $B_{12}$ from the diet. Sickle cell anemia, which occurs mainly in blacks, and Cooley's anemia (also known as thalassemia major), which occurs mainly in people of Mediterranean parentage, are genetically determined defects of hemoglobin formation.

Among the most common anemias in the United States, occurring mainly in women, are those due to deficiency in the diet of iron and the vitamin folic acid.

Anemias also may be associated with other deficiencies and with other symptoms caused by varied disease states:

With growth retardation, darkening of stools from blood pigments: HOOKWORM INFESTATION.

With nausea, diarrhea, retarded growth: WHIPWORM.

With weakness, fatigue, enlarged spleen, vomiting of blood, stools discolored by blood: BANTI'S DISEASE.

With weight loss, repeated infections, bleeding of mucous membranes: MACROGLOBULINEMIA.

With coughing and spitting of blood, breathing difficulty, blood in urine: GOODPASTURE'S SYNDROME.

With diarrhea, appetite and weight loss, weakness, fatigability, muscle cramps: SPRUE, TROPICAL.

With appetite and weight loss, diarrhea, weakness, fever, joint pains and arthritis of knees, wrists and back, nonproductive cough, abdominal and chest pain: WHIPPLE'S DISEASE.

With pain over stomach area, usually more intense after meals, sometimes with one or more other symptoms such as appetite loss, vomiting, weight loss: CANCER OF THE STOMACH.

With intermittent midabdominal cramps, darkening of stools with blood pigments: CANCER OF THE SMALL INTESTINE.

With intermittent lower abdominal cramps, change in stools (from few to many or many to few, sometimes with alterations in size and form): CANCER OF THE COLON.

With irritability, fever, appetite loss, failure to gain weight, in a child: SCURVY.

With yellowish, greasy scaling of scalp, inflammation of tongue, fissuring of lips and angles of mouth: VITAMIN DEFICIENCY (pyridoxine).

## ANKLE

Abnormal bending or flexion, with similar flexion of wrist joints, muscle twitching, cramps, convulsion: TETANY.

Throbbing, crushing pain, appearing suddenly, accompanied by swelling, warmth, redness, shininess of the skin: GOUT.

Swelling with fluid, accompanied by loss of energy, breathing difficulty: CONGESTIVE HEART FAILURE.

## Anus
*The anus is the opening of the rectum on the body surface.*

## ANAL BLISTERS

With red patches, pustules, itching: CANDIDIASIS.

## ANAL DISCHARGE

Purulent, often with skin irritation, recurring abscess formation: FISTULA-IN-ANO.

## ANAL ITCHING (PRURITUS ANI)

The anal area, moist and regularly exposed to fecal material, is susceptible to a scratch-itch cycle. Among possible causes of chronic itching are poor hygiene, irritating soaps and clothing, minor injury from defecation, local diseases such as HEMORRHOIDS, FISSURE, and FISTULA, infectious and parasitic organisms such as fungi and PINWORMS, allergic conditions, DIABETES, and other systemic disorders. Cure is likely if a definite cause can be found and eliminated. Otherwise, treatment may include applications of talc or dusting powder after gentle drying of the skin, avoidance of scratching, and, in severe cases, use of a corticosteroid cream. Conventional anesthetic or other ointments are avoided because they macerate the skin and make it more prone to injury.

## ANAL PAIN

And spasm, intensifying with defecation: FISSURE-IN-ANO.

With red anal swelling, the pain often intensified on walking, sitting, defecation: ANORECTAL ABSCESS.

## APATHY

With one or more of the following symptoms: poor appetite, weight loss, easy fatigue, intolerance of cold, diminished libido, scantiness or absence of pubic and underarm hair, or in women scanty menstruation, failure to lactate after childbirth: HYPOPITUITARISM.

With one or more of the following symptoms: dry cold skin, chilliness, puffiness of hands and face, decreased appetite, weight gain, slowness of speech, drowsiness, constipation, hearing loss, poor memory, and in women excessive or absent menstruation: HYPOTHYROIDISM.

With thick, dry, wrinkled skin, enlarged tongue, thickened lips, broad face, flat nose, puffy feet and hands, dullness, mental retardation, in a child: CRETINISM.

## APPETITE LOSS

Temporary appetite loss, of course, can result from unattractive food, surroundings or company, and emotional states such as anxiety, irritation, anger, and fear. *Chronic* appetite loss, known as *anorexia*, may be a symptom of physical disorders or chronic emotional disturbances; in the latter case it is known as ANOREXIA NERVOSA.

## In childhood infections

With slight fever, headache, backache, rash: CHICKENPOX.

With fever, headache, back pain, gland swelling on either side of the face just below and in front of the ears: MUMPS.

With running nose, sneezing, tearing of the eyes, listlessness, hacking cough at night, rarely fever: WHOOPING COUGH.

## In common infections

With fever, chills, generalized aches and pains that tend to be most pronounced in the back and legs, headache, weakness, sore throat, unproductive cough, mild distress below breastbone, sometimes nasal discharge: INFLUENZA.

With cough, pinkish sputum sometimes becoming rusty, fever often starting with a shaking chill, headache, breathing difficulty, rapid and painful respiration, sometimes with malaise, muscular pain: PNEUMONIA.

With influenzalike symptoms of lassitude, weakness, nausea, drowsiness, abdominal discomfort, fever, headache, sometimes with jaundice: HEPATITIS.

## In other infections

With chills, fever, headache, pain behind eyes, joint and muscle pain, intolerance of light, nausea, vomiting, sore throat, abdominal pain: ROCKY MOUNTAIN SPOTTED FEVER AND OTHER RICKETTSIAL DISEASES.

With chills, fever, severe headache, malaise, occasionally diarrhea—or, alternatively, muscular pain, headache, back pain: BRUCELLOSIS.

With fever, weight loss, fatigue, drowsiness, listlessness, vague pain in chest: TUBERCULOSIS.

With malaise, headache, nosebleeds, backache, diarrhea or constipation, sore throat, fever: TYPHOID FEVER.

With a persistent sore occurring a few days after and at the site of a minor cat scratch, followed within two weeks by gland swellings at sites near the scratch, fever, malaise, headache: CAT-SCRATCH DISEASE.

With cough, purulent sputum, malaise, sweats, chills, fever, sometimes chest pain: LUNG ABSCESS.

With fever, chills, malaise, dry cough becoming productive with mucopurulent sputum: PSITTACOSIS.

With ulcers of mucous membranes of mouth, tongue, nose or

throat, or anus, abdominal discomfort, diarrhea: TUBERCULOSIS OF THE ALIMENTARY TRACT.

## In malignancies

With weakness, fatigue, weight loss, vague upper abdominal distress or heaviness, breastbone tenderness: LEUKEMIA, CHRONIC (myelocytic).

With weakness, fatigue, lymph gland (node) swellings, mild pallor: LEUKEMIA, CHRONIC (lymphocytic).

Following appearance of gland (node) swellings in neck, under arms, and in groin, and itching, sometimes accompanied later by weakness, fever, weight loss: HODGKIN'S DISEASE.

With abdominal mass and pain, blood in urine, fever, nausea, vomiting, in a child: CANCER OF THE KIDNEY (Wilms' tumor).

With upper abdominal distress and pain over stomach area, usually intensified shortly after eating, sometimes with one or more other symptoms such as unexplained weight loss and anemia: CANCER OF THE STOMACH.

With variable abdominal pain, often extending to the back, relieved by sitting up or bending forward, with one or more other symptoms: jaundice, weight loss, nausea, vomiting, constipation or diarrhea, sometimes with vomiting of blood and darkening of stools with blood pigments: CANCER OF THE PANCREAS.

## In deficiency states

With fatigue, lack of energy, aches and pains, sometimes also with irritability, poor memory, sleep disturbances, chest pain, abdominal discomfort, constipation: VITAMIN DEFICIENCY (thiamine).

With fatigue, lack of energy, aches and pains, memory impairment, confusion, sore mouth, scarlet tongue and oral membranes, skin and gastrointestinal disturbances: VITAMIN DEFICIENCY (niacin).

With failure to gain weight, fever, anemia, irritability, in a child: SCURVY.

With swelling of legs, the swelling becoming generalized, digestive disturbances, weight loss, weakness, lethargy: PROTEIN DEFICIENCY (chronic).

With one or more of the following symptoms: apathy, weight loss, easy fatigue, cold intolerance, diminished libido, scantiness or absence of pubic and underarm hair, and, in a woman, scanty menstruation, failure to lactate after childbirth: HYPOPITUITARISM.

With one or more of the following symptoms: chilliness, dry and cold skin, puffiness of hands and face, weight gain, slow speech, mental apathy, drowsiness, constipation, hearing loss, poor memory, and in a woman excessive menstruation or absence of it: HYPOTHYROIDISM.

## In other disorders

With abdominal pain or pressure and one or more other symptoms: malaise, sensation of fullness, nausea, headache, vertigo, vomiting, blood in vomitus: GASTRITIS, ACUTE.

With abdominal pain beginning in umbilical (navel) area and shifting to right lower quadrant, nausea, vomiting, constipation or diarrhea: APPENDICITIS.

With sudden abdominal cramps, malaise, nausea, vomiting, gas sounds in the intestines, diarrhea: GASTROENTERITIS, ACUTE.

With labored breathing, ankle swelling, loss of energy: CONGESTIVE HEART FAILURE.

With fever, chills, malaise, joint pains, lassitude, sometimes tender, small nodules on tips of digits: ENDOCARDITIS, BACTERIAL.

With difficult breathing, deeper and more rapid than normal respiration, coughing and spitting of blood, chest pain, hoarseness, blueness, malaise: SILICOSIS.

With weight loss, breathing difficulty, one or more other symptoms: blueness after exercise, rapid pulse, dry, nonproductive cough, fever, malaise, easy fatigability: PULMONARY GRANULOMATOSES.

With fatigue, lassitude, decreased mental acuity, one or more other symptoms: muscular cramps and twitching, convulsions, nausea, vomiting, yellow-brown skin discoloration, hiccuping, urine smell on breath and sweat, itching: UREMIA.

With diarrhea, weight loss becoming increasingly marked after weeks or months, followed by anemia, weakness, fatigability, muscle cramps: SPRUE, TROPICAL.

With diarrhea, weight loss, anemia, weakness, fever of 100° to 103°, joint pains and arthritis of knees, wrist and back, nonproductive cough, abdominal and chest pain: WHIPPLE'S DISEASE.

With nausea, vomiting, weight loss, malaise, weakness, abdominal discomfort, loss of libido, nasal and other bleeding tendencies, and, in a woman, absence of menstruation: CIRRHOSIS OF THE LIVER.

With nausea, vomiting, excessive urination, excessive thirst, weakness, nervousness, itching: HYPERVITAMINOSIS D.

With increasing weakness, easy fatigability, increased skin pigmentation, black freckles over forehead, face, neck, shoulders, bluish-black discolorations of mucous membranes of lips, mouth and other sites, weight loss, nausea, vomiting, diarrhea, decreased cold tolerance, dizziness, fainting attacks: ADDISON'S DISEASE.

With weakness, nausea, constipation, abdominal pain, thirst, excessive urination, calcium stones in urinary tract: HYPERPARATHYROIDISM.

## ARM

Sudden coldness with numbness, tingling, followed soon by severe pain, blanching or mottling with blue patches: ACUTE ARTERIAL OCCLUSION.

Lameness, with one or more of the following symptoms: fainting attacks or epilepsylike seizures, speech and vision disturbances, transient blindness: AORTIC ARCH SYNDROME.

Stiffness, with stiffness of jaw and neck, swallowing difficulty, fever, sore throat: TETANUS.

Swelling, with increased skin warmth: VENOUS THROMBOSIS.

Swelling, chronic, painless, of whole or part of arm or leg: LYMPHEDEMA.

Swelling, often with swelling of legs, face, torso: NEPHROTIC SYNDROME.

## BACK PAIN

At some time in life, back pain is said to affect about eight out of ten persons severely enough to send them for medical help. A common cause is acute lumbosacral and sacroiliac strain such as may result from lifting a heavy object, twisting the trunk, or bending over. Treatment may include bed rest, massage, aspirin, muscle-relaxant drugs, heat applications. In some cases, including those with sciatica (or pain down a leg), degeneration of spinal disks may be involved. Treatment in the acute phase is the same as for strain, followed by further treatment later which sometimes may include disk surgery. Arthritic changes in the spine may cause back pain, and treatment may include rest on a firm bed, local heat, massage, aspirin, and, if necessary, phenylbutazone or another drug. But back pain, sometimes persistent, sometimes not, may accompany infections and other conditions:

### In infections

With muscle pain, sore throat, nasal discharge, malaise, chilliness, slight fever, nonproductive cough gradually becoming productive of sputum: BRONCHITIS, ACUTE.

On one or both sides of lower back, with urinary frequency and urgency, chills, fever, headache: PYELONEPHRITIS.

With fever, chills, generalized aches and pains, leg pain, headache, weakness, appetite loss, sore throat, nonproductive cough, mild distress under breastbone, sometimes nasal discharge: INFLUENZA.

With swelling of parotid glands just below and in front of ears, fever, headache, appetite loss: MUMPS.

With slight fever, headache, appetite loss, rash: CHICKENPOX.

With joint pain, difficult movement, fever, pink rash, congested eyeballs, flushed face: DENGUE.

With chills, fever, malaise, headache, appetite loss, nosebleeds, diarrhea or constipation: TYPHOID FEVER.

With chills, fever, severe headache, malaise, occasionally diarrhea—or, alternatively, with mild malaise, muscular pain, headache, fever: BRUCELLOSIS.

With swelling of lymph nodes and reddening, swelling, pain in large joints, measleslike spotty rash: RAT-BITE FEVER.

### In other conditions

Persistent back pain, sometimes with pain in chest or pelvis, in a person over 40, with weakness, weight loss, recurrent bacterial infections: MYELOMA, MULTIPLE.

With hoarseness, cough, labored breathing, difficulty in swallowing: ANEURYSM, INTRATHORACIC.

Excruciating, boring: ANEURYSM, ABDOMINAL AORTIC.

Low in the back, with failure to void or marked decline in urination: RENAL FAILURE, ACUTE.

Often from the midback down, frequently with rounding of shoulders, loss of height, vertebral fractures: OSTEOPOROSIS.

## BED-WETTING

Also called *enuresis*, the inability to control urination, especially at night during sleep, occurs often in children who are sound sleepers or who have small bladder capacity. If it persists after age 5 or 6, it may be an indication of emotional or physical disorder. Physical causes, which can be checked for in a urologic examination, include infections and strictures and obstructions in the urinary tract which can be treated with suitable medical and surgical measures. When physical causes are absent, bladder training may be used. In children with small bladder capacity, restriction of urination during the day may help increase the capacity. For sound sleepers, ephedrine or dextroamphetamine may be prescribed. Another drug, imipramine, has been used effectively.

## BELCHING

With one or more of the following symptoms: nausea, heartburn, upper abdominal pain, flatulence, feelings of fullness and abdominal distention during or after a meal: INDIGESTION.

With upper abdominal discomfort, bloating, intolerance of fried foods: GALLSTONES.

Foul-smelling, with vomiting of food eaten in previous meals: stomach outlet obstruction, a complication of PEPTIC ULCER.

## BLADDER CONTROL, LOSS OF (see also URINARY INCONTINENCE)

With loss of bowel control and one or more of the following symptoms: vision disturbances, weakness, fatigue, tremor of limbs, slowing and monotony of speech, impaired balance, unsteady walking, stiff gait: MULTIPLE SCLEROSIS.

## BLEEDING

Excessive, from minor wounds, often with spontaneous hemorrhages under the skin and in the gums, gastrointestinal tract, joints and muscles, sometimes leading to joint stiffening: HEMOPHILIA.

Mild, into skin and mucous membranes, including those of gastrointestinal and genitourinary tracts, often leading to excessive menstruation in women: VON WILLEBRAND'S DISEASE.

Into skin and mucous membranes, with vomiting of blood and darkening of feces by blood pigments: VITAMIN DEFICIENCY (vitamin K).

Into skin and mucous membranes, with purplish-red spots and bruises, and sometimes bleeding into gastrointestinal or genitourinary tract or vagina: PURPURA, IDIOPATHIC THROMBOCYTOPENIC.

Often profuse, from all body openings, with small round purplish-red spots and bruises on the skin from bleeding: DEFIBRINATION SYNDROME.

From bowel, kidneys, mouth, nose, with high fever, infection of mouth, throat or lung, sometimes with joint pains, purplish-red skin spots and bruises, pallor, weakness: LEUKEMIA, ACUTE.

With fever, acute headache, chills, sometimes nausea, vomiting,

jaundice, skin rash, eye inflammation, blood in urine: LEPTO-
SPIROSIS.

## BLOOD, SPITTING OF

With labored breathing: MITRAL STENOSIS.

And coughing of blood, with blueness, clubbing of ends of fingers,
labored breathing on exertion, poor growth, squatting by a young
child after exertion: TETRALOGY OF FALLOT.

## BLINDNESS (see VISION DISTURBANCES)

## BLUENESS (CYANOSIS)

Cyanosis, a dark bluish or purplish coloration of skin and mucous
membranes, is due to inadequate oxygen in the blood. It may occur
in some infections, congenital heart problems, pneumoconioses (pulmonary or lung abnormalities from inhaling dust particles), and other
conditions:

### In infections

After flushing, followed by pallor, with severe breathing difficulty,
high fever, almost constant nonproductive cough, hoarseness: LAR-
YNGOTRACHEOBRONCHITIS, ACUTE.

With fever, appetite and weight loss, breathing difficulty, loss of
strength: COCCIDIOMYCOSIS.

### In congenital heart problems

With clubbing of ends of fingers, coughing and spitting of blood,
labored breathing on exertion, poor growth, squatting by a young
child after exertion: TETRALOGY OF FALLOT.

At birth, becoming progressively more severe: TRANSPOSITION OF
THE GREAT VESSELS.

Of the lower half of the body, with clubbing of the toes: PATENT
DUCTUS ARTERIOSUS.

### In pneumoconioses (from dust particle inhalation)

With labored breathing, deep and rapid respiration, coughing and
spitting of blood, malaise, sleep disturbance, appetite loss, chest
pains, hoarseness: SILICOSIS.

Blueness on exertion, with labored breathing, dry cough: ASBES-TOSIS.

With labored breathing and cough: BERYLLIOSIS.

With labored breathing, cough, blood-flecked sputum: SILO-FILLER'S DISEASE.

### In other conditions

With labored breathing, sometimes pain behind breastbone: EM-PHYSEMA, PULMONARY INTERSTITIAL.

With labored breathing, chest pain, fever, racing pulse: ATELEC-TASIS.

After exercise, with breathing difficulty and one or more of the following symptoms: rapid pulse, dry nonproductive cough, fever, weight and appetite loss, malaise, easy fatigability: PULMONARY GRANULOMATOSES.

With breathing difficulty, cough, asthma, somtimes fainting attacks on exertion, chest pain: COR PULMONALE.

In a child, with chronic cough, rapid breathing rate, large, frequent, foul-smelling stools, protuberant abdomen, barrel-like chest, chronic respiratory infection: CYSTIC FIBROSIS.

### BONE PAIN

Sudden, in a bone anywhere, with fever, tenderness over the bone, painful movement, later swelling: OSTEOMYELITIS.

Persistent, followed by swelling: CANCER OF THE BONE.

Most commonly of pelvis, skull, spine, legs, with softening, thickening, deformity, enlargement, sometimes with hearing impairment from temporal bone involvement: PAGET'S DISEASE.

With spleen or liver enlargement, or both, joint swellings, brown pigmentation of skin: GAUCHER'S DISEASE.

Severe, in back, with joint pain, difficult movement, temperature up to 106°, pink rash, congested eyeballs, flushed face: DENGUE.

### BONE SOFTENING

In a child, with various degrees of deformity, including nodules on the ribs and bending of bones, bowleg, knock-knee, misshapen skull: RICKETS—see under OSTEOMALACIA.

In an adult, with bending, flattening or other deformity of bones in spine, pelvis, legs: OSTEOMALACIA.

With jaundice, itching, deposits of fatty materials in skin and eyelids, high blood-fat levels: CIRRHOSIS, BILIARY.

## BONE TENDERNESS

With heat, swelling, most often of the vertebrae, thighbone, shinbone, sometimes with painful swelling in genital area and skin lesions that begin as small, firm elevations and then become pus-laden abscesses: BLASTOMYCOSIS.

## BOWEL CONTROL, LOSS OF (see also FECAL INCONTINENCE)

With one or more of the following symptoms: loss of bladder control, vision disturbances, weakness, fatigue, tremor of limbs, slowing and monotony of speech, impaired balance, unsteady walking, stiff gait: MULTIPLE SCLEROSIS.

## BOWEL MOVEMENT (see DEFECATION)

## BREAST

Cysts, usually in both breasts, often multiple and of many sizes, giving the breasts a "cobblestone" feel, sometimes with tenderness and premenstrual breast discomfort but often without such symptoms: MASTITIS, CHRONIC CYSTIC.

Lump, firm, well circumscribed, somewhat rubbery in consistency, easily moved about within the breast: FIBROADENOMA, BENIGN.

Lump, small, painless, often in upper, outer portion of breast, slowly growing, with retracted or elevated nipple, often skin dimpling over the lump, distorted breast contour: CANCER OF THE BREAST.

Nipple discharge, clear fluid or bloody: PAPILLOMA, BENIGN INTRADUCTAL.

Pain during the week to ten days before menstruation, with irritability, nervousness, emotional instability, depression, headaches, generalized fluid retention: PREMENSTRUAL TENSION.

Red patches under breasts, with blisters and pustules: CANDIDIASIS.

Male breast enlargement: GYNECOMASTIA.

## BREASTBONE TENDERNESS

With fatigue, appetite or weight loss, vague upper abdominal distress or heaviness: LEUKEMIA, CHRONIC (myelocytic).


## BREATH ODOR

As distinguished from the temporary breath odor that follows eating foods containing garlic or onions, *halitosis*, or chronic bad breath, can be caused by tooth decay and infections of gums, tonsils, nose, or sinuses. Stomach and intestinal disorders may produce it. Also:

With one or more symptoms such as nasal speech, mouth breathing, postnasal discharge, cough, vomiting, change of facial expression: ADENOID HYPERTROPHY.

Urine smell on breath, with lassitude, fatigue, decreased mental acuity, one or more of the following symptoms: muscular cramps and twitching, convulsions, nausea, vomiting, yellow-brown skin discoloration, hiccuping, itching: UREMIA.


## BREATH, SHORTNESS OF

With one or more of the following symptoms: spots before the eyes, ringing in the ears, easy fatigability, weakness, drowsiness, irritability, psychotic behavior, heart pounding: ANEMIA.

With easy fatigability, reduced resistance to respiratory infections: ATRIAL SEPTAL DEFECT.

With easy fatigability, fainting episodes: PULMONARY STENOSIS.


## BREATHING, ABSENCE OF

With unconsciousness, no pulse, no heart sounds: CARDIAC ARREST.


## BREATHING DIFFICULTY (DYSPNEA)

Dyspnea can, of course, occur temporarily after physical exertion. It may be produced by the relative rarity of oxygen at high altitudes. It also accompanies many disease states—infections, dust-produced lung conditions, malignancies, congenital heart defects and other heart problems, and varied other disorders.

### In childhood infections

With a "croaking" sound (stridor), hoarseness, barking cough, spasms of choking: LARYNGITIS, ACUTE OBSTRUCTIVE.

With sore throat, fever, headache, nausea, swallowing difficulty: DIPHTHERIA.

Severe, with violent efforts to breathe, high fever, almost constant nonproductive cough, hoarseness, flushing followed by pallor and blueness: LARYNGOTRACHEOBRONCHITIS, ACUTE.

### In other infections

With rapid, painful respiration, sharp chest pain, cough, pinkish sputum that may become rusty, fever that may start with a shaking chill, headache, sometimes with muscular pain, appetite loss, malaise: PNEUMONIA.

With fever, headache, vomiting, sore throat, pain and stiffness in back and neck, swallowing and speaking difficulty: POLIOMYELITIS.

With breathlessness on exertion, chronic cough (either loose and constant or occurring in spasms lasting several minutes until sputum is brought up): BRONCHITIS, CHRONIC.

### In pneumoconioses (from dust particle inhalation)

With abnormally deep and rapid respiration, sometimes with dry cough, later with malaise, sleep disturbances, appetite loss, chest pain, hoarseness, blueness, coughing and spitting of blood: SILICOSIS.

With dry cough, blueness on exercise: ASBESTOSIS.

With fever, rapid pulse, sometimes faintness: FARMER'S LUNG AND BAGASSOSIS.

With cough and blueness: BERYLLIOSIS.

With blueness, cough, blood-flecked sputum: SILO-FILLER'S DISEASE.

### In malignancies

With wheezing, cough, blood-streaked sputum, chest pain, weakness, weight loss: CANCER OF THE LUNG.

In a child, with firm but not tender abdominal mass, fever, weight loss: NEUROBLASTOMA.

**In congenital heart defects**

With blueness, clubbing of ends of fingers, coughing and spitting of blood, poor growth, frequent squatting by a young child after exertion: TETRALOGY OF FALLOT.

With blueness, growth failure: TRANSPOSITION OF THE GREAT VESSELS.

With fatigue on exertion: VENTRICULAR SEPTAL DEFECT.


**In other conditions**

With fever, joint pains, weight loss, sometimes also with cough, hoarseness: SARCOIDOSIS.

With palpitation, agitation, flushing, itching, ear throbbing, coughing, sneezing: ANAPHYLAXIS.

With vision disturbances, dizziness, headache, itching, sensation disturbances in hands and feet: POLYCYTHEMIA VERA.

With ability to breathe only in upright position, after coughing, wheezing, sometimes a sense of oppression in the chest: PULMONARY EDEMA.

With pallor, weakness, nausea, sweating, chest pain, sometimes coldness and ability to breathe only in upright position: SHOCK.

Quick, shallow breathing, with dull or sharp pain under breastbone or over heart and stomach and radiating to neck or shoulders, fever, chills, weakness, anxiety, sometimes with nonproductive cough: PERICARDITIS.

With difficulty in swallowing, chest or back pain, cough, hoarseness: ANEURYSM INTRATHORACIC.

With chest pain, cough, sometimes with coughing and spitting of blood: PULMONARY EMBOLISM.

With wheezing, chronic, spasmodic, hard, tiring cough brought on by any exertion (even talking), expectoration of thick sputum: EMPHYSEMA, PULMONARY.

With blueness, sometimes pain behind breastbone: EMPHYSEMA, PULMONARY INTERSTITIAL.

On exertion, with dry or slightly productive cough to begin with, later becoming more productive, occurring in the morning, late afternoon, and on retiring: BRONCHIECTASIS.

With wheezing, sense of chest constriction: ASTHMA.

With blueness, chest pain, fever, racing pulse: ATELECTASIS.

With sudden, sharp chest pain that may radiate to a shoulder, across chest, or down over abdomen, and dry, hacking cough: PNEUMOTHORAX.

Rapid, shallow breathing, with sharp, sticking chest pain worse on inhaling, cough, fever, chills: PLEURISY.

With pain on one side of chest, coughing, fever, malaise: EMPYEMA.

Ranging from slight after exercise to progressive and severe, sometimes with blueness after exercise, rapid pulse, dry nonproductive cough, fever, weight and appetite loss, malaise, easy fatigability: PULMONARY GRANULOMATOSES.

Progressively increasing, with productive cough, thick, yellow sputum which may contain bits of firm, yellow-gray material, weight loss, malaise: PULMONARY ALVEOLAR PROTEINOSIS.

Sometimes slight breathing difficulty or difficulty absent at rest, with cough, asthma, blueness, fainting attacks on exertion, chest pain: COR PULMONALE.

Shallow breathing, with agonizing abdominal pain, beads of sweat on forehead, fever, boardlike and tender abdomen: perforation of PEPTIC ULCER.

With sensation of abdominal fullness, pain over stomach area, persistent vomiting or regurgitation of large amounts of bile-stained fluid, severe thirst: GASTRIC DILATION, ACUTE.

With coughing and spitting of blood, anemia, sometimes blood in urine: GOODPASTURE'S SYNDROME.

With fluid accumulation in lungs, ankles, abdomen: AORTIC INSUFFICIENCY.

At first only on severe exertion, later to the point of limiting ability to exercise at all, sometimes with spitting of blood: MITRAL STENOSIS.

With loss of energy, swelling of ankles with fluid, sometimes nausea, appetite loss, abdominal pain, blueness and, in the elderly, confusion: CONGESTIVE HEART FAILURE.

Shallow or irregular, with irritability, prickling or burning sensations in fingers, toes, or lips, muscle cramps: METABOLIC ALKALOSIS.

## Chest
*The chest is the part of the body enclosed by the ribs and the sternum, or breastbone, especially the front aspect of that area.*

### CHEST, BARREL-LIKE

In a child, with chronic cough, rapid breathing, large, frequent and foul-smelling stools, protuberant abdomen, blueness, chronic respiratory infection: CYSTIC FIBROSIS.

## CHEST, FEELING OF CONSTRICTION IN

With wheezing, labored breathing: ASTHMA.

## CHEST, FEELING OF OPPRESSION IN

With cough, wheezing, labored breathing, ability to breathe only in upright position: PULMONARY EDEMA.

## CHEST, FEELING OF "SHOCK" IN

Or feeling of "something turning over in the chest": PREMATURE CONTRACTIONS or ATRIOVENTRICULAR BLOCK.

## CHEST, FLUTTERING SENSATION IN

With fast heartbeats (100 or more per minute), faintness, sometimes nausea: PAROXYSMAL TACHYCARDIA.

## CHEST PAIN

Commonly, a first thought of anyone experiencing chest pain is that the heart may be involved. It may be, of course: real heart disease is a vast enough problem. But it has been estimated that as many as 20 million people in the United States, most of them men and many of them young, are bearing a needless burden. Although they may have some of the symptoms, notably chest pain, there is nothing wrong with their hearts. But they live anxious, often limited lives.

### The chest pain of coronary heart disease

The chest pain of coronary heart disease, also known as coronary artery disease, which may be a forerunner of heart attack, is termed *angina pectoris* (angina meaning choking or suffocating pain, pectoris referring to the chest).

The situation is somewhat comparable to what happens when a car's fuel line corrodes inside, becoming thick with rust deposits so its bore is reduced. Enough fuel may flow through the line from gas tank to engine for slow or moderate speed on a level road. But when the driver tries to speed up or has a hill to climb, the fuel flow is inadequate and the motor sputters as a result. So may the heart in coronary heart disease, producing angina pectoris.

Angina is not like a heart attack in which blood flow to a part of the heart muscle is suddenly restricted severely or cut off entirely, damaging the part of the heart muscle deprived of nourishment. Angina represents protest rather than attack.

It usually comes on during exertion—shoveling snow, climbing stairs, running for a bus, playing tennis. As a rule, it is felt as a constrictive sensation in the midchest, a sensation that often shoots out to the left arm and fingertips. But there are variations: occasionally, the pain appears between the shoulder blades, in the left hand or wrist, in the left arm or shoulder, in the pit of the abdomen, in the jaws and teeth, and/or even in portions of the right arm with no chest pain at all.

Usually, an anginal attack compels the victim to stop whatever he is doing; it is not only painful but frightening, awakening a sense of foreboding, of impending doom.

An attack usually lasts only a few minutes. If the pain persists for more than 15 minutes, it is not likely to be from angina. Angina is usually quickly relieved by rest and also responds readily—within 5 minutes—to a nitroglycerin tablet.

## The chest pain of a heart attack

The hallmark of a heart attack is chest pain. It may range from a slight feeling of pressure to a feeling that the chest is being crushed in a vise.

An angina victim who suffers a heart attack may assume at first that this is angina again. But this time stopping an activity does no good, nor does nitroglycerin. Typically, the pain that occurs with a heart attack lasts for several hours and does not subside until a narcotic such as morphine is administered.

Accompanying the pain almost always is a feeling of grave anxiety, a sense of death being near. Commonly, the face turns ashen gray and there is a cold sweat. Often, there are retching, belching of gas, and vomiting—which is why a heart attack sometimes may be confused with a stomach upset. Shortness of breath is common. Some victims experience palpitation—a sensation that the heart is beating abnormally fast and hard.

*These are some guidelines that may help distinguish the chest pain of a heart attack from angina and from chest pains that have nothing to do with the heart:*

*A heart attack is less likely to be the problem when chest pain is below the nipple and to the left; when the pain is localized COMPLETELY to the left; when the pain is sharp rather than a dull pressure or squeezing sensation; when the pain comes and goes; when it is less when you lie down. If the pain lasts only 1 to 5 minutes, it is probably angina, not a heart attack.*

*Because the first hours and even minutes can be critical in dealing with a heart attack, if pain has persisted for more than 15 minutes and you have the slightest suspicion of a heart attack, ask someone to take you to the nearest hospital or call the rescue squad. And, immediately, in the emergency room, tell personnel there that you may be having a heart attack and insist on being taken to the coronary care unit.*

### Other causes of chest pain

Chest pain can stem from many problems that have nothing to do with the heart itself. They include infectious diseases, malignancies, and a variety of other conditions, some serious, some not.

### In infections

With cough, purulent sputum, malaise, appetite loss, sweats, chills, fever: LUNG ABSCESS.

Sharp pain, with cough, pinkish sputum that may become rusty, fever often starting with a shaking chill, headache, breathing difficulty, rapid and painful respiration, sometimes with muscular pain, appetite loss, malaise: PNEUMONIA.

Vague chest pain, with fever, weight loss, cough, night sweats: TUBERCULOSIS.

With cough, fever, small, hard swelling around the jaw: ACTINOMYCOSIS.

With fever, chills, breathing difficulty, drenching sweats, dry hacking cough: BLASTOMYCOSIS.

### In malignancies

With weakness, weight loss, recurrent bacterial infections, sometimes pain in back or pelvis: MYELOMA, MULTIPLE.

With cough, blood-streaked sputum, breathing difficulty, weight loss, weakness: CANCER OF THE LUNG.

**In other conditions**

Behind the breastbone, with labored breathing, blueness: EMPHY-SEMA, PULMONARY INTERSTITIAL.

With labored breathing, sometimes blueness, fever, racing pulse: ATELECTASIS.

Sudden, sharp, with breathing difficulty, dry hacking cough, and sometimes pain radiating to a shoulder, across the chest or down over the abdomen: PNEUMOTHORAX.

Sharp, sticking, worse on inhaling, with cough, fever, chills, rapid shallow breathing: PLEURISY.

On one side of chest, with breathing difficulty, coughing, fever, malaise: EMPYEMA.

With breathing difficulty, deep and rapid respiration, coughing and spitting of blood, sleep disturbance, malaise, appetite loss, hoarseness, blueness: SILICOSIS.

With breathing difficulty, cough, asthma, blueness, sometimes fainting on exertion: COR PULMONALE.

Under the breastbone, with heartburn, sometimes with swallowing difficulty, vomiting of blood or darkening of stool by blood pigments: HERNIA, HIATAL.

With one or more of the following symptoms: nausea, vomiting sweating, eye tearing, dilation or contraction of pupils, abdominal cramps, diarrhea, thirst, vertigo, confusion, throat constriction, blood-streaked stools and vomitus, limb numbness, itching, muscle weakness, cramps in extremities, collapse: FOOD POISONING, NONBACTERIAL.

With abdominal pain, diarrhea, appetite and weight loss, anemia, fever, weakness, joint pains and arthritis of knees, wrists and back, nonproductive cough: WHIPPLE'S DISEASE.

With fatigue, appetite loss, lack of energy, aches and pains, irritability, poor memory, sleep disturbances, abdominal discomfort, constipation: VITAMIN DEFICIENCY (thiamine).

On exertion, with fatigue, fainting, labored breathing: AORTIC STENOSIS.

With breathing difficulty, nausea, weakness, sweating: SHOCK.

Dull or sharp, under the breastbone or in the region over heart and stomach, radiating to neck or shoulders, often with fever, chills, weakness, anxiety, sometimes with nonproductive cough and quick, shallow breathing: PERICARDITIS, acute.

With labored breathing, difficulty in swallowing, hoarseness, cough: ANEURYSM, INTRATHORACIC.

Severe, much like that of a heart attack: ANEURYSM, DISSECTING AORTIC.

With labored breathing, sometimes coughing and spitting of blood: PULMONARY EMBOLISM.

In the chest wall, severe, throbbing or stabbing: NEURALGIA (intercostal).

Under the breastbone, severe, burning, with difficulty in swallowing, heartburn: ESOPHAGITIS.

Under the breastbone, radiating to the back, severe, occurring after meals, with heartburn, belching, weight and appetite loss: ESOPHAGEAL ULCER.

With any or all of the following: numbness and tingling of arms or fingers, weakness of arms or hands, stiff neck or shoulder, headache, vision blurring, pain in and around the eyes, loss of balance: CERVICAL SYNDROME.

With one or more of the following: belching, breathing difficulty, palpitation: AEROPHAGIA.


## CHILLINESS

With stiff neck, swallowing difficulty, fever, difficulty opening jaws: TETANUS.

With sore throat, nasal discharge, slight fever, back and muscle pain, nonproductive cough gradually producing sputum: BRONCHITIS, ACUTE.

With any or many other symptoms: dry, cold skin, puffiness of hands and face, decreased appetite, weight gain, slow speech, mental apathy, drowsiness, constipation, hearing loss, poor memory, and, in a woman, menstrual disturbances: HYPOTHYROIDISM.

With sweating, flushing or pallor, numbness, hunger, trembling, headache, dizziness, weakness, palpitation, and sometimes faintness, all occurring several hours after meals: HYPOGLYCEMIA.


## CHILLS (see FEVER, a common accompaniment of chills, which are shivering attacks with feelings of coldness and skin pallor)


## CHOKING

Sensation of, possibly with feeling of "shock" or "something turning over" in the chest: PREMATURE CONTRACTIONS.

Spasms of, with hoarseness, "barking" cough, croaking sound during breathing: LARYNGITIS, ACUTE OBSTRUCTIVE.

Spells of, with hacking cough that becomes paroxysmal, sneezing, running nose, tearing of eyes: WHOOPING COUGH.

## COLD, SENSITIVITY TO

With any or many other symptoms: apathy, appetite loss, weight loss, easy fatigue, diminished libido, scantiness or absence of pubic and underarm hair, and in women scanty menstruation, failure to lactate after childbirth: HYPOPITUITARISM.

With any or many other symptoms: dry, cold skin, puffiness of hands and face, decreased appetite, weight gain, slow speech, mental apathy, drowsiness, constipation, hearing loss, poor memory, menstrual disturbance: HYPOTHYROIDISM.

With increased skin pigmentation, black freckles over forehead, face, neck, shoulders, bluish-black discoloration of mucous membranes of lips, mouth, other sites, increasing weakness, easy fatigability, nausea, vomiting, diarrhea, dizziness, fainting attacks: ADDISON'S DISEASE.

## COMA

Coma is a state of profound unconsciousness from which the person cannot be aroused even by powerful stimuli.

With headache, fever, vomiting, stiff neck, muscle twitching, tremors, mental confusion, convulsions: ENCEPHALITIS, VIRAL.

With paralysis of one side of body, speech disturbance, sometimes defective vision: STROKE.

With one or many other symptoms: muscle weakness, failing vision, vomiting, lack of balance and coordination, lethargy, personality changes, headache: CANCER OF THE BRAIN.

With chills, fever, headache, pain behind eyes, joint and muscle pain, intolerance of light, nausea, vomiting, sore throat, abdominal pain: ROCKY MOUNTAIN SPOTTED FEVER.

With fever, restlessness, malaise, uncontrollable excitement, excessive salivation, painful spasms of muscles of throat and larynx: RABIES.

## CONFUSION

With difficult breathing, ankle swelling, energy loss: CONGESTIVE HEART FAILURE.

With one or many other symptoms: nausea, vomiting, tearing of eyes, dilation or contraction of pupils, abdominal cramps, diarrhea, thirst, dizziness, throat constriction, blood-streaked stools and vomitus, limb numbness, itching, muscle weakness, chest pain, cramps in extremities: FOOD POISONING, NONBACTERIAL.

With headache, drowsiness, fever, vomiting, stiff neck, muscle twitching, tremors, convulsions: ENCEPHALITIS, VIRAL.

With headache, vision blurring, depression, agitation, inappropriate speech or dress: CRYPTOCOCCOSIS.

## CONSTIPATION

Constipation—difficulty in emptying the bowel—may result from nervous tension, improper diet, bad toilet habits, insufficient exercise, overuse of laxatives. It is rarely serious unless it accompanies organic disease.

With soft, puttylike, rather than hard, stools, little or no abdominal discomfort, in an older person or in one confined to bed: COLON, INACTIVE.

With abdominal pain beginning in the umbilical (navel) area and shifting to right lower quadrant, nausea, vomiting, appetite loss: APPENDICITIS.

Severe, with low, left-side abdominal pain, distention, nausea, vomiting: DIVERTICULITIS.

Alone or alternating with diarrhea, variable abdominal pain: COLON, IRRITABLE.

In a child, severe, with abdominal distention, vomiting, appetite loss, often anemia and failure to thrive: MEGACOLON.

Sometimes alternating with diarrhea, with cramplike abdominal pain, vomiting which may become fecal in nature, abdominal distention: INTESTINAL OBSTRUCTION.

With variable abdominal pain often extending to the back and relieved by sitting up or bending forward, one or more of the following symptoms: jaundice, weight and appetite loss, nausea, vomiting, sometimes with vomiting of blood and darkening of stool with blood pigments: CANCER OF THE PANCREAS.

With paroxysms of colicky abdominal pain, distention, vomiting, particularly in a woman: PORPHYRIA, ACUTE INTERMITTENT.

With one or many other symptoms: chilliness, dry cold skin, puffiness of hands and face, decreased appetite, weight gain, slow speech, mental apathy, drowsiness, hearing loss, poor memory, excessive or absent menstruation: HYPOTHYROIDISM.

With weakness, appetite loss, nausea, abdominal pain, thirst, ex-

cessive urination, calcium stones in urinary tract: HYPERPARATHY-
ROIDISM.

With fever, chills, headache, nosebleeds, rose spots on chest and
abdomen, appetite loss: TYPHOID FEVER.

With stiffness of jaw and neck, swallowing difficulty, sore throat,
fever, stiff arms or legs: TETANUS.

With abdominal mass and pain, fever, vomiting, emaciation: ACTI-
NOMYCOSIS.

With abdominal pain, slight fever, vague body aches and pains,
painful passage of bloody, mucoid stools: AMEBIASIS.

## CONVULSIONS (see also SEIZURES)

Convulsions are powerful involuntary muscle contractions that
produce contortions of the body. They have many causes, including
excessive use of alcohol, drug overdoses, and brain inflammation associated with some infectious diseases.

With high fever, headache, chills, sometimes vomiting, rash:
SMALLPOX.

With headache, fever, stiff neck, tremors, vomiting, mental confusion: ENCEPHALITIS, VIRAL.

With chills, fever, inflamed painful swellings of lymph nodes in
the groin, vomiting, thirst, generalized pain, headache, mental dullness, delirium: PLAGUE.

With stiffness of jaw and neck, swallowing difficulty, sore throat,
restlessness, stiff arms or legs: TETANUS.

With abnormal bending or flexion of wrist and ankle joints, muscle
twitching, cramps: TETANY.

With sudden severe head pain, nausea, vomiting, neck stiffness,
dizziness: SUBARACHNOID HEMORRHAGE.

With dizziness, faintness: SINOATRIAL EXIT BLOCK.

With "shock in the chest" or "something turning over in the chest"
sensations, sometimes also with dizziness, fainting: ATRIOVENTRICU-
LAR BLOCK.

In an infant, with yellowish greasy scaling of scalp, inflammation
of tongue, fissuring of lips and angles of mouth: VITAMIN DEFICIENCY
(pyridoxine).

With lassitude, fatigue, decreased mental acuity, muscle cramps,
appetite loss, nausea, vomiting, yellow-brown skin discoloration, periods of hiccuping, smell of urine on the breath, itching: UREMIA.

With flushing or pallor, chilliness, numbness, trembling, headache,
dizziness, palpitation, faintness, all several hours after a meal: HY-
POGLYCEMIA.

What to do for convulsions. Although many convulsions end by themselves, call a doctor immediately. As much as possible, keep the person from hurting himself, placing a rolled handkerchief or hard object too large to swallow between his jaws to help prevent biting of tongue or lips. Place him flat on his back, head turned to one side, collar and belt loosened.

## COORDINATION, LACK OF

With one or many other symptoms: lack of balance, headache, muscle weakness, failing vision, vomiting, drowsiness, personality changes: CANCER OF THE BRAIN.

## COUGH

A cough is a sudden noisy expulsion of air from the lungs. It is called *productive* when associated with expectoration of material, *dry* or *nonproductive* when not. In addition to occurring when a foreign body gets into the airways, it accompanies many infections, diseases caused by inhaled particles, and other disorders.

### In childhood infections

With rash covering the body, running nose, slight fever, head and back pain, reddened eyes: MEASLES.

With running nose, sneezing, tearing of eyes, appetite loss, listlessness, rarely fever, the hacking cough often first occurring at night, then during the day as well, becoming paroxysmal in spells of eight to ten in one breath: WHOOPING COUGH.

Almost constant, nonproductive, with high fever, severe breathing difficulty, hoarseness, flushing followed by pallor, blueness: LARYNGOTRACHEOBRONCHITIS, ACUTE.

Barking in nature, with hoarseness, croaking sound during breathing, spasms of choking: LARYNGITIS, ACUTE OBSTRUCTIVE.

### In other common infections

With fever, generalized aches and pains most pronounced in back and legs, headache, sore throat, mild distress below breastbone, weakness, appetite loss, sometimes nasal discharge: INFLUENZA.

Nonproductive, gradually becoming productive, with sore throat, nasal discharge, slight fever, chilliness, back and muscle pain, malaise: BRONCHITIS, ACUTE.

With pinkish sputum that may become rusty, sharp chest pain, high fever usually starting with a shaking chill, headache, often with breathing difficulty, rapid and painful respiration commonly with an expiratory grunt: PNEUMONIA, lobar.

With dryness of throat, tickling sensation, difficult-to-expectorate mucus: PHARYNGITIS.

## In less common infections

With chills, fever, inflamed painful swellings of lymph nodes in groin, vomiting, thirst, generalized pain, headache, mental dullness, sometimes convulsions: PLAGUE.

With fever, weight loss, fatigue, appetite loss, listlessness, vague pains in chest, purulent sputum, night sweats: TUBERCULOSIS.

With small, hard swelling around jaw, sometimes chest pain, fever, abdominal mass and pain, vomiting, diarrhea or constipation: ACTINOMYCOSIS.

With fever, malaise: HISTOPLASMOSIS.

With fever, chest pain, sputum production, sore throat, sometimes arthritislike joint pain and swelling: COCCIDIOMYCOSIS.

Dry, hacking, with fever, chills, drenching sweats, breathing difficulty, sometimes later pus-laden sputum: BLASTOMYCOSIS.

Dry at first, becoming productive with mucopurulent sputum, fever, chills, malaise, appetite loss: PSITTACOSIS.

## In malignancy

New cough, or change in character or severity of a chronic cough, sometimes with wheezing, sputum becoming blood-streaked, chest pain, weakness, breathing difficulty, loss of weight: CANCER OF THE LUNG.

## Foreign body

Cough of varying intensity, sometimes with gagging, shortness of breath, choking, blueness: BRONCHI, FOREIGN BODY IN.

## In pneumoconioses (from dust particle inhalation)

Dry, with labored breathing, blueness on exercise: ASBESTOSIS.
With labored breathing, blueness: BERYLLIOSIS.

With blood-flecked sputum, labored breathing, blueness: SILO-FILLER'S DISEASE.

Dry, with breathing difficulty, abnormally deep and rapid respiration, later with coughing and spitting of blood, chest pain, hoarseness, blueness, appetite loss, sleep disturbances, malaise: SILICOSIS.

## In other disorders

With fever, joint pains, weight loss, sometimes also with hoarseness, breathing difficulty: SARCOIDOSIS.

With itching of nose, roof of mouth, throat, eyes, tearing of eyes, sneezing, nasal discharge, sometimes headaches, irritability, appetite loss, depression, insomnia, wheezing: RHINITIS, ALLERGIC.

With palpitation, agitation, flushing, itching, ear throbbing, sneezing, breathing difficulty: ANAPHYLAXIS.

With spitting of blood, blueness, clubbing of ends of fingers, labored breathing on exertion, squatting by a young child after exertion, poor growth: TETRALOGY OF FALLOT.

Sometimes with wheezing, followed by labored breathing and ability to breathe only in upright position, sense of oppression in chest: PULMONARY EDEMA.

Nonproductive, with dull or sharp chest pain under breastbone or over heart and stomach and radiating to neck or shoulders, fever, chills, weakness, anxiety, sometimes quick, shallow breathing: PERICARDITIS.

With hoarseness, labored breathing, difficulty in swallowing, chest or back pain: ANEURYSM, intrathoracic.

With labored breathing, chest pain, sometimes coughing and spitting of blood: PULMONARY EMBOLISM.

Slight but chronic, aggravated by upper respiratory infections and becoming either loose and constant or appearing in spasms lasting several minutes until sputum is brought up, with increasing difficulty in breathing: BRONCHITIS, CHRONIC.

Chronic, spasmodic, hard, tiring, often precipitated by any exertion including talking, with wheezing, expectoration of thick sputum, labored breathing with even mild exertion: EMPHYSEMA, PULMONARY.

Dry or slightly productive to begin with, becoming more productive, occurring in morning, again late in afternoon, and on retiring, often with relative freedom from cough in between, frequently with coughing of blood, breathing difficulty on exertion: BRONCHIECTASIS.

With purulent sputum, malaise, appetite loss, sweats, chills, fever, sometimes chest pain: LUNG ABSCESS.

With or without a stitch in the side, sometimes with slight fever and, in an asthmatic, increase in asthma severity: LOEFFLER'S SYNDROME.

Dry, hacking, with difficulty in breathing, sudden sharp chest pain that may radiate to shoulder, across chest, or down over abdomen: PNEUMOTHORAX.

With sharp, sticking chest pain worse on inhaling, fever, chills, rapid shallow breathing: PLEURISY.

With chest pain on one side, breathing difficulty, fever, malaise: EMPYEMA.

Dry, nonproductive, with breathing difficulty, blueness after exercise, one or more of the following symptoms: rapid pulse, fever, weight and appetite loss, easy fatigability, malaise: PULMONARY GRANULOMATOSES.

With thick, yellow sputum sometimes containing bits of yellow-gray material, progressive breathing difficulty, weight loss, malaise: PULMONARY ALVEOLAR PROTEINOSIS.

Coughing and spitting of blood, breathing difficulty, blood in urine, anemia: GOODPASTURE'S SYNDROME.

With difficult breathing, asthma, blueness, sometimes fainting attacks on exertion, chest pain: COR PULMONALE.

Nonproductive, with diarrhea, appetite and weight loss, anemia, weakness, fever, joint pains and arthritis of knees, wrists, back, abdominal and chest pain: WHIPPLE'S DISEASE.

With one or more other symptoms: nasal speech, mouth breathing, halitosis, postnasal discharge, vomiting, change of facial expression: ADENOID HYPERTROPHY.

In a child, chronic cough, with rapid breathing rate, delay in regaining birth weight, large, frequent, foul-smelling stools, protuberant abdomen, barrel-like chest, blueness, chronic respiratory infection, susceptibility to heat: CYSTIC FIBROSIS.

## About cough treatment

Any persistent cough should have medical attention. Palliatives—syrups, cough drops, etc.—may temporarily relieve a tickle in the throat, but they do not cure a cough and certainly not the underlying cause. Cough has a useful function, helping to clear breathing passages of irritating substances and usually should not be completely suppressed. A physician can prescribe medication to provide some control of a seriously annoying cough while the underlying cause is sought and treated.

## CYANOSIS (see BLUENESS)

**DEAFNESS** (see HEARING LOSS)


## DEFECATION

Painful, with bleeding from anus: HEMORRHOIDS.

Painful, with bleeding from vagina following coitus, sometimes with painful coitus, watery discharge, urinary frequency and urgency: CANCER OF THE VAGINA.

Intensely painful: FISSURE-IN-ANO.

Repeated urge for, with rectal discomfort, painful diarrhea, blood, mucus and pus in stools: PROCTITIS.


## DELIRIUM

Delirium, a disordered mental state with excitement and illusions, may be caused by alcoholism, insulin shock, drug overdoses, anxiety, exhaustion. Also acute illnesses with very high fever may be responsible.

With stiff neck, violent persistent headache, vomiting, fever, sometimes convulsions in infants: MENINGITIS.

With headache, fever, vomiting, stiff neck, drowsiness, muscle twitching, tremors, mental confusion, convulsions: ENCEPHALITIS, VIRAL.

With chills, fever, headache, pain behind eyes, joint and muscle pain, light intolerance, nausea, vomiting, sore throat, abdominal pain: ROCKY MOUNTAIN SPOTTED FEVER.

With chilly sensations, malaise, headache, fever, rose-colored spots, nosebleeds, backache, diarrhea or constipation, sore throat: TYPHOID FEVER.

With chills, fever, inflamed and painful swellings of lymph nodes in groin, vomiting, thirst, generalized pain, headache, sometimes convulsions: PLAGUE.

With chills, fever, severe headache, vomiting, muscle and joint pain, reddish rash over trunk and extremities followed by rose-colored spots, sometimes jaundice: RELAPSING FEVER.


## DIARRHEA

Diarrhea involves the rapid movement of fecal matter through the intestine, with little time for water to be absorbed from the material, leading to frequent, watery stools. Diarrhea may be associated with emotional upsets that increase gastrointestinal contractions (peristalsis) and secretion of mucus in the colon. It is also associated with many infections, parasitic infestations, some malignancies, and a variety of other disorders that may produce irritation of the intestinal lining.

## In infections

With chills, fever, malaise, headache, appetite loss, nosebleeds, backache, sore throat: TYPHOID FEVER.

With chills, fever, severe headache, malaise—or, alternatively, muscular pain, back pain, headache, rise in evening temperature: BRUCELLOSIS.

With cough, fever, small, hard swelling around the jaw, sometimes with chest pain, abdominal mass and pain, vomiting: ACTINOMYCOSIS.

In children, with sudden fever, drowsiness or irritability, abdominal pain, painful straining at stool and, within 72 hours, blood, pus, and mucus in stools which increase to 20 or more a day, severe weight loss, dehydration: BACILLARY DYSENTERY.

In adults, nonbloody, free of mucus, without fever, sometimes with griping abdominal pain and urgency to defecate and with such episodes increasing, diarrhea becoming severe and stools later containing mucus, pus, and often blood: BACILLARY DYSENTERY.

Painless but severe, with quick dehydration, great thirst, diminished urination, muscle cramps, weakness, wrinkling of skin, eyes sunken, sometimes stupor: CHOLERA.

With abdominal pain, slight fever, vague body aches and pains, painful passage of bloody stools also containing mucus: AMEBIASIS.

With frequent fluid or semifluid stools that may contain blood and mucus, slight fever: AMEBIASIS (DYSENTERY).

With muscular weakness, headache, eye inflammation, weight loss: TOXOPLASMOSIS.

With sudden abdominal cramps, headache, chills, fever, nausea, vomiting: GASTROENTERITIS, FOOD INFECTION or STAPHYLOCOCCUS TOXIN.

## In parasitic infestations

Preceded by a small solid elevated lesion or papule on the skin and accompanied by fever, hives, possibly bladder inflammation: SCHISTOSOMIASIS.

With mucus in stools, abdominal pain, weight loss: GIARDIASIS.
With colicky pains: ROUNDWORM, GIANT INTESTINAL.
With pain in pit of stomach: THREADWORM.
With nausea, anemia, retarded growth: WHIPWORM.
With abdominal discomfort, dizziness, exhaustion: TAPEWORM, DWARF.

## In malignancy

With abdominal pain often extending to the back and relieved by sitting up or bending forward, with one or more of the following symptoms: jaundice, weight and appetite loss, nausea, vomiting, sometimes with blood in vomitus and stools darkened with blood pigments: CANCER OF THE PANCREAS.

## In other disorders

With cramping pain, blood and mucus in stools: POLYPS.

With crampy abdominal pain, nausea, vomiting: GASTROINTESTINAL ALLERGY.

With abdominal pain, weight loss: BOWEL ARTERY ATHEROSCLEROSIS.

With abdominal pain beginning in umbilical (navel) area and shifting to right lower quadrant of abdomen, nausea, vomiting, appetite loss: APPENDICITIS.

With severe, constant, diffused, prostrating abdominal pain, nausea, vomiting, fever, chills: PERITONITIS.

With sudden abdominal cramps, malaise, nausea, vomiting, gas sounds in intestines, appetite loss: GASTROENTERITIS, ACUTE.

Chronic or chronic relapsing diarrhea, with stools loose but free of blood or pus, sometimes containing undigested food residue, mild abdominal pain, nausea, heartburn, fullness after eating, sometimes relieved by belching: DIARRHEA, CHRONIC NONINFLAMMATORY.

With one or more other symptoms: nausea, vomiting, tearing of eyes, dilation or contraction of pupils, abdominal cramps, thirst, dizziness, confusion, collapse, throat constriction, blood-streaked stools and vomitus, limb numbness, itching, muscle weakness, chest pain, cramps in extremities: FOOD POISONING, NONBACTERIAL.

Chronic, with several loose, nonbloody stools daily, abdominal pain, fever, weight loss: REGIONAL ENTERITIS.

Severe, profuse, watery, sometimes bloody, with high fever, abdominal distention, prostration: ENTEROCOLITIS, PSEUDOMEMBRANOUS.

In a series of attacks with the diarrhea bloody but varying in intensity and duration, freedom from symptoms in between attacks, often with urgency to defecate, mild lower abdominal cramps, sometimes progressing later to 10 to 20 bowel movements daily, with severe cramps, sometimes with stools made up almost entirely of blood and pus: COLITIS, CHRONIC ULCERATIVE.

Diarrhea alone, or diarrhea alternating with constipation, and with low-left-side abdominal pain, nausea, vomiting, abdominal distention: DIVERTICULITIS.

Diarrhea alone or alternating with constipation, and with variable abdominal pain: COLON, IRRITABLE.

With appetite loss, weight loss becoming increasingly marked after weeks to months, followed by anemia, weakness, fatigability, muscle cramps: SPRUE, TROPICAL.

With fever, joint pains, arthritis of knees, wrists and back, nonproductive cough, abdominal and chest pain, anemia, weakness, fatigability, appetite and weight loss: WHIPPLE'S DISEASE.

Mild, intermittent, with abdominal pain, nausea, vomiting, massive edema or waterlogging of tissues: LYMPHANGIECTASIA, INTESTINAL.

Painful, with blood, pus and mucus in stools, rectal discomfort, repeated urge to defecate: PROCTITIS.

With nausea, vomiting, abdominal discomfort and distention, sore mouth and tongue, bright scarlet oral membranes, skin disturbances, nervous system disturbances: VITAMIN DEFICIENCY (niacin).

With paroxysms of colicky abdominal pain, distention, vomiting, particularly in a woman: PORPHYRIA, ACUTE INTERMITTENT.

Unyielding, occurring in an infant soon after birth: GLUCOSE-GALACTOSE MALABSORPTION.

With nervousness, weakness, heat sensitivity, sweating, overactivity, restlessness, weight loss, increased appetite, tremor, palpitation, stare, abnormal eye protrusion, sometimes with headache, nausea, abdominal pain: HYPERTHYROIDISM.

With increasing weakness, easy fatigability, increased skin pigmentation, black freckles over forehead, face, neck, shoulders, bluish-black discolorations of mucous membranes of lips, mouth, other sites, weight and appetite loss, nausea, vomiting, decreased cold tolerance, dizziness, fainting: ADDISON'S DISEASE.

Recurrent, with abdominal discomfort, skin flushing precipitated by emotion, food, or alcohol: CARCINOID SYNDROME.

With fever, weight loss, and any or several of the following: severe abdominal pain, diffuse muscle pains, joint pains, wheezing, pneumonia, skin reddening, hives: POLYARTERITIS.

**About treatment for diarrhea**

Mild diarrhea of short duration may be treated with a bland diet, increased liquid intake, use of a kaolin-pectate compound to relieve symptoms. More severe diarrhea, even as necessary diagnostic tests are undertaken, may be treated with antidiarrheal drugs and, when required, by intravenous administration of fluids and electrolytes.

## DIZZINESS

With one or more other symptoms: nausea, vomiting, sweating, dilation or contraction of pupils of eyes, abdominal cramps, diarrhea, thirst, confusion, collapse, throat constriction, blood-streaked stools and vomitus, limb numbness, itching, muscle weakness, chest pain, cramps in extremities: FOOD POISONING, NONBACTERIAL.

With abdominal discomfort, diarrhea, exhaustion: TAPEWORM, DWARF.

With abdominal pain or pressure and any or several other symptoms: nausea, headache, vomiting, blood in vomitus, malaise, appetite loss, sensation of fullness: GASTRITIS.

With faintness, weakness, profuse sweating, later with vomiting of blood or tarry stools: PEPTIC ULCER (hemorrhage).

With headache, nasal and postnasal discharge, sometimes fever to 102° or 103°, toothache, generalized aches, edema or puffiness about the eyes: SINUSITIS.

Episodes of dizziness, with ringing in ears, hearing impairment, nausea, vomiting: MENIERE'S DISEASE.

With sweating, flushing or pallor, chilliness, numbness, hunger, trembling, headache, weakness, palpitation, sometimes faintness several hours after meals: HYPOGLYCEMIA.

With increasing weakness, easy fatigability, increased skin pigmentation, black freckles over forehead, face, neck and shoulders, bluish-black discolorations of mucous membranes of lips, mouth, other sites, weight and appetite loss, nausea, vomiting, diarrhea, fainting: ADDISON'S DISEASE.

With sudden severe head pain, nausea, vomiting, neck stiffness, convulsions: SUBARACHNOID HEMORRHAGE.

With one or many other symptoms: headache, ringing in ears, spots before eyes, easy fatigability, weakness, drowsiness, irritability, pallor, heart pounding, shortness of breath on exertion: ANEMIA.

With headache, visual disturbances, labored breathing, itching, lassitude, sensation disturbances in hands and feet: POLYCYTHEMIA VERA.

With faintness or convulsions: SINOATRIAL EXIT BLOCK.

With "shock in chest" or "something turning over in chest" sensations, sometimes also with faintness, convulsions: ATRIOVENTRICULAR BLOCK.

With one or more other symptoms: fatigue, nervousness, palpitation, insomnia, weakness, headaches: HYPERTENSION.

## DROWSINESS

With fever, headache, sore throat, pain and stiffness of back and neck: POLIOMYELITIS.

With fever, headache, vomiting, stiff neck, muscle twitching, tremors, mental confusion: ENCEPHALITIS, VIRAL.

With fever, abdominal pain, painful straining at stool, stools containing blood, pus, and mucus and increasing to 20 or more a day, severe weight loss, dehydration: BACILLARY DYSENTERY.

With fever, vague pains in chest, purulent sputum, night sweats, weight loss, fatigue, appetite loss, listlessness: TUBERCULOSIS.

With fever, headache, nausea, abdominal discomfort, weakness, sometimes jaundice: HEPATITIS.

With one or more such symptoms as dizziness, headache, ringing in ears, spots before eyes, easy fatigability, weakness, irritability, pallor, heart pounding and shortness of breath on exertion: ANEMIA.

Progressing to stupor and coma: RESPIRATORY ACIDOSIS.

With one or more of the following symptoms: chilliness, dry cold skin, puffiness of hands and face, decreased appetite, weight gain, slow speech, mental apathy, constipation, hearing loss, poor memory, excessive or absent menstruation: HYPOTHYROIDISM.

With one or more of the following symptoms: headache, muscle weakness, failing vision, vomiting, lack of balance and coordination, lethargy, personality changes: CANCER OF THE BRAIN.

## DULLNESS, MENTAL

In a child, with thick, dry, wrinkled skin, enlarged tongue, thickened lips, broad face, flat nose, puffy feet and hands: CRETINISM.

## DYSPEPSIA (see INDIGESTION)

## EAR, DISCHARGE FROM

With itching, redness: DERMATITIS, AURAL ECZEMATOUS.

Chronic, containing pus, sometimes with pain, impaired hearing, ringing in ear, low-grade fever: OTITIS MEDIA, CHRONIC PURULENT.

## EAR, NOISES IN

With one or more of the following symptoms: dizziness, headache, spots before eyes, easy fatigability, weakness, drowsiness, irritability, pallor, heart pounding and shortness of breath on exertion: ANEMIA.

Ringing, with dizziness, gradual hearing loss, rarely pain: OTITIS MEDIA, CHRONIC CONGESTIVE.

Repeated episodes of ringing, with hearing impairment, dizziness, nausea, vomiting, sometimes oscillation of eyeballs: MENIERE'S DISEASE.

**Note.** Noises in the ear (*tinnitus* in medical terminology)—variously described as ringing, hissing, buzzing, whistling, roaring, thumping, either constant or intermittent—may sometimes be associated not only with local ear infections and disorders but with others such as syphilis and meningitis originating elsewhere, with endocrine gland disorders, allergies, heart diseases, high blood pressure, and with use of some drugs such as streptomycin, quinine, and large doses of aspirin and related compounds.

## EAR PAIN

Severe, in outer ear, sometimes with fever and enlargement of neck lymph nodes: OTITIS, ACUTE EXTERNAL.

With fullness, impaired hearing, neck gland swelling: FURUNCULOSIS.

With severe itching, stinging sensation in ear canal: OTOMYCOSIS.

With fullness, ringing, fever, impaired hearing, sometimes with dizziness, vomiting: HERPES ZOSTER, AURAL.

Agonizing, with fever, impaired hearing: MYRINGITIS.

With fullness, impaired hearing, sometimes ringing and dizziness, often with symptoms of the common cold: EUSTACHITIS.

Aching, with fullness, fever, chills, sometimes ringing, hearing impairment: OTITIS MEDIA, ACUTE.

With fullness, deafness, the pain disappearing after a few days but fullness and deafness persisting along with sensation of water in the ear: OTITIS MEDIA, CHRONIC SECRETORY.

Behind ear, over mastoid bone, usually with discharge from ear: MASTOIDITIS, ACUTE.

## EAR, REDNESS OF

Red, scaly, greasy areas on ears, eyelids, scrotum or labia majora, sometimes with dry scaling and fissuring of lips and angles of mouth, tearing of eyes, sensitivity to light: VITAMIN DEFICIENCY (riboflavin).

## EAR, THROBBING IN

With palpitation, agitation, flushing, itching, coughing, sneezing, breathing difficulty: ANAPHYLAXIS.

## EDEMA (FLUID ACCUMULATION)

In edema, an abnormal accumulation of fluid occurs in the spaces between cells in the body. Edema may be localized or generalized throughout the body. It may be caused by local inflammation, poor drainage, other factors:

In ankles with swelling, accompanied by difficult or labored breathing: CONGESTIVE HEART FAILURE.

In ankles with swelling, and fluid accumulation in lungs, abdomen, with labored breathing: AORTIC INSUFFICIENCY.

Generalized, during the week to ten days prior to menstruation, sometimes with breast pain, irritability, nervousness, headaches, disappearing a few hours after onset of menstrual flow: PREMENSTRUAL TENSION.

With abrupt jaundice, fever, fluid in and uncomfortable distention of abdomen: HEPATITIS, ALCOHOLIC.

Beginning in legs, becoming generalized, with digestive disturbances, appetite and weight loss, weakness, lethargy: PROTEIN DEFICIENCY (chronic).

Massive, with abdominal pain, mild intermittent diarrhea, nausea, vomiting: LYMPHANGIECTASIA, INTESTINAL.

About treatment of edema. Local edema due to inflammation or poor drainage may be relieved by elevation of the affected area and application of cold to the area. Generalized edema is treated with diuretic drugs, which increase elimination of fluid in the urine. This is useful symptomatic treatment but not a substitute for determining and treating the cause.

## EJACULATION, PREMATURE

Occurring before or after insertion of the penis in the vagina, premature ejaculation may be the result of inflammatory diseases, such as those of the prostate and urethra, and responsive to effective treatment for the physical causes. Commonly, it is the result of psychic factors that may be best managed through psychotherapy, sometimes through competent medical explanation and reassurance alone. In some cases, use of a local anesthetic jelly, such as 5 percent benzocaine, to desensitize the penis during foreplay may help.

## ELBOW PAIN (see JOINT PAIN)

## EMOTIONAL INSTABILITY

During the week to ten days prior to menstruation, often accompanied by generalized fluid retention, breast pain, headaches: PRE-MENSTRUAL TENSION.

Often with one or more such symptoms as pallor or flushing, chilliness, trembling, numbness, headache, dizziness, weakness, palpitation, faintness, hunger occurring several hours after meals: HYPO-GLYCEMIA.

With one or more other symptoms: appetite loss, lack of energy, aches and pains, chest pain, abdominal discomfort, poor memory, sleep disturbances: VITAMIN DEFICIENCY (thiamine).

With one or more other symptoms: sore mouth, bright scarlet oral membranes, burning of mouth, throat and esophagus, abdominal discomfort and distention, nausea, vomiting, diarrhea: VITAMIN DEFICIENCY (niacin).

With chills, fever, diarrhea, severe headache, insomnia, malaise: BRUCELLOSIS.

## EPILEPTIC SEIZURES (see SEIZURES)

## *Eye* (see also VISION DISTURBANCES)

*The eyeball consists of three coats: The cornea, a clear transparent layer on the front of the eyeball, is a continuation of the sclera, or white of the eye, the tough outer protective coat. The middle coat, the choroid, contains blood vessels. The inner coat, the retina, contains specialized cells (rods and cones) sensitive to light. Behind the cornea and in front of the lens is the iris, a circular pigmented band around the pupil, which, much like the diaphragm of a camera, widens or narrows the pupils for different light conditions. Focusing of light rays on the retina, from which signals can be transmitted via the optic nerve to the brain, is achieved by three structures: a watery material, the aqueous humor, between cornea and lens; the lens, which is just behind the iris; and a jellylike material, the vitreous humor, between lens and retina. The lens focuses with the aid of the ciliary muscle. The eye is protected by the bones of the skull to some extent, by the conjunctival sac which covers the front of the eyeball and lines the upper and lower eyelids, by the eyelids and eyelashes, and by tears from the lacrimal duct that constantly wash the eye to remove foreign materials. Eye disorders include, of course, myopia, or nearsightedness, traceable to an eyeball that is too long so the lens focuses images in front of rather than on the retina; hyperopia, or farsightedess, the result of an eyeball that is too short so the lens focuses images behind the retina; and astigmatism, an impairment of vision caused by an irregularity in the curvature of the cornea or lens. In addition, the eyes may be affected by numerous other defects, disorders, and disturbances.*

## EYE, DEVIATION OF

Also called cross-eye, walleye, squint, appearing early in life: STRABISMUS.

## EYE, EDEMA OF

Puffiness about the eye, with headache, nasal and postnasal discharge, pain, sometimes fever, dizziness, generalized aches, toothache: SINUSITIS.

## EYE, FOREIGN BODY SENSATION IN

With tearing, pain and redness of lid margin, pimplelike area on lid: STY.

With tearing, light sensitivity, blood congestion of the conjunctiva, the delicate membrane lining the lids and covering the eyeball: KERATITIS, DENDRITIC.

## EYE, INFLAMED

With fever, acute headache, chills, sometimes nausea, vomiting, jaundice, skin rash, blood in urine, diminished urination: LEPTOSPIROSIS.

## EYE, ITCHING OF

Sometimes accompanied by excessive tearing, and with redness of the conjunctiva, the delicate membrane lining lids and covering eyeball: CONJUNCTIVITIS, ALLERGIC.

With smarting, worse at night, with reddened conjunctiva and foreign body sensation: CONJUNCTIVITIS, CHRONIC CATARRHAL.

Intense, with tearing, light sensitivity, sticky mucoid discharge: CONJUNCTIVITIS, VERNAL (SPRING).

## EYE, LIGHT SENSITIVITY OF

After injury to one eye, light sensitivity, tearing, vision blurring, pain and tenderness in the other eye: OPHTHALMIA, SYMPATHETIC.

With chills, fever, headache, pain behind eyes, joint and muscle pain, nausea, vomiting, sore throat, abdominal pain: ROCKY MOUNTAIN SPOTTED FEVER.

With pain, inflammation around the cornea: UVEITIS.

With abnormal hair growth, excessive skin pigmentation, sometimes episodes of colicky abdominal pain and neurologic disturbances: PORPHYRIA CUTANEA TARDA.

## EYE, OSCILLATION OF

Involuntary rhythmic movements of eyeball, either horizontal, vertical, or rotatory: NYSTAGMUS.

# EYE PAIN

Behind the eye, with severe headache, back and joint pain, difficulty in movement, fever to as high as 106°, pink rash, blood-congested eyeballs, flushed face: DENGUE.

Behind the eye, with fever, chills, headache, joint and muscle pain, light intolerance, nausea, vomiting, sore throat, abdominal pain: ROCKY MOUNTAIN SPOTTED FEVER.

In the eye, after swelling of upper eyelids, often with one or more other symptoms: light sensitivity, fever, muscle soreness and pain, chills, thirst, profuse sweating, hives, weakness, prostration: TRICHI-NOSIS.

With light sensitivity, inflammation around the cornea: UVEITIS.

In or around the eye, with one or many other symptoms: vision blurring, loss of balance, numbness and tingling of arms or fingers, weakness of arms or hands, stiff neck or shoulder, headache, fainting: CERVICAL SYNDROME.

Severe pain in the orbit, the bony capsule containing the eye, with impaired eye motion, swelling of the lid, edema of the conjunctiva: ORBITAL CELLULITIS.

With redness and swelling about the tear sac, conjunctivitis, inflammation of the edges of the eyelid margins, fever: DACROCYSTI-TIS.

With light sensitivity, tearing, spasm of eye muscle, ulcer on the cornea: CORNEAL ULCER.

With light sensitivity, tearing, diminished vision: KERATITIS, SU-PERFICIAL PUNCTATE.

With swelling of eyelid, blood congestion of the conjunctiva: HERPES ZOSTER, OPHTHALMIC.

Severe, often radiating to forehead, worse at night, with eye unusually red and pupil contracted and sometimes irregular in shape, extreme sensitivity to light, vision blurring, tenderness of the eyeball: IRITIS.

Intense, with rapid vision loss, lid swelling, spread of pus throughout the interior of the eye: PANOPHTHALMITIS.

# EYE, PINK

Reddening of the conjunctiva membrane covering eyeball and lining eyelids, with tearing, watery discharge later containing mucus or pus, sensitivity to light, itching, smarting, burning of the lids, often with discharge sealing the lid margins overnight: CONJUNCTIVITIS, ACUTE CATARRHAL.

Pinkness and swelling of eyelids, edema of conjunctiva, discharge containing pus and mucus: CONJUNCTIVITIS, INCLUSION.

With body rash, running nose, cough, slight fever, pains in head and back: MEASLES.

## EYE PROTRUSION

Protrusion of the eyeball (*exophthalmos*) may result from a wide variety of conditions and requires expert diagnosis.

HYPERTHYROIDISM is one possible cause, in which case the protrusion may be accompanied by one or more such other symptoms as nervousness, weakness, heat sensitivity, sweating, restlessness, weight loss with increased appetite, tremor, palpitation, headache, nausea, abdominal pain, diarrhea.

ORBITAL CELLULITIS, another possible cause, involves inflammation of the orbital tissues that may be caused by spread of infection from the teeth or elsewhere or by injury, with usual symptoms also including severe pain in the orbit, lid swelling, fever, edema of the conjunctiva.

CAVERNOUS SINUS THROMBOSIS, in which a blood clot forms in a venous channel in the brain, may produce protrusion of both eyes, severe headache, convulsions, high temperature.

Other possibilities must be considered. Sudden appearance of protrusion of one eye can be due to hemorrhage of the orbit or sinuses. Appearance over a period of a few weeks may indicate chronic inflammation while slower onset may suggest a tumor. Protrusion of an eye also may be produced by severe nearsightedness of one eye.

## EYE, REDDENING OF

With swelling and sticking together of lids, with lids later becoming pocked and scarred, and with granules (small rounded bodies) forming on interior of eyelid: TRACHOMA.

## EYE, TEARING OF

With dilation or contraction of pupils and with one or many of the following symptoms: abdominal cramps, diarrhea, thirst, dizziness, confusion, throat constriction, blood-streaked stools and vomitus, limb numbness, muscle weakness, chest pain, cramps in extremities: FOOD POISONING, NONBACTERIAL.

Persistent, of one or both eyes: DACRYOSTENOSIS.

With sneezing, running nose, appetite loss, hacking cough, listlessness: WHOOPING COUGH.


## EYE, WHITISH PUPIL OF

In a child, with squinting: RETINOBLASTOMA.


## EYEBROWS, LOSS OF

With sparse, coarse hair, dry rough skin, cracked lips, severe headaches, weakness: HYPERVITAMINOSIS A.


## EYELIDS

Drooping of, with double vision, swallowing and speaking difficulty: MYASTHENIA GRAVIS.

Reddened, scaly, with greasy areas (also of ears, scrotum or labia majora), sometimes with dry scaling and fissuring of lips and angles of mouth: VITAMIN DEFICIENCY (riboflavin).

Painless, slow-growing mass on a lid: CHALAZION.

Edema, or waterlogging: EYELID EDEMA.

Itching, burning, redness of lid margins, swelling of lids, loss of lashes: BLEPHARITIS.

Edema and swelling, followed by one or many other symptoms: pain in eyes, extreme sensitivity to light, fever, muscle soreness and pain, thirst, chills, profuse sweating, hives, weakness, prostration: TRICHINOSIS.

Swelling, with one or many symptoms: headache, fever, chilliness, fatigue, malaise, sore throat, gland swelling, abdominal pain, nausea, jaundice, faintly red skin eruption: MONONUCLEOSIS, INFECTIOUS.

Puffiness, with blood in urine, change in urine color, reduced volume of urine: GLOMERULONEPHRITIS, ACUTE.

Fatty deposits in lids, with similar deposits in the skin, jaundice of long duration, itching, high blood-fat levels, softening of bones: CIRRHOSIS, BILIARY.

## FACE, BROAD

In a child, with flat nose, thickened lips, enlarged tongue, puffy feet and hands, apathy, dullness: CRETINISM.

## FACE, DULL EXPRESSION OF

With one or more other symptoms: nasal speech, mouth breathing, halitosis, postnasal discharge, cough, vomiting: ADENOID HYPERTROPHY.

## FACE, FLUSHING OF (see also FLUSHING)

Of nose, forehead, cheeks, followed by red coloration and appearance of pustules: ACNE ROSACEA.

With palpitation, agitation, itching, ear throbbing, coughing, sneezing, breathing difficulty: ANAPHYLAXIS.

Followed by pallor, blueness, with severe breathing difficulty, fever, almost constant nonproductive cough, hoarseness: LARYNGOTRACHEOBRONCHITIS, ACUTE.

With pain behind eyes, congested eyeballs, severe headache, back and joint pain, difficulty in movement, fever as high as 106°, pink rash: DENGUE.

## FACE, PAIN IN

Severe (stabbing, lightninglike, or shooting) in the face and forehead, lasting in the beginning for a minute or two, with extended periods of freedom from pain lasting weeks or months but with pain-free intervals becoming progressively shorter: NEURALGIA (trigeminal).

In face and in front of ear, with clicking or grating sounds on chewing, limited jaw motion due to pain and spasm: TEMPOROMANDIBULAR JOINT DISORDER.

## FACE, PARALYSIS OF

Usually on one side, with inability to close the mouth, sometimes with inability to close the eye on the affected side: BELL'S PALSY.

## FACE, PUFFINESS OF

With hand puffiness and one or many other symptoms: chilliness, dry cold skin, decreased appetite, weight gain, slow speech, drowsiness, constipation, hearing loss, poor memory, excessive or absent menstruation: HYPOTHYROIDISM.

With blood in urine, change in urine color, reduced urine volume: GLOMERULONEPHRITIS, ACUTE.

Often with swelling of legs, arms, torso: NEPHROTIC SYNDROME.

## FACE, ROUNDED ("MOONFACE")

With weight gain, obesity, fat accumulation in the back ("buffalo hump"), muscle wasting and weakness, easy bruising, menstrual irregularity, sometimes excessive hair growth: CUSHING'S SYNDROME.

## FAINTING (SYNCOPE)

Fainting, or sudden loss of consciousness, often results from inadequate blood supply to the brain, which may be due to a nervous reaction from fear, hunger, pain, or any emotional shock. Fainting also may have physical causes and then is commonly accompanied by other physical symptoms:

With shortness of breath, fatigability: PULMONARY STENOSIS.

With chest pain and labored breathing on exertion, fatigability: AORTIC STENOSIS.

With slow heartbeat (less than 60 per minute): SINUS BRADYCARDIA.

With palpitation, pallor, nausea, weakness: ATRIAL FLUTTER OR FIBRILLATION.

With sensation of "shock in the chest" or "something turning over in the chest," sometimes also with dizziness or convulsions: ATRIOVENTRICULAR BLOCK.

With one or more other symptoms: epilepsylike seizures, arm lameness, speech disturbances, vision disturbances: AORTIC ARCH SYNDROME.

Occurring on exertion, with breathing difficulty, cough, wheezing, blueness, chest pain: COR PULMONALE.

With tingling or burning sensations, lightheadedness, agitation: RESPIRATORY ALKALOSIS.

With increasing weakness, fatigability, increased skin pigmentation, black freckles over forehead, face, neck, shoulders, bluish-black discolorations of mucous membranes of lips, mouth, other sites, weight and appetite loss, nausea, vomiting, diarrhea, dizziness, decreased cold tolerance: ADDISON'S DISEASE.

First aid for fainting. Keep victim lying down, with feet and legs slightly elevated. Loosen tight clothing. Hold smelling salts or aromatic spirits of ammonia under nose until victim revives. Call for medical help if unconsciousness is prolonged beyond five minutes.

## FAINTNESS

With sudden fast heartbeats (100 or more per minute), fluttering sensation in chest, weakness, sometimes nausea: PAROXYSMAL TACHYCARDIA.

With dizziness or convulsions: SINOATRIAL EXIT BLOCK.

With sensation of "shock in the chest" or "something turning over in the chest," sometimes also with dizziness or convulsions: ATRIOVENTRICULAR BLOCK.

With labored breathing, fever, rapid pulse: FARMER'S LUNG AND BAGASSOSIS.

With weakness, dizziness, profuse sweating, followed later by vomiting of blood, or tarry stools: PEPTIC ULCER (hemorrhage).

With sweating, flushing or pallor, chilliness, numbness, trembling, headache, dizziness, weakness, palpitation: HYPOGLYCEMIA.

First aid for faintness. If possible, a person about to faint should lie down with legs somewhat elevated, collar and clothing loosened. If this is not possible, lower head between knees for about five minutes.

## FATIGUE

A feeling of tiredness or exhaustion, fatigue is normal during or after intense physical activity, emotional strain, or lack of rest. A tendency to easy fatigability can result from poor physical condition, poor diet, or other poor living habits. Tiredness also can result from boredom with work or daily routine. Fatigue that is not relieved by rest can also be associated with an oncoming or already present disease state:

## In infections

With fever, malaise, headache, one or more other symptoms of sore throat, gland swelling, severe weakness, abdominal pain, nausea, jaundice, eyelid swelling, faintly red skin eruption: MONONUCLEOSIS, INFECTIOUS.

With fever, weight and appetite loss, vague pains in chest, purulent sputum, night sweats: TUBERCULOSIS.

With abdominal pain and sometimes slight fever, vague body aches and pains, painful passage of stools containing blood and pus: AMEBIASIS.

## In deficiency states

With appetite loss, lack of energy, aches and pains, irritability, poor memory, sleep disturbances, chest pain, abdominal discomfort, constipation: VITAMIN DEFICIENCY (thiamine).

With appetite loss, lack of energy, aches and pains, memory impairment, confusion, sore mouth, scarlet tongue and oral membranes, skin and gastrointestinal disturbances: VITAMIN DEFICIENCY (niacin).

## In malignancies

With weakness, appetite loss, weight loss, vague upper abdominal distress or heaviness, breastbone tenderness: LEUKEMIA, CHRONIC (myelocytic).

With appetite loss, mild pallor, lymph gland (node) swellings: LEUKEMIA, CHRONIC (lymphocytic).

## In heart defect conditions

With labored breathing on exertion: VENTRICULAR SEPTAL DEFECT.

With shortness of breath, fainting episodes: PULMONARY STENOSIS.

With labored breathing and chest pains on exertion, fainting: AORTIC STENOSIS.

With breathing difficulty on exertion and sometimes at night, weight loss: MITRAL INSUFFICIENCY.

## In other conditions

With joint pains, malaise, repeated mild or severe infections: PRIMARY SPLENIC NEUTROPENIA.

With enlarged spleen, increasingly severe anemia, weakness, vomiting of blood, discoloration of stools with blood: BANTI'S DISEASE.

With one or more other symptoms of headache, ringing in ears, spots before eyes, weakness, drowsiness, irritability, heart pounding, shortness of breath on exertion: ANEMIA.

With overpowering weakness, followed in a few days by sudden malaise, chills, high fever, sore throat, swallowing difficulty, mouth ulcers, prostration: AGRANULOCYTOSIS.

Sometimes with nervousness, dizziness, palpitation, insomnia, weakness, headache: HYPERTENSION.

With breathing difficulty, one or more other symptoms of blueness after exercise, rapid pulse, dry nonproductive cough, fever, weight and appetite loss, malaise: PULMONARY GRANULOMATOSES.

With lassitude, decreased mental acuity, and later one or more other symptoms: muscle twitching and cramps, convulsions, nausea and vomiting, yellow-brown skin discoloration, hiccuping, urine smell on breath and sweat, itching: UREMIA.

With diarrhea, appetite loss, weight loss becoming increasingly marked after weeks to months, weakness, muscle cramps: SPRUE, TROPICAL.

With fever, diarrhea, appetite and weight loss, anemia, joint pains and arthritis of knees, wrists and back, nonproductive cough, abdominal and chest pain: WHIPPLE'S DISEASE.

With one or many other symptoms: apathy, appetite and weight loss, cold intolerance, diminished libido, scantiness or absence of pubic and underarm hair, scanty menstruation, failure to lactate after childbirth: HYPOPITUITARISM.

With increasing weakness, increased skin pigmentation, black freckles over forehead, face, neck and shoulders, bluish-black discolorations of mucous membranes of lips, mouth and other sites, weight loss, appetite loss, nausea, vomiting, diarrhea, decreased cold tolerance, dizziness, fainting: ADDISON'S DISEASE.

With one or many other symptoms: vision disturbances, weakness, tremor or shaking of limbs, slowing and monotony of speech, impaired balance, unsteady walking, stiff gait, loss of bladder and bowel control: MULTIPLE SCLEROSIS.

## FECAL INCONTINENCE

Loss of ability to control defecation can be caused by injury to the anal sphincters, the circular muscles that open for defecation and remain closed until voluntarily opened. Other possible causes include congenital defects of the anorectal area or nervous system; local disease such as rectal prolapse; neurologic diseases such as diabetes, stroke, brain tumor, multiple sclerosis; anal cancer; irritable colon or ulcerative colitis. Surgery sometimes can correct defects, and treatment for underlying disease often may overcome fecal incontinence. In some cases, drugs, including codeine, may be helpful.

## FEET

Pain in the arch, extending to calf muscles and sometimes to knee, hip, lower back, with discomfort increased by extended walking or standing: FLATFOOT.

Pain in the arch, which may extend to calf, with restricted ankle movement: ACHILLES TENDON CONTRACTURE.

Pain in heel: HEEL PAIN.

Pain in big toe joint: BUNION.

Pain in big toe or instep, throbbing, crushing, appearing suddenly, with swelling, warmth, redness, shininess of skin: GOUT.

Burning pain in the feet with redness, sometimes also involving the hands: ERYTHROMELALGIA.

Swelling of foot, after appearance of small solid elevated lesion (papule) or abscess that ruptures and produces a fistula or tubelike passage: MADUROMYCOSIS.

Itching between toes, with reddish patches, often scaly or blistered: ATHLETE'S FOOT (Section Three, Missed Diagnoses).

Thickening of soles, sometimes disabling: PLANTAR KERATOSIS.

Puffy feet, often with puffy hands, in a child, with thick dry wrinkled skin, enlarged tongue, thickened lips, broad face, flat nose, dullness, apathy, mental retardation: CRETINISM.

## FEVER (PYREXIA)

Fever, or abnormal rise in temperature, is an important indication of a disturbance in normal processes in the body. Temporary elevations of temperature are normal, however, after sports or other vigorous activity, emotional excitement, and in women at the time of ovulation. Since normal temperature varies from person to person, what should be considered an abnormal rise can vary, and it is advisable for a person to establish what is normal in the individual case by taking a number of readings over a period of time and averaging them. Some allowance, too, should be made for minor elevations. A mouth temperature of 99° does not necessarily indicate fever even though it is above the 98.6° arrow on the thermometer. When a temperature is 100° or more by mouth or 101° or above by rectum, fever is likely to be present.

Although fever brings discomfort, it may, in the view of some physicians, be a valuable protective device because some disease-causing organisms are destroyed at temperatures above body normal. Prolonged or very high fever, however, usually requires control, sometimes before the underlying cause can be determined. For this purpose, aspirin or another antipyretic drug may be used. Another measure that may be prescribed: sponging parts of the body and arms and legs with cool water or a mixture of alcohol and water.

Commonly present in almost all infectious diseases, fever may also accompany some parasitic diseases, some malignancies, and a considerable variety of other conditions:

### In childhood infections

With rash covering body, running nose, cough, pains in head and back, reddened eyes: MEASLES.

Temperature of 103°–104° for three or four days, often with convulsions, with temperature then falling, followed by pink-reddish rash on chest and abdomen, mildly on face, arms, and legs: ROSEOLA.

Mild at first, sometimes remaining so, sometimes climbing to 104° by the second day, with appearance, sometimes delayed for hours or days, of joint swellings and tenderness, often a rash on body, sometimes spasmodic twitching movements: RHEUMATIC FEVER.

With bright red rash, sore throat, swelling of lymph nodes of neck, sometimes headache, nausea, vomiting: SCARLET FEVER.

With breathing and swallowing difficulty, sore throat, headache, nausea: DIPHTHERIA.

High fever, with severe breathing difficulty and violent efforts to breathe, almost constant nonproductive cough, hoarseness, flushing followed by pallor, blueness: LARYNGOTRACHEOBRONCHITIS, ACUTE.

To 105° or 106°, with sore throat, pain in tonsil area especially during swallowing, headache, malaise, sometimes with stiff neck: TONSILLITIS.

### In other common infections

With malaise, eruption of blisters along the course of a sensory nerve, most often in the chest: HERPES ZOSTER.

With blisterlike, measleslike, or scarlet-feverlike rash, malaise, headache, sore throat: MONONUCLEOSIS, INFECTIOUS.

In a child, rarely in an adult, accompanied by sneezing, nasal discharge, scratchy throat, malaise: COLD, COMMON.

With generalized aches and pains that may be most pronounced in back and legs, headache, weakness, appetite loss, moderate sore throat, nonproductive cough, mild distress below breastbone, sometimes nasal discharge: INFLUENZA.

Slight, with chilliness, sore throat, nasal discharge, back and muscle pain, nonproductive cough gradually producing sputum, malaise: BRONCHITIS, ACUTE.

Sometimes to 105°, beginning with shaking chill, accompanied by sharp chest pain, cough, pinkish sputum sometimes becoming rusty, headache, breathing difficulty, rapid and painful respiration, sometimes malaise, appetite loss, muscular pain: PNEUMONIA.

With chills, frequency and urgency of and pain and burning on urination, nausea, vomiting, general muscle aches, lassitude: URINARY TRACT INFECTION.

With chills, frequency and urgency of urination, headache, sometimes pain in one or both sides of lower back: PYELONEPHRITIS.

With chills, severe, constant, diffuse and prostrating abdominal pain, nausea, vomiting, sometimes diarrhea: PERITONITIS.

With chills, sudden abdominal cramps, nausea, vomiting, diarrhea: GASTROENTERITIS, FOOD INFECTION or STAPHYLOCOCCUS TOXIN.

With headache, nausea, lassitude, drowsiness, weakness, abdominal discomfort, sometimes jaundice: HEPATITIS.

To 102° or 103°, with headache, nasal and postnasal discharge, dizziness, toothache, generalized aches, puffiness about eyes: SINUSITIS.

With small, hard sore on genital area, swelling of lymph nodes in groin area, sometimes skin rash, joint inflammation: LYMPHOGRANULOMA VENEREUM.

## In less common infections

With headache, sore throat, pain and stiffness in back and neck: POLIOMYELITIS.

With drowsiness, headache, vomiting, stiff neck, muscle twitching, tremors, mental confusion: ENCEPHALITIS, VIRAL.

With violent, persistent headache, stiff neck, vomiting: MENINGITIS.

With restlessness, uncontrollable excitement, excessive salivation, painful spasms of muscles of larynx and throat: RABIES.

With headache, muscle aches, yellowing of skin, darkening of urine, vomiting with blood in vomitus: YELLOW FEVER.

With severe headache, pain behind eyes, back and joint pain, pink rash, flushed face, congested eyeballs: DENGUE.

With chills or chilly sensations, headache, pain behind eyes, joint and muscle pain, intolerance of light, nausea, vomiting, sore throat, abdominal pain, rash on wrists and ankles spreading to trunk and limbs: ROCKY MOUNTAIN SPOTTED FEVER.

With abdominal pain, painful straining at stool, blood, pus and mucus in stools which increase to 20 or more a day, severe weight loss, dehydration: BACILLARY DYSENTERY.

With chilly sensations, malaise, headache, nosebleeds, backache, diarrhea or constipation, sore throat, rose spots on chest and abdomen: TYPHOID FEVER.

Sudden, acute, with chills, severe headache, malaise, occasionally diarrhea—or beginning with mild malaise, muscular pain, headache, pain in back, rise in evening temperature, later fever up to 105°, profuse sweating: BRUCELLOSIS.

Sudden, with chills, headache, nausea, vomiting, severe weakness, small ulcerated sore, generalized red rash: TULAREMIA.

Sudden, with chills, fever to 106°, inflamed painful lymph node swellings in groin, vomiting, thirst, generalized pain, headache, delirium: PLAGUE.

With stiffness of jaw, neck, arms or legs, sore throat, swallowing difficulty, restlessness, irritability, constipation, convulsions: TETANUS.

With vague pains in chest, purulent sputum, night sweats, weight loss, appetite loss, listlessness, fatigue: TUBERCULOSIS.

Sudden, with chills, high fever, severe headache, vomiting, muscle and joint pain, reddish rash followed by rose-colored spots, sometimes jaundice: RELAPSING FEVER.

With acute headache, chills, sometimes nausea and vomiting, sometimes subsequently jaundice, skin rash, bleeding into skin, eye inflammation, blood in urine, diminished urination: LEPTOSPIROSIS.

High fever alternating with normal temperature at 24- to 48-hour intervals, lymph node swelling, reddening, swelling and pain in large joints, back pain, measleslike spotty rash: RAT-BITE FEVER.

With solid elevated red-brown skin lesion (papule) which enlarges, reddens, and blisters, malaise, muscle pain, headache, nausea, vomiting: ANTHRAX.

With either chest pain and cough or abdominal mass and pain, vomiting, diarrhea or constipation: ACTINOMYCOSIS.

With cough, malaise, other symptoms somewhat like those of influenza: HISTOPLASMOSIS.

With one or more other symptoms: cough, chest pain, chills, sputum production, sore throat, pain and swelling of joints: COCCIDI-OMYCOSIS.

With chills, drenching sweats, cough, breathing difficulty, pus-laden and blood-streaked sputum: BLASTOMYCOSIS.

Slight fever, with abdominal pain, sometimes fatigue, vague body aches and pains, painful passage of blood and mucus in stools: AMEBIASIS.

Slight fever, with pain or discomfort over liver in upper right part of abdomen especially with movement and sometimes radiating to right shoulder, sometimes with sweats, nausea, vomiting, chills, weakness, weight loss: AMEBIASIS (HEPATITIS).

Following a few hours after chills, temperature reaching as high as 104° or 105°, then subsiding and followed by profuse perspiration, with headache, nausea, body pains, the attacks lasting four to five hours and recurring at regular intervals: MALARIA.

Mild, with swelling of neck and underarm glands (nodes), malaise, muscle pains, somtimes mild anemia, low blood pressure: TOXO-PLASMOSIS.

High fever, with chills, skin rash, prostration: TOXOPLASMOSIS (acute fulminating).

After swelling of upper eyelids, pain in eyes, often accompanied by one or more other symptoms: sensitivity to light, muscle soreness and pain, thirst, profuse sweating, hives, weakness, prostration: TRICHINOSIS.

With persistent sore that appears within a few days after and at the site of a minor cat scratch, followed by gland (node) swellings at sites near scratch, headache, appetite loss, malaise: CAT-SCRATCH DISEASE.

With cough, purulent sputum, malaise, appetite loss, chills, sweats, sometimes chest pain: LUNG ABSCESS.

With chills, dry cough becoming productive, sputum containing pus and mucus, malaise, appetite loss: PSITTACOSIS.

## In parasitic disease

Preceded by small solid elevated lesion (papule) on skin, with one or more other symptoms: hives, diarrhea, bladder inflammation: SCHISTOSOMIASIS.

## In vitamin deficiency

With irritability, failure to gain weight, appetite loss, anemia, in a child: SCURVY.

## In malignancies

Often high and abrupt, with mouth, throat or lung infection, joint pains, small purplish-red skin spots, bleeding from mouth, nose, bowel, kidneys: LEUKEMIA, ACUTE.

Fever appearing after neck gland swellings, swelling of underarm and groin glands (lymph nodes), itching, sometimes later accompanied by weakness, weight and appetite loss: HODGKIN'S DISEASE.

With gland (lymph node) enlargement in neck, underarms, or groin, usually on one side, sweating, debility: LYMPHOSARCOMA.

In a child, with abdominal mass and pain, blood in urine, nausea, vomiting, appetite loss: CANCER OF THE KIDNEY (Wilms' tumor).

With abdominal mass and pain, blood in urine: CANCER OF THE KIDNEY.

In a child, with firm but not tender abdominal mass, weight loss, obstruction of urine flow or breathing difficulty: NEUROBLASTOMA.

## In other disorders

With joint pains, weight loss, sometimes also with cough, breathing difficulty, hoarseness: SARCOIDOSIS.

Mild, lasting a day or two, with hives or skin rash, joint pains, gland (lymph node) swelling: SERUM SICKNESS.

With red skin spots that become purple, itching, malaise, sometimes joint and abdominal pain: PURPURA, ALLERGIC.

Sudden, high, after two or three days of fatigue and extreme weakness, accompanied by malaise, chills, sore throat, swallowing difficulty, mouth ulcers, prostration: AGRANULOCYTOSIS.

With chills, malaise, joint pains, lassitude, appetite loss, sometimes tender small nodules about the tips of the digits: ENDOCARDITIS, BACTERIAL.

With dull or sharp pain under breastbone or over heart and stomach radiating to neck or shoulders, weakness, anxiety, quick, shallow breathing, sometimes nonproductive cough: PERICARDITIS.

With labored breathing, sometimes blueness, chest pain, racing pulse: ATELECTASIS.

Slight fever, with cough with or without a stitch in the side, and, in an asthmatic, increase in asthma severity: LOEFFLER'S SYNDROME.

With chills, sharp, sticking chest pain worse on inhaling, rapid, shallow breathing, cough: PLEURISY.

With chest pain on one side, breathing difficulty, cough, malaise: EMPYEMA.

With labored breathing, rapid pulse, sometimes faintness: FARMER'S LUNG AND BAGASSOSIS.

With breathing difficulty, one or more other symptoms of blueness after exercise, rapid pulse, dry nonproductive cough, weight and appetite loss, easy fatigability: PULMONARY GRANULOMATOSES.

With recurrent attacks of pain in kidney region, sometimes with blood and pus in urine: HYDRONEPHROSIS.

With agonizing abdominal pain, shallow breathing, beads of sweat on forehead, boardlike and tender abdomen: PEPTIC ULCER (perforation).

With abdominal pain that may be mild or severe, constant or intermittent, beginning in stomach area and sometimes radiating to back and left shoulder, sometimes with jaundice: PANCREATITIS, CHRONIC.

With chronic diarrhea (several loose, nonbloody stools daily), abdominal pain, weight loss: REGIONAL ENTERITIS.

High, with severe, profuse, watery, sometimes bloody diarrhea, abdominal distention, prostration: ENTEROCOLITIS, PSEUDOMEMBRANOUS.

With diarrhea, appetite and weight loss, anemia, weakness, fatigability, joint pains and arthritis of knees, wrists and back, nonproductive cough, abdominal and chest pain: WHIPPLE'S DISEASE.

With abrupt onset, jaundice, fluid accumulation in and distention of abdomen, edema of tissues elsewhere: HEPATITIS, ALCOHOLIC.

With chills, pain in upper right quadrant of abdomen extending into right shoulder, severe and remaining steadily severe for hours, nausea, abdominal distention, sometimes jaundice: CHOLECYSTITIS, ACUTE.

Intermittent fever, with chills, jaundice, abdominal pain: CHOLANGITIS, ASCENDING.

With weight loss, one or more other symptoms: severe abdominal pain, diffuse muscle pain, joint pain, bloody diarrhea, wheezing, skin reddening, hives, pneumonia: POLYARTERITIS.

To 106° or higher, with flushing, hot dry skin, sometimes with muscular twitching or cramps, convulsions: HEAT HYPERPYREXIA.

## FINGER

Attacks of pallor and blueness of fingers, sometimes of toes as well: RAYNAUD'S DISEASE.

Burning, tingling, numbness beginning in fingers and toes, often extending elsewhere: POLYNEURITIS.

Clubbing (bulbous enlargement of the tips), with blueness, coughing and spitting of blood, labored breathing on exertion, poor growth, frequent squatting after exertion by a young child: TETRALOGY OF FALLOT.

Small, tender nodules about the tips, with fever, chills, joint pains, lassitude, malaise, appetite loss: ENDOCARDITIS, BACTERIAL.

Small, red to violet spots on fingertip skin, often bleeding spontaneously or after trivial injury: TELANGIECTASIA, HEREDITARY HEMORRHAGIC.

Small solid skin lesions (nodules) on the finger that enlarge slowly and break down into ulcers: SPOROTRICHOSIS.

Burning or prickling sensations in fingers, toes, or lips, with irritability, shallow or irregular breathing, muscle cramps: METABOLIC ALKALOSIS.

Pain, numbness, tingling of fingers: CARPAL TUNNEL SYNDROME.

Numbness and tingling of fingers or of arms, with any or many other symptoms: weakness of arms or hands, stiff neck or shoulders, headaches, "knots" in muscles of neck, shoulder or arm, swelling and stiffness of fingers, blurred vision, loss of balance, pain around the eyes, fainting: CERVICAL SYNDROME.

## FINGERNAIL

Painful, red, inflamed swelling: CANDIDIASIS.

Inflammation around nail, sometimes with pus: PARONYCHIAL INFECTIONS.

Thickening, with loss of nail luster, separation of nail plate, sometimes destruction of nail: RINGWORM.

## FLATULENCE

Flatulence is an uncomfortable accumulation of air or gas in stomach or intestines. Excessive intake of carbonated beverages or excessive swallowing of air are common causes of flatulence in the stomach. Intestinal flatulence may follow eating gas-producing foods such as many raw fruits and vegetables, large amounts of sugar, beans, fried foods, nuts.

With one or more other symptoms: heartburn, nausea, upper abdominal discomfort, feelings of fullness and abdominal distention during or after a meal: INDIGESTION.

## FLUSHING (see also FACE, FLUSHING OF)

With sweating, chilliness, numbness, hunger, trembling, headache, dizziness, weakness, palpitation, sometimes faintness several hours after meals: HYPOGLYCEMIA.

Precipitated by food, alcohol, emotion, with abdominal discomfort, recurrent diarrhea: CARCINOID SYNDROME.

With fever to 106° or higher, hot, dry skin, muscular twitching or cramps, convulsion: HEAT HYPERPYREXIA.

## FRIGIDITY

Frigidity—the partial or complete inability of a woman to be aroused sexually or to experience orgasm—may be due to poor general health, malnutrition, infection, injury, or physical abnormalities. More often, it is the result of psychologic influences such as conscious or unconscious feelings of guilt associated with sex, fear of pregnancy or pain, resentment of the partner for some reason. In such cases, psychiatric counseling may be needed.

## GAIT

Shuffling, stooped, with back bent forward, with one or more other symptoms: tremor of hands, nodding of head, slow movements, loss of mobility in face: PARKINSON'S DISEASE.

Stiff, with unbending knees, one or many other symptoms: vision disturbances, weakness, fatigue, tremor of limbs, slowing and monotony of speech, impaired balance, loss of bladder and bowel control: MULTIPLE SCLEROSIS.

## GAS SOUNDS (BORBORYGMUS)

All bowels rumble as the result of contractions of the intestinal wall and movement of gas and liquid within the intestinal channel. The onomatopoetic term, *borborygmus*, has been used in medicine for centuries to indicate the rumblings. Normally, there are soft, gurgling sounds. With excessive gas or FLATULENCE there may be rushing, crackling noises, louder, more turbulent than normal. Discernible by an experienced physician using a stethoscope, distinctive changes in the sounds are associated with various disorders and often can be helpful to the physician in diagnosis. For example, with an obstruction between stomach and small intestine, there may be loud, high-pitched sounds similar to those of water splashing in a partially filled container. With an obstruction in the colon, there often are explosive staccato pops.

## GENITALS (see also PENIS, SCROTUM, VAGINA, VULVA)

The genitals, or reproductive organs, are also called the genitalia. In a woman, the internal organs consist of ovaries, uterine tubes, uterus, and vagina. The external, collectively known as the vulva, consist of mons pubis, labia majora, labia minora, clitoris, vestibule of the vagina, vulvovaginal glands, and bulb of the vestibule. The male genitalia consist of the testes, seminiferous (semen-carrying) tubules, epididymides (cordlike structures along the back border of the testes with ducts in which sperm are stored), ductus deferens (the excretory duct of the testes, also known as the vas deferens), which joins the excretory duct of the seminal vesicles to form the ejaculatory duct, the seminal vesicles which produce secretions that go into the semen, the prostate, bulbourethral glands, and glans penis.

Small, hard sore in genital area 7 to 12 days or longer after sexual contact, with groin lymph nodes swelling soon afterward, sometimes to walnut size, sometimes accompanied by fever, rash, joint inflammation, and, in women, enlargement of the vulva and narrowing of rectum: LYMPHOGRANULOMA VENEREUM.

One or more small sores on or near external genitalia three to five days after sexual contact, with the sores soon developing into ulcers with irregular edges, and red swollen surrounding areas: CHANCROID.

## GLAND SWELLING, LYMPH

The *lymph glands,* also called *lymph nodes,* are part of the lymphatic system, a network of vessels that collect fluids from tissues and return them to the blood by way of two veins in the neck area. The nodes or glands, small masses of spongy tissue, which occur at intervals throughout the lymphatic system, are especially numerous in the neck, armpits, and groin. They act as filters, removing bacteria and other particles, and produce antibodies and other agents to combat infections. With their increased activity during infections, they may become swollen and painful.

Painful swelling of nodes under jaw, sometimes under arms and in groin, with fever, chilliness, headache, fatigue, malaise, sore throat, sometimes abdominal pain, nausea, jaundice, faintly red skin eruption, eyelid swelling: MONONUCLEOSIS, INFECTIOUS.

Swelling of neck and underarm nodes, with irregular mild fever, muscle pain, malaise, mild anemia; or, in some cases, high fever, chills, skin rash, prostration; in still other cases, muscular weakness, headache, diarrhea, eye inflammation: TOXOPLASMOSIS.

With sore at site of minor cat scratch, with fever, malaise, headache, appetite loss: CAT-SCRATCH DISEASE.

Generalized swelling, with increasing weakness, fatigue, appetite loss, mild pallor: LEUKEMIA, CHRONIC (lymphocytic).

Painless enlargement, usually first on one side of neck, then the other, and later under the arms and in the groin, often with severe itching and, later, sweating, weakness, fever, loss of weight and appetite: HODGKIN'S DISEASE.

Enlargement in neck, under arms, or in groin, usually on one side, later with fever, sweating, loss of strength, debility: LYMPHOSARCOMA.

Swelling usually in groin, with chills, fever, vomiting, thirst, generalized pain, headache, sometimes convulsions: PLAGUE.

With fever alternating with normal temperature, redness, swelling and pain in large joints, back pain, measleslike spotty rash: RAT-BITE FEVER.

## GLAND SWELLING, PAROTID

The parotid is the largest of the three main pairs of salivary glands located on either side of the face, just below and in front of the ears.

Increasing parotid swelling for two or three days, first on one side, than the other (sometimes both sides swell simultaneously or occasionally the second side does not swell), with headache, back pain, appetite loss, fever: MUMPS.

## GROIN

The groin is the junction of abdomen and thighs.

Red patches, with blisters, small pustules: CANDIDIASIS.

Swelling of lymph nodes in groin after appearance of small hard sore in genital area, sometimes accompanied by fever, rash, joint inflammation: LYMPHOGRANULOMA VENEREUM.

## GROWTH RETARDATION

Many factors, alone or in combination, may contribute to slowing normal growth of a child. They include nutritional deficiencies (of vitamins, minerals, or protein); malabsorption problems that prevent adequate use of nutrients in the diet; varied chronic diseases. Also:

With stool darkening from blood pigments, anemia: HOOKWORM.

With anemia, nausea, diarrhea: WHIPWORM.

With blueness, clubbing of ends of fingers, coughing and spitting of blood, labored breathing on exertion, frequent squatting in a young child after exertion: TETRALOGY OF FALLOT.

With blueness, great breathing difficulty: TRANSPOSITION OF THE GREAT VESSELS.

Stunting of growth, dwarfism: HYPOPITUITARISM.


## GUMS

Swelling, redness, bleeding: GINGIVITIS.

Abrupt pain, with bleeding, ulceration, painful swallowing and talking, unpleasant breath, excessive salivation: GINGIVOSTOMATITIS, NECROTIZING ULCERATIVE.

Swollen, bleeding, with muscle and joint aches, black and blue spots on skin, lassitude, weakness, irritability, weight loss: SCURVY.

Recession of, with bleeding when teeth are brushed, sometimes with acute gum infection: PERIODONTITIS.


## HAIR

Excessive (hirsutism), with excessive skin pigmentation, light sensitivity, sometimes episodes of colicky abdominal pain: PORPHYRIA CUTANEA TARDA.

Excessive, with "moon" or rounded face, obesity, fat accumulation in the back (buffalo hump), muscle wasting and weakness, easy bruising, menstrual irregularities: CUSHING'S SYNDROME.

Progressively more excessive on face, with acne, absence of or infrequent scanty menstruation, infertility: POLYCYSTIC OVARY SYNDROME.

Loss of body hair, pink or brown patches on skin, loss of sensation in parts of the body, small solid swellings (nodules), fever: LEPROSY.

Scantiness or absence of pubic and underarm hair, with one or many other symptoms: apathy, appetite and weight loss, easy fatigue, cold intolerance, diminished libido, scanty menstruation, failure to lactate after childbirth: HYPOPITUITARISM.

Sparse, coarse, with loss of eyebrows, dry rough skin, cracked lips, severe headaches, generalized weakness: HYPERVITAMINOSIS A.

**HALITOSIS** (see BREATH ODOR)

## HALLUCINATIONS

Hallucinations—sight, touch, sound, smell, or taste impressions unrelated to any actual external stimuli—may result from mental illness, drugs, alcohol, or an organic illness such as brain tumor. They may also sometimes occur with exhaustion. Hallucinations also may be associated with a less well-known but far from uncommon condition:

Occurring at the beginning of sleep, almost invariably associated with attacks of overpowering sleepiness a few to many times a day: NARCOLEPSY.

## HAND

Attacks of burning pain, with redness: ERYTHROMELALGIA.

Puffiness, also with facial puffiness, and one or many other symptoms: chilliness, dry cold skin, decreased appetite, weight gain, slow speech, drowsiness, constipation, hearing loss, poor memory, excessive or absent menstruation: HYPOTHYROIDISM.

Puffiness, also with puffiness of feet, in a child, with thick dry wrinkled skin, enlarged tongue, thickened lips, broad face, flat nose, apathy, dullness: CRETINISM.

Weakness and wasting of hand muscles, later spreading to forearms and shoulders, with weakness and spasticity of legs: AMYOTROPHIC LATERAL SCLEROSIS.

Weakness, with one or many other symptoms: numbness and tingling of arms or fingers, stiff neck or shoulders, headache, "knots" in neck, shoulder or arm muscles, swelling and stiffness of fingers, blurred vision, loss of balance, pain in and around eyes, fainting: CERVICAL SYNDROME.

## HEAD

Sudden, severe head pain, with nausea, vomiting, stiffness of neck, dizziness, convulsions: SUBARACHNOID HEMORRHAGE.

## HEADACHE

Piercing, throbbing, pounding, splitting or dull, headaches seem to be universal. An estimated seven of every ten adults in the United

States resort to analgesics for headaches at least once a month, and in one of every dozen cases headache is a chronic problem.

Most headaches are not related to organic disease. The most common: psychogenic (tension) headaches and migraine. Also numerous: cluster headaches and depression headaches.

**Psychogenic.** Often arises in back part of head and spreads over entire head, may produce viselike constriction, a kind of "hatband" head pain, tends to be long-lasting, may respond to aspirin alone or aspirin combined with a mild tranquilizing agent or a mild sedative such as phenobarbital.

**Migraine.** Pain may be generalized or confined to one side of head, sometimes preceded by a brief period of irritability, restlessness, depression, or appetite loss and, in a few cases, by visual disturbances, and often accompanied by nausea, vomiting, light sensitivity. May respond, in mild cases, to aspirin, otherwise to ergotamine tartrate preparations. Recent studies suggest that some patients may respond well to propranolol, others to an antidepressant drug such as amitriptyline.

**Cluster.** Excruciatingly painful, one-sided, involving eye, temple, neck, and face, called "cluster" because a headache may appear suddenly, recur repeatedly for days or weeks, disappear suddenly, then return in another clustered batch. A recent study suggests that three to six inhalations, 15 to 20 minutes apart, of epinephrine in aerosol form may break the cyclic pattern and minimize severity of the headaches.

**Depression.** Often a constant steady headache that may be present all day long, usually worse in the morning, generalized over the entire head, often associated with sleep disturbance (frequent awakening during the night and early awakening in morning), sometimes with one or more other complaints of constipation, chest pain, gastrointestinal disturbances, loss of interest in work and sex. Often responds to antidepressant drug treatment, which also may relieve other symptoms.

Headache, along with other symptoms, also accompanies many infections and a variety of other diseases:

### In malignancy

With one or many other symptoms: muscle weakness, failing vision, vomiting, lack of balance and coordination, drowsiness, lethargy, personality changes, sometimes coma: CANCER OF THE BRAIN.

## In childhood infections

With slight fever, rash, backache, appetite loss: CHICKENPOX.

With bright red rash, sore throat, swelling of neck lymph nodes, nausea, vomiting: SCARLET FEVER.

With sore throat, nausea, swallowing and breathing difficulty: DIPHTHERIA.

With swelling of glands below and in front of ears, fever, appetite loss, back pain: MUMPS.

## In other common infections

With fever, chills, malaise, sore throat, blisterlike, measleslike, or scarlet-feverlike rash: MONONUCLEOSIS, INFECTIOUS.

With fever, generalized aches and pains most pronounced in back and legs, sore throat, mild distress below breastbone, weakness, appetite loss, sometimes nasal discharge: INFLUENZA.

With scratchy throat, sneezing, nasal discharge, malaise, sometimes fever: COLD, COMMON.

With sharp chest pain, cough, pinkish sputum becoming rusty, shaking chill followed by fever, breathing difficulty, rapid and painful respiration, sometimes with malaise, appetite loss, muscular pain: PNEUMONIA.

With frequency and urgency of urination, fever, chills, sometimes pain in one or both sides of lower back: PYELONEPHRITIS.

With fever, nausea, abdominal discomfort, drowsiness, lassitude, weakness, appetite loss, sometimes jaundice: HEPATITIS.

With nasal and postnasal discharge, sometimes fever to 102°, dizziness, toothache, generalized aching, puffiness about the eyes: SINUSITIS.

With sore throat, pain in tonsil area especially during swallowing, chills, fever to 106°, malaise, sometimes stiff neck: TONSILLITIS.

## In less common infections

With fever, pain and stiffness in back and neck, sore throat, drowsiness: POLIOMYELITIS.

With stiff neck, fever, vomiting, muscle twitching, tremor, mental confusion: ENCEPHALITIS, VIRAL.

With chills, fever, malaise, appetite loss, nosebleeds, backache, diarrhea, sore throat: TYPHOID FEVER.

With chills, fever, depression, sometimes back pain, diarrhea: BRUCELLOSIS.

With chills, fever, cough, inflamed painful swellings of lymph nodes usually in groin, vomiting, thirst, generalized pain, mental dullness, sometimes convulsions: PLAGUE.

With pain behind eyes, back and joint pain, difficulty in movement, fever to 106°, pink rash, congested eyeballs, flushed face: DENGUE.

With pain behind eyes, chills, fever, joint and muscle pain, intolerance of light, nausea, vomiting, sore throat, abdominal pain: ROCKY MOUNTAIN SPOTTED FEVER.

With fever, eye inflammation, chills, sometimes nausea, vomiting, jaundice, skin rash, blood in urine, diminished urination: LEPTOSPIROSIS.

With chills, fever, delirium, vomiting, muscle and joint pain, reddish rash over trunk and extremities followed by rose-colored spots, sometimes jaundice: RELAPSING FEVER.

With fever, chills, rash, sometimes vomiting, convulsions: SMALLPOX.

With fever, muscle aches, flushed face, congested gums, red and pointed tongue, nausea, vomiting, constipation, jaundice: YELLOW FEVER.

With chills, fever, nausea, vomiting, red rash, severe weakness: TULAREMIA.

With red-brown elevated skin lesion that enlarges, reddens, and blisters, muscle pain, malaise, fever, nausea, vomiting: ANTHRAX.

With vision blurring, sometimes confusion, depression, agitation or other mental disturbance: CRYPTOCOCCOSIS.

With muscular weakness, diarrhea, weight loss, eye inflammation, sometimes swelling of lymph glands (nodes), cough, breathing difficulty: HISTOPLASMOSIS.

With chills, fever to 104° or 105°, profuse perspiration, nausea, body pains, exhaustion: MALARIA.

With a persistent sore a few days after and at site of a minor cat scratch, followed by gland (lymph node) swellings at sites near scratch, fever, malaise, appetite loss: CAT-SCRATCH DISEASE.

Violent, persistent headache, with stiff neck, fever, vomiting: MENINGITIS.

### In other disorders

With itching of nose, roof of mouth, throat and eyes, tearing of eyes, sneezing, nasal discharge, sometimes coughing, wheezing, insomnia: RHINITIS, ALLERGIC.

With one or more other symptoms: dizziness, ringing in ears, spots before eyes, easy fatigability, weakness, drowsiness, irritability, pallor, heart pounding and shortness of breath on exertion: ANEMIA.

With dizziness, vision disturbances, labored breathing, itching, lassitude, disturbances of sensations in hands and feet: POLYCYTHEMIA VERA.

Sometimes with nosebleeds: COARCTATION OF THE AORTA.

Sometimes with one or more other symptoms: fatigue, nervousness, dizziness, palpitation, insomnia, weakness: HYPERTENSION.

With abdominal pain or pressure, one or more other symptoms: nausea, dizziness, vomiting, blood in vomitus, sensation of fullness, appetite loss, malaise: GASTRITIS.

With sudden abdominal cramps, chills, fever, nausea, vomiting, diarrhea: GASTROENTERITIS, FOOD INFECTION or STAPHYLOCOCCUS TOXIN.

During week to ten days before menstruation, sometimes with breast pain, generalized fluid retention, irritability, nervousness, depression: PREMENSTRUAL TENSION.

With nasal obstruction, breathing difficulty, sometimes nasal discharge: POLYPS.

Severe, with coarse and sparse hair, loss of eyebrows, dry rough skin, cracked lips, weakness: HYPERVITAMINOSIS A.

With sweating, flushing or pallor, chilliness, numbness, trembling, dizziness, weakness, palpitation, hunger, sometimes faintness, all occurring several hours after meals: HYPOGLYCEMIA.

With weakness, sometimes malaise and abdominal pain, nausea, vomiting: METABOLIC ACIDOSIS.

With nervousness, weakness, heart sensitivity, sweating, overactivity, restlessness, weight loss with increased appetite, tremor, palpitation, stare, sometimes nausea, abdominal pain, diarrhea: HYPERTHYROIDISM.

With palpitation, pallor, sweating, nausea, apprehension, high blood pressure, pain over stomach area: PHEOCHROMOCYTOMA.

With pain and tenderness of temporal arteries in head, sometimes vision disturbance: TEMPORAL ARTERITIS.

With one or many other symptoms: numbness and tingling of arms or fingers, weakness of arms or hands, stiff neck or shoulder, "knots" in neck, shoulder or arm muscles, swelling and stiffness of fingers, blurring of vision, loss of balance, pain in and around eyes, fainting: CERVICAL SYNDROME.

## HEARING LOSS

Episodes of, with ringing in ears, vertigo, nausea, vomiting: MEN-
IERE'S DISEASE.

With one or many other symptoms: chilliness, dry cold skin, puffiness of hands and face, decreased appetite, weight gain, slow
speech, mental apathy, drowsiness, constipation, poor memory: HY-
POTHYROIDISM.

### Other causes

Hearing loss, ranging from partial to complete, may be induced by
many factors.

In one form, *conductive* deafness, anything that interferes with
conduction of sound to the inner ear can be responsible—including
excessive wax in the ear, a boil, a perforation or inflammation of the
eardrum, a middle ear inflammation. Commonly in children excessive adenoidal tissue about the opening of the eustachian tube in the
mouth can block the tube and prevent normal middle ear ventilation,
causing hearing loss. In young adults, otosclerosis is the most common cause; it involves the formation of spongy bone in the inner ear
that may prevent free movement of the bones that transmit sound. An
early symptom of otosclerosis is ringing in the ears, but the most
noticeable is progressive loss of hearing. Of unknown cause, otosclerosis strikes women about twice as often as men. Most patients benefit from surgery in which the stirrup bone (stapes) in the inner ear is
freed or replaced with grafted body tissue attached to a plastic or
stainless steel wire tube. Treatment for other types of conductive
deafness is aimed at eliminating the wax, perforation, or other cause.

Hearing loss also may be *perceptive*, or *sensory-neural*, involving
disorders of the inner ear, nerve of hearing, brain pathways, or auditory center in the brain. Such structures may be affected by mumps,
measles, and other infections, tumors, injury from skull fracture, and
injury sometimes from drugs to which an individual may be sensitive, including aspirin and similar compounds, quinine, antibiotics,
alcohol. Treatment is for the underlying cause if possible. If the
cause cannot be overcome, audiometric studies may be done and
hearing aids evaluated.

## HEARTBEAT

Stopping of the beat, absence of breathing: CARDIAC ARREST.

**First Aid**

In some cases, if the heart is not severely damaged and action can be taken rapidly, the heart can be stimulated to resume beating.

**Closed-chest heart massage.** While having medical aid summoned, place both hands, one on top the other, on the lower portion of victim's chest, at the bottom of the breastbone. Apply pressure through the heel of your bottom hand, pushing firmly but not more than about two inches downward. Repeat 60 times a minute. *In addition:*

**Breathing.** Rescue breathing as well as heart massage will be needed. If another rescuer is available, he or she should proceed simultaneously, as you do heart massage, to lift up the victim's neck with one hand and push the forehead down with the other. This opens the airway and breathing may start. If not, pinch victim's nostrils shut with fingers of one hand and, mouth-to-mouth, blow air in. When the victim's chest moves up, take mouth away and allow chest to go down by itself. Beginning rescue breathing should include four quick full breaths without waiting for full deflation of lungs between breaths.

**The combination.** If there is only one rescuer, he must carry out both breathing and massage in this ratio: after 15 chest compressions at a rate of 80 per minute, administer 2 very quick lung inflations. With two rescuers, 5 chest compressions at a rate of 60 per minute should be carried out, then 2 lung inflations, then compressions again, repeating the cycle.

Abnormally fast (more than 100 per minute) heartbeat, also abnormally forceful: SINUS TACHYCARDIA.

Sudden fast beats (100 per minute or more) with fluttering sensation in chest, weakness, faintness, sometimes nausea: PAROXYSMAL TACHYCARDIA.

Skipped beats, sometimes with feeling of "something turning over in chest" or "shock in chest": PREMATURE CONTRACTIONS.

Slow beats (less then 60 per minute), sometimes with faintness or dizziness: SINUS BRADYCARDIA.

**HEARTBURN**

Heartburn, a burning sensation in the esophagus (gullet) or below the breastbone in the region of the heart, occurs when the stomach regurgitates part of its contents, forcing them upward into the esophagus. Since the material is acid, it acts as an irritant. Emotional disturbance, excitement, and nervous tension are frequent causes; they may affect both the motion and secretions of the stomach. Heartburn may also be associated with other symptoms and disturbances:

With one or more other symptoms: nausea, upper abdominal pain, flatulence, belching, feelings of fullness and abdominal distention during or after a meal: INDIGESTION.

Sometimes with swallowing difficulty, gastrointestinal bleeding manifested as vomiting of blood or darkening of stools by blood pigments: HERNIA, HIATAL.

With chronic or chronic relapsing diarrhea, stools loose but free of blood or pus and sometimes containing undigested food residue, mild abdominal pain, nausea, fullness after meals: DIARRHEA, CHRONIC NONINFLAMMATORY.

## HEAT SENSITIVITY

With one or many other symptoms: nervousness, weakness, sweating, restlessness, weight loss with increased appetite, tremor, palpitation, stare, abnormal eye protrusion, sometimes headache, nausea, abdominal pain, diarrhea: HYPERTHYROIDISM.

## HICCUP (SINGULTUS)

Hiccups involve involuntary contractions of the diaphragm leading to uncontrolled inhalations which, because air passages are partially closed, produce the unique noise of hiccuping. Transient hiccuping is common, sometimes the result of rapid eating but often of unknown cause. Hiccuping also may accompany serious conditions such as UREMIA, HEPATITIS, PANCREATITIS, PNEUMONIA, with other accompanying symptoms. It may also be associated with alcoholism and emotional disturbances.

**Treatment.** Any of a variety of simple measures may work to stop hiccups: a series of deep, regular breaths; drinking a glass of water rapidly; pulling on the tongue; swallowing dry bread or crushed ice; rebreathing into a paper bag which, by increasing carbon dioxide content of lungs and blood, may cause brain breathing centers to call for stronger, deeper breathing, making diaphragm contractions more regular and stopping hiccups. In unyielding cases, an often-successful measure is the insertion by a physician of a plastic or rubber tube through the nose to stimulate the pharynx.

## HIVES

Also called *urticaria* and *angioedema*, hives consists of an eruption of slightly elevated patches on the skin, redder or paler than surrounding areas, often accompanied by itching.

With crampy abdominal pain, nausea, vomiting, diarrhea: GASTROINTESTINAL ALLERGY.

With fever, joint pains, skin rash, gland (lymph node) swelling: SERUM SICKNESS.

After swelling of upper eyelids, pain in eyes, often accompanied by one or many other symptoms: light sensitivity, fever, muscle soreness and pain, thirst, chills, profuse sweating, weakness, prostration: TRICHINOSIS.

Preceded by a papule or small, solid skin elevation, fever, with chronic diarrhea, sometimes bladder inflammation: SCHISTOSOMIASIS.

**Other causes.** Hives also may appear with or follow some streptococcal and viral infections, insect stings or bites, and may be caused by allergy to some drugs as well as foods.

**Treatment.** Acute hives usually subsides within one to several days and may be relieved by an oral antihistamine drug. Angioedema, a more severe reaction, may include swelling of under-skin tissue in hands, feet, eyelids, lips, genitalia, or upper airway producing wheezing and breathing difficulty and may be treated with a cortisonelike drug such as prednisone.

## HOARSENESS

Hoarseness can result from shouting or prolonged excessive use of the voice. It may accompany many upper respiratory infections such as the common cold, influenza, and diphtheria. Other causes:

With throat tickling and rawness, constant effort to clear the throat: LARYNGITIS, ACUTE.

With burning, dryness or lump in throat, chills, fever, swallowing difficulty: PHARYNGITIS.

With "barking" cough, croaking sound during breathing, spasms of choking: LARYNGITIS, ACUTE OBSTRUCTIVE.

With severe breathing difficulty, high fever, almost constant but nonproductive cough, flushing followed by pallor and blueness: LARYNGOTRACHEOBRONCHITIS, ACUTE.

Chronic: POLYPOSIS OF THE VOCAL CORDS.

Persistent, without pain, especially in anyone over the age of 40: CANCER OF THE LARYNX.

With cough, labored breathing, difficulty in swallowing, chest or back pain: ANEURYSM, INTRATHORACIC.

With fever, joint pains, weight loss, sometimes also cough, breathing difficulty: SARCOIDOSIS.

## HUNGER, EXCESSIVE

With excessive urination, thirst, itching, weakness, weight loss, dryness of the skin: DIABETES.

Beginning several hours after meals, accompanied by one or more other symptoms: sweating, flushing or pallor, chilliness, numbness, trembling, headache, dizziness, palpitation, weakness, sometimes faintness: HYPOGLYCEMIA.

## IMPOTENCE

Impotence—inability to attain or maintain a satisfactory erection—may result from physical and psychic causes. Almost invariably, when physical causes are involved, other symptoms are present. Physical causes include anatomic faults in the urethra, inflammatory disease of the genitalia, alcoholism, DIABETES, SYPHILIS, aortic ANEURYSM, MULTIPLE SCLEROSIS, STROKE. Commonly, impotence may be overcome once underlying problems are controlled. Psychic factors are often responsible and include fear of inducing pregnancy, anxiety over contracting venereal disease, inhibitions resulting from religious scruples, and other influences, often helped by psychotherapy. In some older men who experience increasing impotence unrelated to disease or psychic causes, testosterone, the male sex hormone, may sometimes be useful.

## INFECTIONS, REPEATED

Repeated occurrences of meningitis, middle ear infections, pneumonia, purulent skin infections: HYPOGAMMAGLOBULINEMIA.

Mild or severe, with malaise, fatigability, joint pains, or chronic ill health: PRIMARY SPLENIC NEUTROPENIA.

With weakness, weight loss, persistent pain especially in back, chest, or pelvis: MYELOMA, MULTIPLE.

With weakness, weight loss, anemia, bleeding of mucous membranes: MACROGLOBULINEMIA.

With shortness of breath, fatigability: ATRIAL SEPTAL DEFECT.

With chronic cough, rapid breathing rate, large, frequent, foul-smelling stools, protuberant abdomen, barrel-like chest, blueness: CYSTIC FIBROSIS.

## INFERTILITY

About 10 percent of American couples have infertility problems. Recent studies suggest that in about 40 percent of the cases, infertility or relative infertility in the male is a major factor; in about 60 percent, the major difficulty may lie with the female—although in some cases relative infertility in both partners may be involved and can be treated.

Factors in a man include impaired sperm production, obstruction of the seminal tract, defective delivery of sperm into the vagina. Sperm production may be impaired as the result of infection or injury of the testes, drug toxicity, hydrocele (a scrotal mass with fluid), underfunctioning of thyroid (HYPOTHYROIDISM) or pituitary gland (HYPOPITUITARISM), tumor of the adrenal gland. Obstruction of the seminal tract may result from inflammatory conditions such as PROSTATITIS and URETHRITIS. Defective delivery of sperm may result from premature ejaculation, prostate surgery, stricture or narrowing of the urethra, or hypospadias (opening of the urethra on the underside of the penis). Medical or surgical treatment often can be effective, with even sperm production failure sometimes responding to treatment with chorionic gonadotropins or methyltestosterone.

Factors in a woman that require investigation include failure of ovulation, hostile mucus, abnormalities of such structures as cervix and tubes.

## INSOMNIA

Insomnia—the inability to fall asleep readily or remain asleep throughout the night—may, of course, accompany various disease conditions such as HYPERTENSION and BRUCELLOSIS. But it has many other causes, ranging from sensitivity to noise, to the caffeine in coffee, tea and cola drinks consumed late in the day, to heavy meals consumed shortly before bedtime, to carrying to bed personal problems and anxieties about job, finances, family matters. Drug dependency, too, recent sleep research laboratory studies indicate, is a common cause of insomnia. Some estimates indicate use of sleeping pills by 25 to 50 percent of all Americans. Although at first the pills may increase sleep time, almost without exception they eventually make insomnia worse. Depression is another relatively common cause of insomnia. Its recognition and adequate treatment with antidepressant medication may lead to relief of the insomnia and other symptoms associated with the depressed state.

One newer approach to treating insomnia is based on the concept that in many cases it is a matter of misuse of the bed and bad sleeping habits. This method calls for the individual to actually go to bed only when tired, never otherwise; once in the bedroom to avoid TV viewing, reading or worrying; to stay in bed to sleep, not stew, and if sleep does not come within a short time to leave the bed and the room and return only when ready to try to fall asleep again—and, again, if sleep does not come readily, to leave bed and room, and keep repeating the process until sleep comes quickly after return to bed. Moreover, no matter how little sleep obtained this way during early stages, the alarm should be set for the same time every morning, since the body needs rest and a regular schedule will help to get it.

### INSTABILITY, EMOTIONAL (see EMOTIONAL INSTABILITY)

### INTERCOURSE, PAINFUL (DYSPAREUNIA)

With bleeding afterward, sometimes watery discharge, urinary frequency and urgency, painful defecation: CANCER OF THE VAGINA.

Much more commonly, pain during or after intercourse may be due to vaginal spasm, inadequate lubrication, or genital tract problems. Lack of adequate lubrication may be the result of insufficient foreplay. Genital tract problems include tears of the hymen, inflammatory conditions, overtight episiotomy repair in childbirth, endometriosis, any of which requires treatment.

### IRRITABILITY

Irritability, of course, is not abnormal under circumstances of fatigue or frustration. It also is an accompaniment of mental disorder and distressing physical disease. It may be particularly pronounced in some diseases:

In early infancy, with epileptic seizures, vomiting: PHENYLKETON-URIA.

During the week to ten days prior to menstruation, with one or more other symptoms: breast pain, nervousness, depression, headache, generalized fluid retention: PREMENSTRUAL TENSION.

With one or more other symptoms: pallor, dizziness, headache, ringing in the ears, spots before the eyes, easy fatigability, weakness, drowsiness, heart pounding and shortness of breath on exertion: ANEMIA.

With fatigue, lack of energy, appetite loss, aches and pains, often poor memory, sleep disturbances, chest pain, abdominal discomfort, constipation: VITAMIN DEFICIENCY (thiamine).

In a child, with appetite loss, failure to gain weight, fever, anemia: SCURVY.

With shallow or irregular breathing, prickling or burning sensations in fingers, toes, or lips, muscle cramps: METABOLIC ALKALOSIS.

With chills, fever, headache, pain behind eyes, joint and muscle pain, light intolerance, nausea, vomiting, sore throat, abdominal pain: ROCKY MOUNTAIN SPOTTED FEVER.

With chills, fever, headache, diarrhea, malaise: BRUCELLOSIS.

With fever, abdominal pain, painful straining at stool, blood and pus in stools which increase to 20 or more a day: BACILLARY DYSEN-TERY.

With stiffness of jaw, neck, arms, or legs, swallowing difficulty, fever, sore throat: TETANUS.


## ITCHING (see also SKIN, ITCHING)

With hives, fever, joint pains, skin rash, gland swelling: ANAPHY-LAXIS.

With vision disturbances, dizziness, headache, labored breathing, sensation disturbances in hands and feet: POLYCYTHEMIA VERA.

With red skin spots that turn purple, often with fever, malaise, sometimes joint pain, bouts of abdominal pain: PURPURA, ALLERGIC.

With lassitude, fatigue, decreased mental acuity, muscular twitching and cramps, convulsions, nausea, vomiting, yellow-brown skin discoloration, hiccuping, urine smell on breath and sweat: UREMIA.

With one or many other symptoms: nausea, vomiting, sweating, eye tearing, dilation or contraction of pupils, diarrhea, abdominal cramps, thirst, dizziness, confusion, throat constriction, blood-streaked stools and vomitus, limb numbness, muscle weakness, chest pain, cramps in extremities: FOOD POISONING, NONBACTERIAL.

With jaundice, deposits of fatty substances in skin and eyelids, softening of bones, high blood-fat levels: CIRRHOSIS, BILIARY.

With appetite loss, nausea, vomiting, excessive urination and thirst, weakness, nervousness: HYPERVITAMINOSIS D.

With excessive urination, thirst, hunger, weakness, weight loss, dryness of skin: DIABETES.

Intense, worse at night, with slightly elevated grayish white lines sometimes visible on close inspection, sometimes with blisters and pustules: SCABIES.

With painless enlargement of lymph glands (nodes) in neck, underarms and groin, later with sweating, fever, weakness, loss of appetite and weight: HODGKIN'S DISEASE.

Of anus: CANDIDIASIS.

Around anal and perineal area (the area between anal opening and vagina or scrotum): PINWORMS.

Of nose, roof of mouth, throat and eyes, with eye tearing, sneezing, nasal discharge, sometimes headache, irritability, coughing, wheezing: RHINITIS, ALLERGIC.

Of some area of skin, followed by eruption of slightly elevated patches, redder or paler than surrounding skin: HIVES.

With hives, fever, joint pains, rash, gland (lymph node) swelling: SERUM SICKNESS.

**Treatment.** Effective treatment requires determining and combating the cause of itching. Treatment of the symptom itself, as a temporary measure, may include use of starch baths, an antihistamine such as cyproheptadine, and, when required, topical corticosteroid preparations.

### JAUNDICE

A yellowness of skin and eyes, jaundice is produced by an excess of a normal bile pigment, *bilirubin*. Bilirubin is derived from the hemoglobin released from worn-out red blood cells which are normally replaced by new red cells, and normally the liver absorbs the pigment and secretes it along with other constituents of bile. Jaundice can occur when the liver is diseased, or bile flow is obstructed, or, as in some anemias, red blood cell destruction is excessive.

Chronic, with itching, high blood-fat levels, deposits of fatty substances in the skin and eyelids, softening of bones: CIRRHOSIS, BILIARY.

Abrupt, with fever, fluid accumulation in and distention of abdomen, edema or waterlogging of tissues elsewhere: HEPATITIS, ALCOHOLIC.

With pain in right upper abdominal quadrant, extending into right shoulder, severe, remaining steadily severe for hours, sometimes with fever, chills, nausea, abdominal distention: CHOLECYSTITIS, ACUTE.

With intermittent fever and chills, abdominal pain: CHOLANGITIS, ASCENDING.

With fever, headache, nausea, drowsiness, appetite loss, lassitude, weakness: HEPATITIS.

With abdominal pain that may be constant or intermittent, mild or severe, beginning in stomach area and sometimes radiating to back and left shoulder, sometimes with fever: PANCREATITIS, CHRONIC.

With fever, headache, chilliness, fatigue, malaise, one or more other symptoms of sore throat, gland (lymph node) swelling, severe weakness, occasionally abdominal pain, nausea, eyelid swelling, faintly red skin eruptions: MONONUCLEOSIS, INFECTIOUS.

With acute headache, fever, chills, sometimes nausea, vomiting, skin rash, blood in urine, diminished urination: LEPTOSPIROSIS.

With episodes of joint pain, fever, severe abdominal pain with vomiting: ANEMIA, SICKLE CELL.

With spleen enlargement, pallor, lack of energy, sometimes episodes of chills, fever, aching in abdomen and in back and legs: ANEMIA, HEMOLYTIC.

With fluid accumulation in and distention of abdomen, often with tender, rapidly enlarging liver: CANCER OF THE LIVER.

With variable abdominal pain often extending to the back and relieved by sitting up or bending forward, often with other symptoms such as weight and appetite loss, nausea, vomiting, constipation or diarrhea, sometimes with vomiting of blood and darkening of stools: CANCER OF THE PANCREAS.

## JAW

Small, hard swelling, with or without pain, around the jaw or under the mucous membrane of the mouth or the skin of the neck, sometimes also affecting other parts of the head, breaking down and discharging little yellowish granules: ACTINOMYCOSIS.

Limited motion, often with clicking or grating sounds on chewing and with pain in the face and in front of the ear: TEMPOROMANDIBULAR JOINT DISORDERS.

Stiffness, with stiff neck, swallowing difficulty, stiff arms or legs, fever, sore throat, constipation, sometimes convulsions: TETANUS.

## JOINT PAIN

Joints, which are junctions of two or more bones, have complex structures. In addition to ends of bones, they include ligaments, tough fibers that bind bones together; cartilage, a tissue that covers and cushions bone ends; an articular capsule to enclose bone ends; synovial membrane, lining the capsule and producing a lubricating fluid; and, in many cases, bursae (fluid-filled cushioning sacs). Commonly, joints are subject to great stress in normal living. They are also subject to wrenches, sprains, dislocations, and painful inflammation caused by injury or disease.

### In arthritic disorders

Morning stiffness of one or more joints of hands, feet, wrist, elbow, ankle becoming swollen, painful, inflamed, with malaise, fever, weight loss: ARTHRITIS, RHEUMATOID.

Pain, less severe than in rheumatoid arthritis, most often in weight-bearing joints in knees and hips, sometimes in joints in neck, spine, fingers: ARTHRITIS (OSTEOARTHRITIS).

Joint pain flare-ups, similar in severity to those of rheumatoid arthritis but paralleling flare-ups of the skin disease psoriasis: ARTHRITIS, PSORIATIC.

Throbbing, crushing pain appearing suddenly in big toe or other joint in ankle, instep, knee, wrist, elbow, with swelling, warmth, redness, shininess of overlying skin: GOUT.

### In infections

Acute pain in many joints, similar to that of rheumatoid arthritis, with redness, exquisite tenderness, pain on motion, formation or discharge of pus particularly at knee, wrist, ankle, commonly with urinary frequency and other symptoms of PROSTATITIS in a man, vaginal discharge in a woman: ARTHRITIS, GONOCOCCAL.

With pain behind eyes, headache, back pain frequently accompanying other joint pain, difficulty in movement, fever to 106°, pink rash, flushed face: DENGUE.

With muscle pain, pain behind eyes, chills, fever, sore throat, abdominal pain, nausea, vomiting: ROCKY MOUNTAIN SPOTTED FEVER.

With chills, fever, muscle pain, headache, vomiting, reddish rash over trunk and extremities followed by rose-colored spots, sometimes jaundice: RELAPSING FEVER.

With chills, fever, headache, malaise, sometimes diarrhea: BRUCELLOSIS.

With fever, tiredness, vague pain in limbs, pain, swelling and tenderness of joints, with pain often disappearing in one group of joints and starting up in another: RHEUMATIC FEVER.

With redness and swelling of large joints, back pain, fever alternating with normal temperature, swelling of lymph nodes, spotty rash: RAT-BITE FEVER.

With swelling and one or more other symptoms: fever, cough, sputum production, sore throat: COCCIDIOMYCOSIS.

With chills, fever, malaise, lassitude, appetite loss, sometimes tender small nodules about the tips of digits: ENDOCARDITIS, BACTERIAL.

In legs, with swelling, limp: TUBERCULOSIS (of bones and joints).

In the spine, with painful muscle spasm, limitation of movement, followed by curvature of spine and abscess formation: TUBERCULOSIS (of bones and joints).

## In malignancy

With high fever, infection of mouth, throat or lung, sometimes small purplish-red spots and bruises on skin, bleeding from mouth, nose, bowel, kidneys: LEUKEMIA, ACUTE.

## In other disorders

Episodes of joint pain with fever, severe abdominal pain, vomiting, jaundice: ANEMIA, SICKLE CELL.

With fever, weight loss, sometimes also cough, breathing difficulty, hoarseness: SARCOIDOSIS.

With fever lasting a day or two, hives, skin rash, itching, gland (lymph node) swelling: SERUM SICKNESS.

With red skin spots that turn purple, itching, fever, malaise, sometimes abdominal pain: PURPURA, ALLERGIC.

With joint stiffening, excessive bleeding from minor injuries: HEMOPHILIA.

With fatigability, malaise, chronic ill health, repeated mild or severe infections: PRIMARY SPLENIC NEUTROPENIA.

Of shoulder, knee, elbow, sudden and severe, with limitation of motion: BURSITIS.

With muscle pain, tenderness, stiffness, occurring suddenly, usually following injury, strain, exposure to damp or cold, sometimes infection: FIBROMYOSITIS.

With stiffness, often with reddening and puffiness of face and skin over elbows, knees, other joints, sometimes with painful swollen

muscles, swallowing difficulty, gastrointestinal disturbances: DERMA-
TOMYOSITIS.

With fever, weight loss, one or more other symptoms: severe abdominal pain, diffuse muscle pains, bloody diarrhea, heart failure,
wheezing, pneumonia, skin reddening, hives: POLYARTERITIS.

Of knees, wrists, back, with diarrhea, appetite and weight loss,
anemia, weakness, fever to 103°, nonproductive cough, abdominal
and chest pain: WHIPPLE'S DISEASE.

Vague joint and muscle aches, lassitude, weakness, irritability,
weight loss, swollen and bleeding gums, small black and blue spots
on skin: SCURVY.

## KIDNEY PAIN

The kidneys, two glandular, almost bean-shaped organs, each
about 4 inches long, 2 inches wide, and 1 inch thick in an adult, are
located behind the abdominal cavity, on either side of the backbone,
just underneath the rib cage.

Recurrent attacks of pain in kidney area, either dull and nagging or
sharp, sometimes with fever and with blood and pus in the urine:
HYDRONEPHROSIS.

Excruciating intermittent pain usually starting in kidney area and
radiating across abdomen into genital area and inner aspects of thigh,
sometimes with nausea, vomiting, chills, fever, frequency of urination: URINARY CALCULI (STONES).

Episodic pain, with blood in urine, abdominal discomfort: POLY-
CYSTIC KIDNEY DISEASE.

## KNEE

*Knock-knee* is an inward curving of the knees and sometimes a
rubbing together of the knees during walking. Once a common
symptom of rickets, knock-knee today is more often caused by irregular bone growth or weak ligaments, with milder cases in young children often disappearing as bones, muscles and ligaments strengthen
after early childhood. More serious cases may be corrected by special strengthening exercises and expert joint manipulation.

Swelling and tenderness of a knee, with pain on bending, is called
*housemaid's knee.* A form of BURSITIS, it involves injury to the bursa
in front of the kneecap as the result of prolonged kneeling on hard
surfaces. It may be alleviated with medical treatment and avoided

thereafter by use of a thick, soft pad when working in kneeling position.

*Water on the knee,* with the knee swollen from accumulated fluid, may follow a knee injury, infection or acute arthritis, and commonly improves with rest for the joint and, when infection or arthritis is involved, appropriate treatment.

*Trick knee,* often occurring in athletes after a blow or twisting violent enough to weaken or tear ligaments or other structures of the knee, is highly susceptible to further trouble because of weakness and may require use of an elastic bandage during vigorous activity.

Throbbing, crushing pain in a knee, appearing suddenly, with swelling, warmth, redness, shininess of overlying skin: GOUT.

## LACTATION

Failure of, after childbirth, with one or many other symptoms: apathy, appetite and weight loss, easy fatigue, cold intolerance, diminished libido, scantiness or absence of underarm and pubic hair, scanty menstruation: HYPOPITUITARISM.

Inappropriate lactation in childless women and in men may be due to a pituitary tumor or to some drugs such as reserpine, meprobamate, other tranquilizers and methyldopa or to other conditions such as ENCEPHALITIS, DIABETES. Lactation due to drugs stops when the drugs are stopped. Lactation due to other causes may respond when the underlying problem is diagnosed and treated. Inappropriate lactation of unknown cause may sometimes respond to treatment with a combination of female hormones estrogen and progestin.

## LASSITUDE

With dizziness, headache, vision disturbances, labored breathing, itching, sensation disturbances in hands and feet: POLYCYTHEMIA VERA.

With fever, chills, malaise, joint pains, appetite loss, sometimes tender small nodules about the tips of the digits: ENDOCARDITIS, BACTERIAL.

With muscle cramps and twitching, nausea, vomiting, yellow-brown discoloration of skin, hiccuping, itching, urine smell on breath and sweat: UREMIA.

With urinary frequency, urgency, pain and burning, often with chills, fever, nausea, vomiting, general muscle aches: URINARY TRACT INFECTIONS.

With fever, headache, abdominal discomfort, appetite loss, nausea, drowsiness, sometimes jaundice: HEPATITIS.

With weakness, irritability, weight loss, vague muscle and joint aches, swollen and bleeding gums, small black and blue spots on the skin: SCURVY.

## LEG

Some bowing, or outward curvature of one or both legs (*bowleg*), is normal in infants, but disappears in healthy babies as bones develop. If dietary deficiencies cause the bones to remain pliable instead of developing normally, permanent bowing may develop with walking. In adults, bowing may occur in association with a disease affecting the bones: OSTEOMALACIA.

Muscle cramps in, leg muscle fatigability, soreness in calf muscles, sometimes with ankle swelling that may disappear overnight, sometimes itching, scaly skin: VARICOSE VEINS.

Coldness, numbness, tingling or burning, sometimes followed by pain or tightness after exertion: BUERGER'S DISEASE.

Sudden coldness, numbness, tingling, followed by severe pain, with blanching or mottling with blue patches: ACUTE ARTERIAL OCCLUSION.

Pain, beginning in buttock and extending down back of thigh and leg to ankle: SCIATICA.

Pain and aching episodes in legs, abdomen, back, with chills, fever, malaise, spleen enlargement, jaundice: ANEMIA, HEMOLYTIC.

Pain on walking, with weakness, intensifying until walking is impossible, disappearance of symptoms after leg rest: INTERMITTENT CLAUDICATION.

Swelling, pain or tenderness in a leg, sometimes with noticeably increased warmth and dilation of veins: VENOUS THROMBOSIS.

Chronic swelling, painless, of whole or part of leg: LYMPHEDEMA.

Swelling with fluid (edema), followed by generalized edema, digestive disturbances, weight loss, appetite loss, weakness, lethargy: PROTEIN DEFICIENCY (chronic).

Swelling with fluid, sometimes enormous, with swelling then affecting arms, face, torso: NEPHROTIC SYNDROME.

Stiffness, with stiffness of jaw, neck, sore throat, swallowing difficulty, fever, restlessness: TETANUS.

Weakness and spasticity of legs, with weakness and wasting of hand muscles, forearms, shoulders: AMYOTROPHIC LATERAL SCLEROSIS.

## LETHARGY

With swelling of legs that becomes generalized, digestive disturbances, appetite and weight loss, weakness: PROTEIN DEFICIENCY (chronic).

With one or many other symptoms: headache, muscle weakness, failing vision, vomiting, loss of balance and coordination, drowsiness, personality changes: CANCER OF THE BRAIN.

With pain behind eyes, chills, fever, headache, joint and muscle pain, intolerance of light, nausea, vomiting, sore throat, abdominal pain: ROCKY MOUNTAIN SPOTTED FEVER.

With headache, fever, chilliness, fatigue, severe weakness, sore throat, sometimes abdominal pain, nausea, jaundice, faintly red skin eruption, eyelid swelling: MONONUCLEOSIS, INFECTIOUS.

With one or more other symptoms: dry cold skin, puffiness of hands and face, decreased appetite, weight gain, slow speech, mental apathy, constipation, hearing loss, poor memory, menstrual disturbance: HYPOTHYROIDISM.

## LIBIDO, REDUCED

With appetite loss, nausea, vomiting, weight loss, malaise, weakness, abdominal discomfort, nose and other bleeding tendencies and, in women, absence of menstruation: CIRRHOSIS OF THE LIVER.

With skin pigmentation, diabetes, liver disease, sometimes heart failure: HEMOCHROMATOSIS.

With one or many other symptoms: apathy, appetite and weight loss, easy fatigue, cold intolerance, scantiness or absence of pubic and underarm hair and, in women, scanty menstruation, failure to lactate after childbirth: HYPOPITUITARISM.

## LIGHTHEADEDNESS

With burning or tingling sensations, agitation, fainting: RESPIRATORY ALKALOSIS.

## LIGHT SENSITIVITY (see EYE)

## LIMBS, NUMBNESS OF (see also NUMBNESS)

Numbness, with one or more other symptoms: limb cramps, nausea, vomiting, sweating, eye tearing, dilation or contraction of pupils, abdominal cramps, diarrhea, thirst, dizziness, confusion, throat constriction, blood-streaked stools and vomitus, itching, muscle weakness, chest pain: FOOD POISONING, NONBACTERIAL.

## LIPS

Cracked, with sparse and coarse hair, eyebrow loss, dry rough skin, severe headaches, weakness: HYPERVITAMINOSIS A.

Dry scaling and fissuring of lips and angles of mouth: CHEILOSIS.

Dry scaling and fissuring of lips and angles of mouth, with red, scaly, greasy areas on ears, eyelids, scrotum or labia majora, sometimes also with tearing of eyes and sensitivity to light: VITAMIN DEFICIENCY (riboflavin).

Small red to violet spots on lips that may bleed spontaneously or after trivial injury: TELANGIECTASIA, HEREDITARY HEMORRHAGIC.

Itching or stinging sore: FEVER BLISTER (COLD SORE).

Thickened, in a child with thick, dry, wrinkled skin, enlarged tongue, broad face, flat nose, puffy feet and hands, dullness: CRETINISM.

Sore or blister, nonhealing, easy to bleed: CANCER OF THE LIP.

Prickling or burning sensations of lips, fingers, or toes, with irritability, shallow or irregular breathing, muscle cramps: METABOLIC ALKALOSIS.

## LISTLESSNESS (see also LETHARGY)

With hacking cough, running nose, tearing of eyes, sneezing, appetite loss: WHOOPING COUGH.

With fever, weight loss, vague pains in chest, purulent sputum, night sweats, fatigue, drowsiness, appetite loss: TUBERCULOSIS.

## LIVER

Located on the right side of the abdominal cavity, just under the diaphragm, the liver is a large four-lobed organ that stores nutrients, makes bile, purifies the blood by removing toxic materials, waste products, worn-out red blood cells. The liver can be damaged by viruses (HEPATITIS, YELLOW FEVER), bacterial infections (BRUCEL-

LOSIS and others), parasites (AMEBIASIS), toxic substances (carbon tetrachloride), and excessive alcohol, which may produce CIRRHOSIS with chronic inflammation and degeneration of liver cells. Often a first symptom of liver damage or disease is JAUNDICE. Other symptoms include vomiting of blood and passing of bloody, gray, or black, tarlike stools. In some cases, pain, discomfort or enlargement of the liver may be a symptom.

Enlargement, also with spleen enlargement, sometimes bone pain, joint swellings, brown pigmentation of skin: GAUCHER'S DISEASE.

Pain or discomfort over liver, especially with movement, sometimes radiating to right shoulder, with one or more other symptoms: fever, sweats, chills, nausea, vomiting, weakness, weight loss: AMEBIASIS (HEPATITIS).

## LYMPH NODE SWELLING (see GLAND SWELLING, LYMPH)

## MALAISE

A general feeling of uneasiness, indisposition, or feeling unwell, malaise is a symptom that may precede or accompany many illnesses:

### In oommon infcctions

With fcvcr, chills, blisterlike, measleslike or scarlet-feverlike rash, headache, sore throat: MONONUCLEOSIS, INFECTIOUS.

With scratchy throat, sneezing, nasal discharge: COLD, COMMON.

With sore throat, nasal discharge, chilliness, slight fever, back and muscle pain, nonproductive cough gradually producing sputum: BRONCHITIS, ACUTE.

With cough, pinkish sputum sometimes becoming rusty, sharp chest pain, high fever usually starting with shaking chill, headache, often with breathing difficulty and rapid, painful respiration, muscular pain, appetite loss: PNEUMONIA.

With sudden abdominal cramps, nausea, vomiting, appetite loss, gas sounds in intestines, diarrhea: GASTROENTERITIS, ACUTE.

With sore throat, pain in tonsil area especially on swallowing, chills, fever to 106°, headache, sometimes stiff neck: TONSILLITIS.

### In other infections

With chills, fever, headache, depression: BRUCELLOSIS.

With chilly sensations, headache, fever, appetite loss, nosebleeds, backache, diarrhea or constipation, sore throat: TYPHOID FEVER.

With fever, excessive salivation, extremely painful spasms of muscles of larynx and throat, restlessness: RABIES.

With eruption of blisters along the course of a sensory nerve, most often in the chest, fever, chills: HERPES ZOSTER.

With red-brown elevated skin lesion that enlarges, reddens, and blisters, muscle pain, fever, chills, headache, nausea, vomiting: ANTHRAX.

With fever, cough, grippelike (flulike) feelings: HISTOPLASMOSIS.

With irregular mild fever, swelling of neck and underarm glands (lymph nodes), muscle pain: TOXOPLASMOSIS.

With fever, chills, joint pains, lassitude, appetite loss, sometimes small tender nodules about the tips of the digits: ENDOCARDITIS, BACTERIAL.

With cough, purulent sputum, appetite loss, sweats, chills, fever, sometimes chest pain: LUNG ABSCESS.

With fever, chills, dry cough becoming productive with sputum containing pus and mucus, appetite loss: PSITTACOSIS.

## In other conditions

Episodes of malaise, chills, fever, aching in abdomen, back, legs, jaundice, spleen enlargement: ANEMIA, HEMOLYTIC.

With a persistent sore appearing within a few days and at site of a minor cat scratch, later gland (lymph node) swellings at sites near the scratch, fever, headache, loss of appetite: CAT-SCRATCH DISEASE.

With red skin spots that turn purple, itching, fever, sometimes joint and abdominal pain: PURPURA, ALLERGIC.

After two or three days of fatigue and overpowering weakness, with chills, high fever, sore throat, swallowing difficulty, mouth ulcers: AGRANULOCYTOSIS.

With fatigability, joint pains, repeated mild or severe infections: PRIMARY SPLENIC NEUTROPENIA.

With chest pain on one side, breathing difficulty, cough, fever: EMPYEMA.

With labored breathing, rapid breathing, dry cough, sleep disturbance, appetite loss, chest pains, hoarseness, blueness, coughing and spitting of blood: SILICOSIS.

With breathing difficulty, one or more other symptoms: blueness after exercise, rapid pulse, dry nonproductive cough, fever, weight and appetite loss, easy fatigability: PULMONARY GRANULOMATOSES.

With progressively increasing breathing difficulty, cough, thick yellow sputum that may contain bits of firm, yellow-gray material, weight loss: PULMONARY ALVEOLAR PROTEINOSIS.

With abdominal pain or pressure, any or many other symptoms:

appetite loss, sensation of fullness, nausea, dizziness, headache, vomiting with blood in vomitus: GASTRITIS, ACUTE.

With appetite loss, nausea, vomiting, weight loss, weakness, abdominal discomfort, loss of libido, nose and other bleeding tendencies, and, in a woman, absence of menstruation: CIRRHOSIS OF THE LIVER.

With headache, weakness, sometimes abdominal pain, nausea, vomiting: METABOLIC ACIDOSIS.

## MEMORY IMPAIRMENT

Impairment of memory has many possible causes, ranging from hearing difficulties to mental illness, from lack of attention to brain injuries, from habitual use of some drugs (sleeping pills, bromides) to overdoses of vitamin D, from severe infections such as encephalitis and meningitis to anemia, hardening of brain arteries, and more. Almost invariably, when memory is associated with some disorder, other more-commanding symptoms will be present and help to pinpoint the underlying problem. For example, when memory impairment is associated with HYPOTHYROIDISM, other symptoms may include chilliness, dry cold skin, puffiness of hands and face, slow speech, drowsiness; when the impairment is associated with VITAMIN DEFICIENCY (thiamine), other symptoms may include general aches and pains, chest pain, abdominal discomfort, constipation, fatigue, appetite loss.

## MENSTRUATION (see also UTERINE BLEEDING)

Absence of, not occurring as normal at puberty or developing after previous menstruation: AMENORRHEA.

Absence of, with abdominal discomfort, loss of libido, nose and other bleeding tendencies, nausea, vomiting, weight loss, weakness, malaise: CIRRHOSIS OF THE LIVER.

Absent or excessive, with one or more other symptoms: chilliness, dry cold skin, puffiness of hands and face, decreased appetite, weight gain, slow speech, mental apathy, constipation, drowsiness: HYPOTHYROIDISM.

Excessive, sometimes with painful menstruation, vaginal discharge or frequent urination: UTERUS, MYOMA OF.

Excessive, sometimes with low backache before menstruation, discomfort especially after coitus: CERVICITIS.

Irregular, often with discharge after coitus, vaginal bleeding or spotting: CANCER OF THE CERVIX.

Irregular, with heavy flow sometimes followed by none, often accompanied by vaginal bleeding, odorous discharge: CANCER OF THE UTERUS.

Painful, with pain appearing up to 48 hours before flow and persisting for a variable period: DYSMENORRHEA.

Excessive, with bleeding into skin and mucous membranes: VON WILLEBRAND'S DISEASE.

Irregularities, with moon or rounded face, weight gain, fat accumulations in the back ("buffalo hump"), muscle wasting, weakness, easy bruising: CUSHING'S SYNDROME.

Scanty, with one or more other symptoms: apathy, appetite and weight loss, easy fatigue, cold intolerance, diminished libido, scantiness or absence of pubic and underarm hair: HYPOPITUITARISM.


## MOUTH

Breathing through mouth, sometimes with nasal speech, halitosis, postnasal discharge, cough, vomiting, change of facial expression: ADENOID HYPERTROPHY.

Bleeding from mouth and often from nose, bowel, kidneys, with one or many other symptoms: throat or lung infection, high fever, sometimes joint pains, small purplish-red spots on skin, bruises, pallor, weakness: LEUKEMIA, ACUTE.

Bleeding from mouth or nose, with waxy pallor of skin and mucous membranes, sometimes severe sore throat: ANEMIA, APLASTIC.

Dry scaling and fissuring of angles of mouth and lips, sometimes with red, scaly, greasy areas on ears, eyelids, scrotum or labia majora, sensitivity to light, eye tearing: VITAMIN DEFICIENCY (riboflavin).

Blisters, multiple in mouth, with eroded areas throughout mouth, fever to 104° or 105°, crusted lips: ERYTHEMA MULTIFORME (oral).

Fissuring of angles of mouth and lips, inflammation of tongue, greasy scaling of scalp, anemia and, in infants, convulsions: VITAMIN DEFICIENCY (pyridoxine).

Painful recurring ulcer or ulcers of mouth: STOMATITIS, RECURRENT APHTHOUS.

Ulcers, following two or three days of fatigue and overpowering weakness, accompanied by chills, high fever, sore throat, swallowing difficulty, extreme prostration: AGRANULOCYTOSIS.

Open-mouthedness, with one or several other symptoms: tremors, drooling, speaking difficulty, incoordination, rigidity, behavior changes: WILSON'S DISEASE.

Redness and swelling of mouth tissues which may become sore especially during eating, sometimes with unpleasant mouth odor, dryness of mouth or excessive salivation, ulcers: STOMATITIS.

White patches on a red, moist inflamed surface in mouth, often on tongue or inner cheeks: CANDIDIASIS.

Itching or stinging sore in mouth or on lips: FEVER BLISTER (COLD SORE).

Yellowish-white leathery patches in the mouth: LEUKOPLAKIA (oral).

Sore on gum, palate, tongue, or floor of mouth which fails to heal within two weeks, sometimes with burning: CANCER OF THE MOUTH.

Sore, with bright scarlet tongue and mouth membranes, sometimes with ulcerations on undersurface of tongue, burning of mouth, throat and esophagus, abdominal discomfort and distention, nausea, vomiting, diarrhea: VITAMIN DEFICIENCY (niacin).

Roughness or itching of inner surface of cheek, with bluish-white lines on cheek and tongue which increase in size and sometimes become painful and ulcerated: LICHEN PLANUS.

## MUSCLE ACHES AND PAINS

With sore throat, nasal discharge, malaise, chilliness, slight fever, back pain, nonproductive cough gradually producing sputum: BRONCHITIS, ACUTE.

With irregular mild fever, swelling of neck and underarm glands (lymph nodes), malaise, sometimes anemia: TOXOPLASMOSIS.

After swelling of upper eyelids and pain in eyes, often accompanied by one or more of the following symptoms: sensitivity to light, fever, thirst, profuse sweating, hives, weakness, prostration: TRICHINOSIS.

With cough, pinkish sputum sometimes becoming rusty, sharp chest pain, high fever often starting with shaking chill, headache, breathing difficulty: PNEUMONIA.

With urination frequency, urgency, pain and burning, often with chills and fever, nausea, vomiting, lassitude: URINARY TRACT INFECTIONS.

With chills, fever, headache, pain behind eyes, joint pain, intolerance of light, sore throat, abdominal pain, nausea, vomiting: ROCKY MOUNTAIN SPOTTED FEVER.

With chills, fever, headache, malaise, sometimes diarrhea: BRUCELLOSIS.

With fever, headache, flushed face, red tongue, severe prostration, jaundice: YELLOW FEVER.

With reddish rash, fever, chills, joint pain, headache, vomiting: RE-LAPSING FEVER.

With red-brown elevated skin lesion that enlarges, reddens, blisters, malaise, headache, fever, nausea, vomiting: ANTHRAX.

With fever, weight loss, and any or many other symptoms: joint pains, severe abdominal pain, bloody diarrhea, wheezing, skin reddening, hives, pneumonia, heart failure: POLYARTERITIS.

Painful swelling of muscles or gradual weakness, with reddening and puffiness of skin on face, about eyes, over elbows, knees, other joints, joint pain and stiffness, swallowing difficulty, gastrointestinal disturbances: DERMATOMYOSITIS.

Vague muscle aches, with vague joint aches, lassitude, weakness, weight loss, swollen and bleeding gums, small black and blue spots on skin: SCURVY.

Muscle and joint pain, tenderness, stiffness, occurring suddenly and aggravated by movement, usually following injury, strain, exposure to cold or dampness, sometimes after infection: FIBROMYOSITIS.

## MUSCLE CRAMPS AND SPASMS

With episodic weakness, burning or tingling sensations, transient paralysis, excessive urination and thirst, blood pressure elevation: HYPERALDOSTERONISM.

Excruciatingly painful cramps, most often of arm and leg muscles, coming on suddenly and in spasms, with relative comfort between spasms: HEAT CRAMP.

With fever to 106° or higher, flushing, hot dry skin, sometimes with convulsions: HEAT HYPERPYREXIA.

With diarrhea, appetite loss, weight loss becoming increasingly marked after weeks to months, anemia, weakness, fatigability: SPRUE, TROPICAL.

With diarrhea, thirst, diminished urination, weakness: CHOLERA.

With lassitude, fatigue, decreased mental acuity, nausea, vomiting, yellowish-brown discoloration of skin, hiccuping, urine smell on breath and sweat, itching: UREMIA.

With abnormal bending or flexion of wrist and ankle joints, convulsions: TETANY.

With irritability, shallow or irregular breathing, burning or prickling sensations of fingers, toes, or lips: METABOLIC ALKALOSIS.

## MUSCLE WEAKNESS (see also WEAKNESS)

With headache, diarrhea, weight loss, eye inflammation: TOXO-PLASMOSIS.

With double vision, drooping of upper eyelids, swallowing and speaking difficulty: BOTULISM.

With one or many other symptoms: nausea, vomiting, sweating, eye tearing, dilation or contraction of pupils, abdominal cramps, diarrhea, dizziness, thirst, confusion, throat constriction, blood-streaked stools and vomitus, numbness of limbs, itching, chest pain, cramps in extremities: FOOD POISONING, NONBACTERIAL.

And wasting, with abdominal distention, malodorous stools, vomiting, failure to thrive: CELIAC DISEASE.

Sometimes with paralysis, breathing difficulty, failure of muscular contraction in the bowel leading to abdominal pain and distention: HYPOKALEMIA.

And wasting with moon or rounded face, obesity, fat accumulations in the back ("buffalo hump"), easy bruising, menstrual irregularities in women: CUSHING'S SYNDROME.

And wasting of muscles of pelvis, shoulder, legs and in some cases the eyes: MUSCULAR DYSTROPHIES.

With one or several other symptoms: headache, failing vision, vomiting, loss of balance and coordination, drowsiness, lethargy, personality changes: CANCER OF THE BRAIN.

## NASAL SPEECH

With mouth breathing, halitosis, postnasal discharge, cough, sometimes vomiting, change of facial expression: ADENOID HYPERTROPHY.

## NAUSEA AND VOMITING

Nausea and vomiting commonly go together although there may sometimes be nausea without the vomiting. A distressing sickness at the stomach, a feeling that vomiting may occur, nausea is usually felt when nerve endings in the stomach, esophagus, and other parts of the body are sufficiently irritated so they transmit impulses to a brain center that controls vomiting. When the nerve irritation becomes intense, vomiting follows. Nausea, which may be accompanied by faintness, weakness, dizziness, headache and sweating, may follow distention of the stomach or lower esophagus or impairment of normal forward movement of food in the duodenum, the first part of the small intestine. It may also be provoked by strong emotions, unpleasant odors, or pain anywhere in the body.

Along with other symptoms, nausea and vomiting may be associated with many infections and numerous other disorders, some relatively minor, some more serious:

### In congenital disorders in infancy

With unusual irritability, epileptic seizures: PHENYLKETONURIA.

With growth failure, abnormal fluid accumulation (edema): GALACTOSEMIA.

### In childhood infections

With bright red rash, fever, sometimes sore throat, swelling of lymph nodes in neck: SCARLET FEVER.

With fever, sore throat, swallowing difficulty, headache, prostration: DIPHTHERIA.

With paroxysms of coughing, running nose, sneezing, appetite loss: WHOOPING COUGH.

### In other common infections

With fever, chilliness, headache, sore throat, gland (lymph node) swelling, fatigue, malaise, sometimes abdominal pain, jaundice, faintly red skin eruption, eyelid swelling: MONONUCLEOSIS, INFECTIOUS.

With urinary frequency, urgency, pain and burning, chills, fever, general muscle aches, lassitude: URINARY TRACT INFECTIONS.

With sudden abdominal cramps, headache, chills, fever, diarrhea: GASTROENTERITIS, FOOD INFECTION or STAPHYLOCOCCUS TOXIN.

### In less common infections

With chills, fever of 104° or 105°, profuse perspiration, headache, body pains: MALARIA.

With chills, fever, headache, pain behind eyes, joint and muscle pain, intolerance of light, sore throat, abdominal pain: ROCKY MOUNTAIN SPOTTED FEVER.

With chilly sensations, malaise, headache, appetite loss, fever, nosebleeds, backache, diarrhea or constipation, sore throat: TYPHOID FEVER.

With fever, acute headache, chills, jaundice, skin rash, blood in urine, diminished urination: LEPTOSPIROSIS.

With chills, fever, headache, red rash, severe weakness: TULARE-MIA.

With red-brown skin elevation that enlarges, reddens, and blisters, fever, malaise, headache, muscle pain: ANTHRAX.

With pain or discomfort over liver in upper right part of abdomen, especially with movement, sometimes radiating to right shoulder, with one or more other symptoms of fever, sweats, chills, weakness, weight loss: AMEBIASIS (HEPATITIS).

With chills, fever, inflamed painful swellings of lymph nodes in groin, thirst, generalized pain, headache, sometimes convulsions: PLAGUE.

With chills, fever, headache, muscle and joint pain, reddish rash over trunk and extremities followed by rose-colored spots, sometimes jaundice: RELAPSING FEVER.

With headache, fever, stiff neck, muscle twitching, tremors, mental confusion: ENCEPHALITIS, VIRAL.

With fever, headache, muscle aches, prostration, yellowing of skin, blood in vomitus: YELLOW FEVER.

With high fever, rash, headache, chills, sometimes convulsion: SMALLPOX.

### In parasitic infestation

With diarrhea, anemia, retarded growth: WHIPWORM.

### In malignancies

In a child, with abdominal mass and pain, fever, blood in urine, appetite loss: CANCER OF THE KIDNEY (Wilms' tumor).

With variable abdominal pain often extending to the back and relieved by sitting up or bending forward, one or more other symptoms: jaundice, weight loss, appetite loss, constipation or diarrhea, vomiting of blood, stools darkened with blood pigments: CANCER OF THE PANCREAS.

With upper abdominal distress and pain over stomach area, usually but not necessarily intensified shortly after eating, sometimes with one or more other symptoms: appetite loss, unexplained weight loss, anemia: CANCER OF THE STOMACH.

With one or many other symptoms: headache, muscle weakness, failing vision, loss of balance and coordination, drowsiness, lethargy, personality changes: CANCER OF THE BRAIN.

## In vitamin-related disorders

With abdominal discomfort and distention, diarrhea, scarlet-colored tongue and mouth membranes, sore mouth, skin and nervous system disturbances: VITAMIN DEFICIENCY (niacin).

With appetite loss, excessive urination and thirst, itching, weakness, nervousness: HYPERVITAMINOSIS D.

## In other disorders

With any or several other symptoms: heartburn, upper abdominal pain, flatulence, belching, feelings of fullness and abdominal distention during or after a meal: INDIGESTION.

In waves, with cold sweating, yawning, pallor, sometimes dizziness, headache: MOTION SICKNESS.

With sudden fast heartbeats (100 or more per minute), fluttering sensation in the chest, faintness, weakness: PAROXYSMAL TACHYCARDIA.

With pallor, palpitation, fainting, weakness: ATRIAL FLUTTER OR FIBRILLATION.

With breathing difficulty, ankle swelling with fluid, loss of energy: CONGESTIVE HEART FAILURE.

With chest pain, breathing difficulty, sweating, weakness: SHOCK.

With chronic or chronic relapsing diarrhea, stools loose but free of blood or pus, sometimes containing undigested food residue, heartburn and fullness after eating: DIARRHEA, CHRONIC NONINFLAMMATORY.

With fever, headache, abdominal discomfort, lassitude, weakness, appetite loss, drowsiness, sometimes jaundice: HEPATITIS.

With pain in right upper abdominal quadrant, extending into right shoulder, severe and remaining steadily severe for hours, sometimes with fever, chills, abdominal distention, jaundice: CHOLECYSTITIS, ACUTE.

With nervousness, weakness, heat sensitivity, sweating, overactivity, restlessness, weight loss with increased appetite, tremor, palpitation, stare, abnormal eye protrusion, sometimes with headache, abdominal pain, diarrhea: HYPERTHYROIDISM.

With palpitation, pallor, headache, apprehension, abdominal pain over stomach area, high blood pressure: PHEOCHROMOCYTOMA.

With weakness, appetite loss, constipation, abdominal pain, thirst, excessive urination, urinary stones: HYPERPARATHYROIDISM.

With crampy abdominal pain, diarrhea: GASTROINTESTINAL ALLERGY.

With lassitude, fatigue, one or several other symptoms: muscular cramps and twitching, yellow-brown skin discoloration, hiccuping, urine smell on breath and sweat, itching: UREMIA.

With vomitus sometimes containing blood, abdominal pain or pressure, one or more other symptoms: headache, dizziness, appetite loss, sensation of fullness, malaise: GASTRITIS.

With pain over stomach region usually one to three hours after meals and usually relieved by eating or an antacid drug: PEPTIC ULCER.

With abdominal pain beginning in umbilical (navel) area and shifting to right lower quadrant of abdomen, appetite loss, constipation or diarrhea: APPENDICITIS.

With severe, constant, diffused, prostrating abdominal pain, fever, chills, sometimes diarrhea: PERITONITIS.

With severe, steady, boring abdominal pain, sharpest in stomach area, extending to back and chest, often partially relieved by sitting up: PANCREATITIS.

With sudden abdominal cramps, gas sounds in intestine, diarrhea, appetite loss: GASTROENTERITIS, ACUTE.

With one or many other symptoms: abdominal cramps, diarrhea, thirst, dizziness, tearing of eyes, dilation or contraction of pupils, sweating, sense of constriction in throat, blood-streaked stools and vomitus, itching, limb numbness, chest pain, cramps in extremities: FOOD POISONING, NONBACTERIAL.

With low, left-sided abdominal pain, distention, severe constipation or diarrhea (or one alternating with the other): DIVERTICULITIS.

With abdominal pain, mild intermittent diarrhea, massive edema or waterlogging: LYMPHANGIECTASIA, INTESTINAL.

With appetite and weight loss, malaise, weakness, abdominal discomfort, nose and other bleeding tendencies, loss of libido, absence of menstruation: CIRRHOSIS OF THE LIVER.

Episodes of nausea and vomiting, with dizziness, ringing in ears, hearing impairment: MENIERE'S DISEASE.

With weakness, headache, malaise, abdominal pain: METABOLIC ACIDOSIS.

With increasing weakness, easy fatigability, increased skin pigmentation, black freckles over forehead, face, neck, shoulders, bluish-black discolorations of mucous membranes of lips, mouth, other sites, weight and appetite loss, diarrhea, decreased cold tolerance, dizziness, fainting attacks: ADDISON'S DISEASE.

With sudden severe head pain, neck stiffness, dizziness, convulsions: SUBARACHNOID HEMORRHAGE.

With blood in vomitus, discoloration of stools with blood, enlarged spleen, increasing anemia, weakness, fatigue: BANTI'S DISEASE.

With blood in vomitus, sometimes with heartburn, swallowing difficulty, chest pain under breastbone, darkening of stools with blood pigments: HERNIA, HIATAL.

With blood in vomitus, after early symptoms of faintness, weakness, dizziness, profuse sweating: PEPTIC ULCER (hemorrhage).

Vomiting of food eaten in previous meals, with foul belching: PEPTIC ULCER (stomach outlet obstruction).

Persistent, vomitus containing large amounts of bile-stained fluid, severe thirst, breathing difficulty, pain over stomach area, sensation of abdominal fullness: GASTRIC DILATION, ACUTE.

With intermittent cramplike pain in abdomen, vomiting sometimes becoming fecal in nature, abdominal distention (in some cases with no passage of gas or feces, in others with diarrhea or constipation or one alternating with the other): INTESTINAL OBSTRUCTION.

With malodorous stools, abdominal distention, muscle wasting and weakness: CELIAC DISEASE.

With nasal speech, mouth breathing, halitosis, postnasal discharge, cough, change of facial expression: ADENOID HYPERTROPHY.

With paroxysms of colicky abdominal pain, distention, diarrhea or constipation, particularly in a woman: PORPHYRIA, ACUTE INTERMITTENT.

## NECK, MASS IN

Usually neither tender nor painful: CANCER OF THE THYROID.

## NECK PAIN

With stiffness, also pain and stiffness in back, fever, headache, vomiting, sore throat, drowsiness: POLIOMYELITIS.

Radiating to jaw, arms or chest, sometimes with low-grade fever: THYROIDITIS, SUBACUTE GRANULOMATOUS.

## NECK, STIFF

With persistent, violent headache, vomiting, fever, and in an infant convulsions: MENINGITIS.

With sudden severe head pain, nausea, vomiting, dizziness, convulsions: SUBARACHNOID HEMORRHAGE.

Commonly without other symptoms: from *muscle spasm* caused by sleeping in bad position, chill, unusual exercise, sudden twisting of neck, and often relieved by aspirin, hot moist applications, massage.

With stiff arms or legs, sore throat, swallowing difficulty, chilliness, restlessness: TETANUS.

With one or many other symptoms: numbness and tingling of fingers or arm, weakness of arms or hands, stiff shoulder, headache, "knots" in neck, shoulder or arm muscles, swelling and stiffness of fingers, blurred vision, loss of balance, pain in and around eyes, sometimes fainting: CERVICAL SYNDROME.

With headache, drowsiness, fever, vomiting, muscle twitching, tremors, mental confusion, sometimes convulsions, coma: ENCEPHALITIS, VIRAL.

With sore throat, pain in tonsil area especially during swallowing, headache, malaise, chills, fever to 105° or 106°: TONSILLITIS.

## NECK SWELLING

In front, from thyroid gland enlargement (goiter), often with fullness in throat, sometimes with symptoms of HYPOTHYROIDISM: THYROIDITIS, HASHIMOTO'S.

In front, from thyroid gland enlargement: GOITER.

## NECK, "WRY" OR TWISTED

Twisting of head to one side, sometimes developing suddenly but more usually gradually, either sustained or intermittent with repeated jerky movements of head to one side: TORTICOLLIS, SPASMODIC.

## NERVOUSNESS

Commonly, nervousness is associated with worry or fear over financial, family, or other matters. It may also accompany worry over health and in some cases may be a symptom of disease:

With one or more other symptoms: dizziness, palpitation, fatigue, insomnia, headache, weakness: HYPERTENSION.

During the week to ten days prior to menstruation, sometimes with breast pain, irritability, headache, generalized fluid retention: PREMENSTRUAL TENSION.

With appetite loss, nausea, vomiting, excessive urination and thirst, itching, weakness: HYPERVITAMINOSIS D.

With heat sensitivity, sweating, restlessness, weakness, weight loss with increased appetite, tremor, palpitation, stare, abnormal eye protrusion, sometimes headache, nausea, abdominal pain, diarrhea: HY-PERTHYROIDISM.

## NODES, LYMPH (see GLAND SWELLING, LYMPH)

## NOSE, DISCHARGE FROM

With postnasal discharge, headache, pain, sometimes fever to 102° or 103°, dizziness, toothache, generalized aches, puffiness about eyes: SINUSITIS.

Postnasal, with one or more other symptoms: nasal speech, mouth breathing, halitosis, cough, vomiting, change of facial expression: AD-ENOID HYPERTROPHY.

With itching of nose, roof of mouth, throat and eyes, tearing of eyes, sneezing, sometimes headache, coughing, wheezing: RHINITIS, ALLERGIC.

With sore throat, malaise, chilliness, slight fever, back and muscle pain, nonproductive cough gradually producing sputum: BRONCHI-TIS, ACUTE.

With sneezing, appetite loss, tearing of eyes, hacking cough, list-lessness: WHOOPING COUGH.

With rash covering body, cough, slight fever, pains in head and back, reddened eyes: MEASLES.

With fever, generalized aches and pains most pronounced in back and legs, headache, sore throat, weakness: INFLUENZA.

With scratchy throat, sneezing, malaise, sometimes fever: COLD, COMMON.

## NOSE, FLAT

In a child with thick dry wrinkled skin, enlarged tongue, thick-ened lips, broad face, puffy feet and hands, dullness, apathy: CRETIN-ISM.

## NOSE, OBSTRUCTED BREATHING THROUGH

Sometimes with headache, postnasal discharge: DEVIATED SEP-TUM.

With continuous discharge, sometimes postnasal drip, throat tickle, dry lips, coated tongue, intermittent headache: RHINITIS, CHRONIC.

With crust formation, offensive nasal odor, dryness and irritation within nose, disturbances in smell: RHINITIS, ATROPHIC.

With headache, sometimes nasal discharge: POLYPS.


## NOSE PATCHES OR NODULES

Sometimes dark purple or ivory, growing in size: RHINOSCLEROMA.


## NOSEBLEEDS

Bleeding from the nose is a common problem, most often due to some direct injury, picking of the nose, or foreign body in the nose. Sometimes it occurs as the result of excessive sneezing or coughing. Some people, too, have blood vessels in the nose that are more delicate, more easily ruptured. Nosebleeds do, however, accompany some systemic diseases:

With small, round, purplish-red spots and bruises on the skin: PURPURA, IDIOPATHIC THROMBOCYTOPENIC.

With high fever, infection of mouth, throat or lungs, sometimes joint pains, small purplish-red skin spots and bruises, bleeding also from mouth, bowel, kidneys: LEUKEMIA, ACUTE.

With elevated blood pressure in arms, lower pressure in the legs, sometimes with headache: COARCTATION OF THE AORTA.

With abdominal discomfort, nausea, vomiting, appetite and weight loss, malaise, weakness, loss of libido, absence of menstruation: CIRRHOSIS OF THE LIVER.

With chilly sensations, headache, backache, sore throat, fever, appetite loss, diarrhea or constipation: TYPHOID FEVER.

With fever, vague pain in limbs, joint pains, tiredness: RHEUMATIC FEVER.

Treatment. A slight nosebleed usually stops by itself. If it continues or bleeding is severe, place the person in a chair, loosen any tight clothing around neck, apply cold compresses to nose and back of neck. Often effective is pressing the skin on the outside of the nostril against the bony cartilage so as to largely close off the bleeding nostril for about five minutes. The bleeding nostril also can be plugged with sterile cotton. If bleeding continues, call for medical help.

**NUMBNESS** (see also LIMBS, NUMBNESS OF)

Numbness and tingling of arms or fingers, with one or more of the following symptoms: weakness of hands or arms, stiff neck and pain with movement, stiff shoulder, headache, "knots" in muscles of neck, shoulders or arms, finger swelling and stiffness, vision blurring, loss of balance, pain in or around the eyes, fainting: CERVICAL SYNDROME.

Numbness occurring several hours after meals, with one or more of the following symptoms: flushing or pallor, chilliness, hunger, trembling, headache, dizziness, weakness, palpitation, faintness, sometimes convulsions: HYPOGLYCEMIA.

Numbness and tingling, or pain, which may begin in fingers and toes and extend elsewhere: POLYNEURITIS.

Numbness and tingling sensations, with one or more of the following symptoms: headache, dizziness, breathing difficulty, vision disturbances, itching, lassitude: POLYCYTHEMIA VERA.

Numbness, with pallor and blueness of fingers and sometimes toes, followed by redness and throbbing pain: RAYNAUD'S DISEASE.

Numbness with tingling sensations of toes, fingers, nose or ears, followed by burning, itching and swelling: FROSTBITE.

Numbness and tingling of legs and fingers, with one or more of the following symptoms: red, sore tongue, difficulty in swallowing, pale lemon skin color, unsteady gait, impaired memory: ANEMIA.


**PAIN** (see also ABDOMINAL PAIN, BACK PAIN, CHEST PAIN, EAR PAIN, EYE PAIN, FACE, PAIN IN, HEADACHE, HEEL PAIN [in Diseases Section], JOINT PAIN, KIDNEY PAIN, NECK PAIN)

Describing pain is difficult. It can be extremely variable, ranging from slight to severe, dull to acute, spasmodic to constant.

Among the most common types of pain are cramps, constant ache, intermittent colicky pain, and constant colicky pain.

Cramps are short-term, episodic, and poorly localized.

Constant ache is pain that steadily rises in intensity, as pain of a toothache.

Intermittent colicky pain increases to a maximum, then suddenly decreases or disappears. After a short or long period of time, the cycle is repeated.

Constant colicky pain varies in intensity but some pain is always present.

Pain may also be described as paroxysmal (appearing suddenly, periodically); griping (severe, in the bowels); intermittent (ceasing at intervals); recurrent (returning at intervals).

## PALLOR

With one or more of the following symptoms: easy fatigability, drowsiness, shortness of breath on exertion, headache, dizziness, ringing in the ears, spots before the eyes, heart pounding on exertion: ANEMIA.

Waxy, of skin and mucous membranes, sometimes with severe sore throat, brown skin pigmentation, bleeding into skin and mucous membranes, along with one or more other general symptoms of anemia (above): ANEMIA, APLASTIC.

With nausea, palpitation, weakness, fainting: ATRIAL FLUTTER OR FIBRILLATION.

Mild, with gland (lymph node) swelling, appetite loss, weakness, fatigue: LEUKEMIA, CHRONIC (lymphocytic).

With moist, cool skin, racing pulse, apathy or agitation, sometimes with nausea, sweating: SHOCK.

After flushing, followed by blueness, with severe breathing difficulty, high fever, almost constant nonproductive cough, hoarseness: LARYNGOTRACHEOBRONCHITIS, ACUTE.

With palpitation, sweating, headache, nausea, pain over stomach area, high blood pressure, apprehension: PHEOCHROMOCYTOMA.

With sweating, chilliness, numbness, hunger, trembling, headache, dizziness, weakness, palpitation several hours after meals: HYPOGLYCEMIA.

## PALPITATIONS

Palpitations are heartbeats so unusually rapid (usually over 120 per minute), strong or irregular as to call attention to themselves. Commonly, palpitations result from excitement or nervousness or strong exertion. They may, however, be linked with disease:

With pallor, sweating, headache, nausea, pain over the stomach area, high blood pressure, apprehension: PHEOCHROMOCYTOMA.

With breathing difficulty, flushing, itching, throbbing in the ears, coughing, sneezing, agitation: ANAPHYLAXIS.

With pallor, nausea, weakness, fainting: ATRIAL FLUTTER OR FIBRILLATION.

Sometimes with one or more other symptoms: headache, fatigue, nervousness, dizziness, weakness, insomnia: HYPERTENSION.

With sweating, flushing or pallor, chilliness, numbness, hunger, trembling, headache, dizziness, weakness, sometimes faintness a few hours after meals: HYPOGLYCEMIA.

With nervousness, weakness, heat sensitivity, sweating, restlessness, weight loss with increased appetite, tremor, stare, abnormal protrusion of the eye, sometimes with headache, nausea, abdominal pain, diarrhea: HYPERTHYROIDISM.

## PARALYSIS

Paralysis—the complete or partial loss of ability to move muscles in some part or parts of the body—usually is caused by disease or injury of some part of the nervous system but may in some cases result from a muscle disorder.

Of one side of the body, with speech disturbance, sometimes defective vision, deep coma: STROKE.

Of any part of the body, after one or many other symptoms: vision disturbances, weakness, fatigue, tremor of limbs, slowing and monotony of speech, impaired balance, unsteady walking, stiff gait, loss of bladder and bowel control: MULTIPLE SCLEROSIS.

With headache, fever, vomiting, stiff neck, muscle twitching, tremors: ENCEPHALITIS, VIRAL.

Partial, in a child, with lack of muscle coordination, sometimes visual, hearing, and speech defects: CEREBRAL PALSY.

Transient, with episodes of weakness, burning or tingling sensations, muscle spasms and cramps, excessive urination and thirst, blood pressure elevation: HYPERALDOSTERONISM.

Following early symptoms of fever, headache, vomiting, sore throat, pain and stiffness in back and neck: POLIOMYELITIS.

Of skeletal muscles: HYPERKALEMIA.

Momentary, of the limbs, especially in connection with anger, fear or other emotional reactions, usually with attacks of overpowering sleepiness a few to many times a day: NARCOLEPSY.

## PENIS

Containing the urethra, a common duct for urine and semen, which runs through its length, the penis has at the end a cone-shaped body, the glans penis, which is partially covered by a fold of skin, the foreskin.

Inflammation of glans penis and foreskin: BALANOPOSTHITIS.

Area of reddish pigmentation on the glans: ERYTHROPLASIA OF QUEYRAT.

Area of redness on glans or prepuce developing into a papule or painless ulcerated lesion, generally appearing about three weeks after infection through sexual contact: a chancre, the primary lesion of SYPHILIS.

Discharge of whitish fluid or pus, with painful burning sensation during urination: GONORRHEA.

Watery, whitish discharge, often slight and unnoticed, with exacerbations and remissions, sometimes with mild pain on urination, lower abdominal pain: URETHRITIS, NONGONOCOCCAL.

Painful, persistent erection without sexual excitement: PRIAPISM.

Deviation of erect penis to one side, sometimes with painful erection, inability to engage in coitus: PEYRONIE'S DISEASE.

At birth, opening of the urethra at a point short of the tip of the penis: HYPOSPADIAS.

## PERSONALITY CHANGES

With one or many other symptoms: headache, muscle weakness, failing vision, vomiting, loss of balance and coordination, drowsiness, lethargy: CANCER OF THE BRAIN.

With irascibility, obstinacy, spitefulness, irregular jerky movements of face, neck and arms, speech disturbances, shuffling gait, memory and judgment impairment: HUNTINGTON'S CHOREA.

## PERSPIRATION (see SWEATING)

## PHOTOPHOBIA (see EYE, LIGHT SENSITIVITY)

## PROSTRATION (EXTREME EXHAUSTION)

With high fever, chills, skin rash: HISTOPLASMOSIS.

With severe, profuse, watery, sometimes bloody diarrhea, high fever, abdominal distention: ENTEROCOLITIS, PSEUDOMEMBRANOUS.

After swelling of upper eyelids, pain in eyes, often accompanied by one or several other symptoms: sensitivity to light, fever, muscle soreness and pain, thirst, chills, profuse sweating, hives: TRICHINOSIS.

Sudden, extreme, after two or three days of fatigue and overpowering weakness, accompanied by chills, high fever, sore throat, swallowing difficulty, mouth ulcers: AGRANULOCYTOSIS.

With cold, ashen, damp skin, profuse sweating, semicomatose condition: HEAT PROSTRATION.

With sore throat, fever, headache, nausea, swallowing difficulty: DIPHTHERIA.

With fever, headache, muscle aches, yellowing of skin: YELLOW FEVER.

## RASH (see also SKIN)

### In common childhood infections

Pink spots, each about one-fourth inch in diameter, commonly starting at hairline and behind the ears and spreading downward to cover the body in about 36 hours, with the spots separate at first but some, later, running together to give a blotchy look, fading after three or four days, with running nose, cough, slight fever, pains in head and back, reddened eyes: MEASLES.

Rash much like that of measles (above) but spots usually do not coalesce, fades after two or three days, with slight cold, sore throat: MEASLES, GERMAN.

Pinkish, lasting a few days, appearing after three or four days of fever, usually just as the fever is beginning to decline: ROSEOLA.

Small red spots on back and chest, enlarging within a few hours, with a fluid-filled blister appearing in center of each spot, the fluid turning yellow after a day or two, with formation of a crust or scab that peels off in five to twenty days, often accompanied by severe itching: CHICKENPOX.

Bright red rash, fading within a week, sometimes with only mild fever, sore throat, swelling of lymph nodes in neck, sometimes with temperature as high as 105°, chills, headache, nausea, vomiting: SCARLET FEVER.

### In other infections

Faintly red eruptions, with one or many other symptoms: malaise, fatigue, headache, fever, chilliness, sore throat, gland (lymph node) swelling, severe weakness, occasionally abdominal pain, nausea, jaundice, eyelid swelling: MONONUCLEOSIS, INFECTIOUS.

Red, flat, creeping from one part of body to another, brief, sometimes lasting less than a day, with fever, vague pain in limbs, nosebleeds, nodules below skin at elbows, knees, wrists, swollen, tender joints: RHEUMATIC FEVER.

Pale pink, spotty, particularly on face, with pain behind eyes, severe headache, back and joint pain, fever, difficulty in movement, congested eyeballs: DENGUE.

Red spots, small at first, becoming larger, beginning on extremities and spreading to trunk, with chills, fever, headache, pain behind eyes, joint and muscle pain, light intolerance, nausea, vomiting, sore throat, abdominal pain: ROCKY MOUNTAIN SPOTTED FEVER.

Pinkish, over body, with high fever, headache, body aches: ROCKY MOUNTAIN SPOTTED FEVER AND OTHER RICKETTSIAL DISEASES (typhus).

Crops of rounded rose spots on chest and abdomen, with chilly sensations, malaise, headache, nosebleeds, backache, appetite loss, diarrhea or constipation, sore throat: TYPHOID FEVER.

Generalized red rash, following a small sore that becomes ulcerated, with fever, headache, nausea, vomiting, severe weakness: TULAREMIA.

Reddish, followed by rose-colored spots over trunk and extremities, with chills, fever, severe headache, muscle and joint pain: RELAPSING FEVER.

Measleslike spotty rash (above, under Common Childhood Infections), following a fluid-filled sore, with high fever alternating with normal temperature, swollen lymph nodes, swollen and painful large joints, back pain: RAT-BITE FEVER.

Red pustules (pus-containing lesions), small, first on face, then arms, wrists, hands, legs, reaching trunk in about 24 hours, with the lesions deep in the skin and commonly leaving pits after healing, with chills, high fever, prostration, sometimes headache, backache, muscular pains: SMALLPOX.

Crops of blisters along the course of a sensory nerve, most often in the chest, with great pain, often preceded for three or four days by chills, fever, malaise: HERPES ZOSTER (SHINGLES).


**RECTUM** (see also ANUS, ANAL BLISTERS, ANAL DISCHARGE, ANAL ITCHING, ANAL PAIN)

Discomfort, with repeated urge to defecate, painful diarrhea with blood, mucus, and pus in stools: PROCTITIS.

Protrusion of rectal mucous membrane through the anus: PROLAPSE OF THE RECTUM.

Bleeding from, with painful defecation, sense of rectal fullness: HEMORRHOIDS.

## RESTLESSNESS

With weakness, heat sensitivity, sweating, overactivity, weight loss with increased appetite, tremor, palpitation, stare, abnormal eye protrusion, sometimes with headache, nausea, abdominal pain, diarrhea: HYPERTHYROIDISM.

With fever, mental depression, malaise, excessive salivation, painful spasms of muscles of larynx and throat, great thirst: RABIES.

With stiffness of jaw, neck, arms, legs, swallowing difficulty, fever, sore throat: TETANUS.

With itching about the anal area: PINWORMS.

## SCALP

Yellowish, greasy scaling of skin of scalp, with itching, sometimes spreading to face, neck, central part of trunk, underarm areas: DERMATITIS, SEBORRHEIC.

Yellowish, greasy scaling of scalp, with inflammation of tongue, fissuring of lips and angles of mouth, anemia, and, in infants, convulsions: VITAMIN DEFICIENCY (pyridoxine).

## SCROTAL MASS

A scrotal mass may develop as the result of inflammation of the scrotal wall or scrotal contents, malignancy, or mechanical abnormality.

In *hydrocele,* the most common mass, fluid accumulates as the result of inflammation of a testis that leads to fluid overproduction or reduced resorption because of obstruction. Treatment is surgical.

In *spermatocele,* which resembles hydrocele, there is a cyst containing sperm, which can be removed surgically.

In *varicocele,* there is a collection of congested varicose veins in the scrotum which sometimes may diminish in size or disappear but can be removed if it is painful or large or if it leads to infertility through interference with sperm production.

An inguinal HERNIA may extend into the scrotum, producing a mass. Surgical repair is needed.

*Lymphedema,* or swelling with excessive lymph fluid, may result from many possible causes, including compression of a vein in the abdomen, cirrhosis, abdominal tumor. Thorough evaluation is needed and in some cases surgery may be required.

In *urethral stricture,* there is abnormal narrowing of the canal from bladder to outside, often as the result of gonococcal or other infection, and urine may seep into the scrotum. In treatment, antibiotics are used along with drainage when necessary; in some cases, surgery may be required to divert the urine.

In *epididymoorchitis,* the testis and epididymis (the cordlike structure along the back border of the testis containing ducts in which sperm are stored) are inflamed as a complication of infection. In treatment, suitable antibacterial agents are used along with rest, ice bags, and scrotal support.

In CANCER OF THE TESTIS, the scrotal mass progressively increases in size and sometimes may be associated with pain.

## SCROTUM

Red, scaly, greasy areas, also commonly on ears, eyelids, with dry scaling and fissuring of lips and angles of mouth, sometimes also with eye tearing and sensitivity to light: VITAMIN DEFICIENCY (riboflavin).

## SEIZURES (see also CONVULSIONS)

Outcry, followed by falling, unconsciousness, contraction of muscles of arms, legs, trunk and head, often with urinary and fecal incontinence, an attack lasting up to five minutes, often followed by deep sleep: EPILEPSY (grand mal).

Clouding of consciousness for seconds, without falling, often involving only cessation of any activity during an attack and resumption immediately afterward, occurring most often in children: EPILEPSY (petit mal).

Staggering without falling, purposeless movement, unintelligible sounds, lasting one to two minutes: EPILEPSY (psychomotor).

## SKIN, ABNORMAL PATCHES OF

Pinkish oval, which may be accompanied by mild to moderate itching, usually on trunk, sometimes affecting mostly the arms: PITYRIASIS ROSEA.

Pimplelike, violaceous on wrists, front and back leg surfaces, trunk, genital area, often with severe itching: LICHEN PLANUS.

Itching, oozing, round, of various sizes, appearing suddenly on arms, legs, sometimes on back, buttocks or much of body: DERMATITIS, NUMMULAR.

Round or oval, enlarging, spreading, becoming swollen, tender, red, with skin hot to the touch, often accompanied by fever, headache, vomiting, malaise: ERYSIPELAS.

Reddish, often scaly or blistered, on scalp, body, genital area, nails, or between toes, sometimes becoming ring-shaped as the infection spreads out, with itching, soreness: RINGWORM.

Pink or brown, with loss of sensation, small solid swellings, often with fever, sometimes loss of body hair, open sores on face, forehead, ear lobes: LEPROSY.

## SKIN, ABNORMAL PIGMENTATION OF

Excessive, with excessive hairiness, light sensitivity, sometimes episodes of colicky abdominal pain: PORPHYRIA CUTANEA TARDA.

With diabetes, liver disease, loss of libido, sometimes heart failure: HEMOCHROMATOSIS.

Brown, with joint swelling, bone pain, spleen or liver enlargement or both: GAUCHER'S DISEASE.

With black freckles over forehead, face, neck, shoulders, bluish-black discoloration of mucous membranes of lips, mouth, other sites, increasing weakness, easy fatigability, weight loss, nausea, vomiting, diarrhea, decreased cold tolerance, dizziness, fainting: ADDISON'S DISEASE.

Patchy losses of pigmentation: VITILIGO.

## SKIN, BEARD AREA, PAIN OF

Pain, itching when hairs are touched or moved as in shaving, with pustules in hair follicles: FOLLICULITIS.

## SKIN, BLACK SPOTS OF

With chills, fever, inflamed painful lymph node swelling usually in groin, vomiting, thirst, generalized pain, headache: PLAGUE.

## SKIN, BLACK AND BLUE SPOTS OF

With lassitude, weakness, irritability, weight loss, vague muscle and joint aches, swollen and bleeding gums: SCURVY.

## SKIN, BLISTERS OF

After pinhead-size, itching eruptions, pale or red, on chest, back, waistline, underarms, sometimes other areas: MILIARIA (HEAT RASH).

Clusters of large "water blisters" which may appear first near nose and mouth, sometimes inside them, gradually spreading over rest of body, bursting, leaving patches of raw, tender skin, with itching, burning, offensive odor: PEMPHIGUS.

## SKIN, BLUENESS OFF (see also BLUENESS)

With running nose, sneezing, hacking cough, appetite loss, listlessness: WHOOPING COUGH.

With wrinkling of skin, diarrhea, great thirst, diminished urination, muscle cramps, weakness, stupor: CHOLERA.

## SKIN CANCER

Skin CANCER, the most common of all malignancies, must be suspected, unless another diagnosis can be made, whenever a pigmented area of the skin present for years changes size, color, or appearance, or when any other skin change occurs and fails to heal promptly.

## SKIN, COOL OR COLD

Also moist, with apathy or agitation, pallor, racing pulse: SHOCK.

Also ashen and damp, with profuse sweating, semicomatose or unconscious condition: HEAT PROSTRATION.

## SKIN, FATTY DEPOSITS IN

Also with similar deposits in eyelids, jaundice, itching, bone softening: CIRRHOSIS, BILIARY.

Pinkish-yellow, with abdominal pain, exacerbated by large amounts of fats in the diet: HYPERLIPOPROTEINEMIA, TYPE 1.

## SKIN, HOT

Also dry, flushed, with fever to 106° or higher, sometimes with muscular twitching or cramps, convulsions: HEAT HYPERPYREXIA (also known as *sunstroke* or *heatstroke*).

## SKIN, ITCHING (see also ITCHING)

Intense, worse at night, with slightly elevated grayish white lines sometimes visible on close inspection, sometimes with blisters and pustules: SCABIES.

Intense, of scalp or skin on shoulders, buttocks, abdomen, with small red marks: PEDICULOSIS (lice infestation).

Peculiar itching eruption with a winding trail of inflammation: CREEPING ERUPTION, also known as *cutaneous larva migrans*.

With redness, sometimes crustiness, blisters, watery discharges, or other changes of skin: DERMATITIS, CONTACT.

Without blisters or other lesions, although scratching and rubbing may cause outbreaks and thickening of skin: DERMATITIS, ATOPIC.

Sudden outbreaks of itching, burning swellings or hives: ALLERGY, PHYSICAL (HEAT OR COLD).

## SKIN LUMP

Inflamed, on and under the skin, with a core: boil or FURUNCLE.

Boil-like lumps, often in the underarm area: HIDRADENITIS SUP-PURATIVA.

## SKIN MASS

Slow-growing, firm, movable, nontender, with cheesy contents, on face, ears, scalp, back or scrotum: CYST, SEBACEOUS (or wen).

Small solid masses, often on finger, enlarging slowly, breaking down into ulcers: SPOROTRICHOSIS.

## SKIN NODULES (SMALL SWELLINGS)

On body, often with fever, pink or brown spots on skin, loss of sensation in parts of body: LEPROSY.

# SKIN PAPULE (SMALL SOLID ELEVATED LESION)

Followed by fever, hives, sometimes bladder inflammation or chronic dysentery: SCHISTOSOMIASIS.

Multiple, spreading slowly, developing into pus-laden abscesses: BLASTOMYCOSIS.

Red-brown, enlarging, reddening, blistering, with fever, malaise, nausea, vomiting, headache, muscle pain: ANTHRAX.

Persistent, at site of and within a few days after a minor cat scratch, with later gland (lymph node) swellings at sites near scratch, fever, headache, malaise, appetite loss: CAT-SCRATCH DISEASE.

# SKIN, PENILE SORE OF

Painless, generally appearing about three weeks after infection through sexual contact, resembling blister, pimple, or ulcerated open sore: chancre of SYPHILIS.

# SKIN PUSTULES (PUS-FILLED ELEVATIONS)

With blackheads, on face, neck, upper part of trunk: ACNE.

Rupturing and crusting within a few hours to several days, sometimes spreading all over body, usually occurring in infants and young children but occasionally in adults: IMPETIGO.

# SKIN, REDDENING OF

Accompanied by blister formation, crusting, thickening, scarlet-colored tongue and oral membranes, gastrointestinal and nervous system disturbances: VITAMIN DEFICIENCY (niacin).

Mottled reddening, followed after months or years by hardening and immobility of the skin, usually beginning in hands and feet, spreading to other areas: SCLERODERMA.

With puffiness of the skin on face, about eyes, elsewhere, fever, sometimes painful swollen muscles or gradual muscle weakness, joint pain and stiffness, swallowing difficulty, gastrointestinal disturbances: DERMATOMYOSITIS.

Reddening or hives, or both, with fever, weight loss, one or more other symptoms: severe abdominal pain, diffuse muscle pain, joint pains, bloody diarrhea, wheezing, pneumonia: POLYARTERITIS.

With maceration, burning, itching, in underarm, groin, anal areas, spaces between fingers and toes, underbreast area: INTERTRIGO (CHAFING).

After brief exposure to sunlight, sometimes with hives, large watery blisters: PHOTOSENSITIVITY.

Painful, after tingling, numbing sensations, sometimes followed by burning, itching, swelling: FROSTBITE.

## SKIN, RED ERUPTION OF

Shaped somewhat like a butterfly, usually on nose and cheek, sometimes elsewhere, with itching scaling: LUPUS ERYTHEMATOSUS (chronic discoid).

## SKIN, RED SPOTS OF (see also RASH)

Gradually darkening, becoming purple, with itching, often fever, malaise, sometimes joint and abdominal pain: PURPURA, ALLERGIC.

Small, red to violet, on skin and mucous membranes, often bleeding spontaneously after trivial injury: TELANGIECTASIA, HEREDITARY HEMORRHAGIC.

Purplish-red, small, round, with bruises, from bleeding into skin: PURPURA, IDIOPATHIC THROMBOCYTOPENIC.

Purplish-red, small, with bruises, high fever, infections of mouth, throat or lungs, sometimes bleeding from mouth, nose, bowel, kidneys: LEUKEMIA, ACUTE.

## SKIN, ROUGH, SCALY, DRY

Over elbows, knees, upper arms, thighs, sometimes the face and elsewhere; in severe cases, with thickening, fissures, redness: ICHTHYOSIS.

## SKIN, SCALING OF

With fissuring, maceration, in toe webs, genital area, underarms, sometimes trunk and extremities: ERYTHRASMA.

Silvery scales, over bright red patches, most often on knees, elbows, scalp, chest, abdomen, backs of arms and legs, palms of hands, soles of feet, sometimes dot-shaped marks on fingernails: PSORIASIS.

## SKIN, ULCERS OF

Or, sometimes, acnelike outbreaks, with headache, vision blurring, sometimes confusion, agitation: CRYPTOCOCCOSIS.

## SKIN, WRINKLING OF

Also thick, dry, in a child, with enlarged tongue, thickened lips, broad face, flat nose, puffy feet and hands, dullness, apathy: CRETIN-ISM.

With blueness, sunken eyes, diarrhea, thirst, diminished urination, muscle cramps, weakness: CHOLERA.

## SKIN, YELLOWING OF

With fever, headache, muscle aches, prostration: YELLOW FEVER.

Yellow-brown, with fatigue, lassitude, and one or several other symptoms: muscular cramps and twitching, convulsions, nausea, vomiting, hiccuping, urine smell on breath and sweat: UREMIA.

## SLEEP ATTACKS

A few to many a day, lasting minutes to hours, while working, eating, driving, sometimes with weakness or momentary paralysis of limbs: NARCOLEPSY.

## SNEEZING

With scratchy throat, nasal secretions, malaise, moderate headache: COLD, COMMON.

With running nose, hacking cough, appetite loss, listlessness: WHOOPING COUGH.

With itching of nose, roof of mouth, throat, eyes, tearing of eyes, nasal discharge, sometimes headache, irritability, appetite loss, insomnia, coughing, wheezing: RHINITIS, ALLERGIC.

With palpitation, agitation, flushing, ear throbbing, coughing, breathing difficulty: ANAPHYLAXIS.

## SPEECH DISTURBANCES

Difficulty in speaking, with double vision, drooping of upper eyelids, swallowing difficulty, muscle weakness: BOTULISM.

Difficulty in speaking, with one or several other symptoms: tremors, drooling, incoordination, open-mouthedness, rigidity, behavioral changes: WILSON'S DISEASE.

Difficulty in speaking, with swallowing difficulty, eyelid drooping, double vision: MYASTHENIA GRAVIS.

Slow speech, with one or many other symptoms: chilliness, dry cold skin, puffiness of hands and face, decreased appetite, weight gain, mental apathy, drowsiness, constipation, hearing loss, poor memory, excessive or absent menstruation: HYPOTHYROIDISM.

Slowing and monotony of speech, with one or many other symptoms: vision disturbances, unusual fatigue, weakness, tremor of limbs, impaired balance, unsteady walking, stiff gait, loss of bladder and bowel control: MULTIPLE SCLEROSIS.

Speech disturbances, with one or several other symptoms: headache, vomiting, convulsions, coma, paralysis of arm or leg: STROKE.


## SPINE STIFFENING (see also BACK PAIN)

With movement increasingly difficult and painful, sometimes with breathing difficulty: ANKYLOSING SPONDYLITIS.


## SQUATTING

By a young child after exertion, often with blueness, clubbing of ends of fingers, coughing and spitting of blood, labored breathing on exertion, poor growth: TETRALOGY OF FALLOT.


## STERILITY (see INFERTILITY)


## STOOLS

Darkened from blood pigments, with retarded growth, anemia: HOOKWORM.

Darkened from blood pigments, with one or more other symptoms: heartburn, pain under breastbone, swallowing difficulty, vomiting of blood: HERNIA, HIATAL.

Darkened from blood pigments, with intermittent midabdominal cramps, anemia: CANCER OF THE SMALL INTESTINE.

Darkened from blood pigments, with variable abdominal pain often extending to the back and relieved by sitting up or bending forward, one or more other symptoms: jaundice, weight and appetite loss, nausea, vomiting, constipation or diarrhea, sometimes vomiting of blood: CANCER OF THE PANCREAS.

Blood in, with cramping lower abdominal pain, diarrhea: POLYPS (intestinal).

Blood in, often with one or more other symptoms: sense of fullness at anus, painful defecation: HEMORRHOIDS.

Blood-streaked, with one or many other symptoms: nausea, vomiting, sweating, tearing of eyes, dilation or contraction of pupils, abdominal cramps, diarrhea, thirst, dizziness, confusion, collapse, throat constriction, limb numbness, itching, muscle weakness, chest pain, cramps in extremities: FOOD POISONING, NONBACTERIAL.

Blood and mucus in, with abdominal pain, sometimes fatigue, slight fever, vague body aches and pains: AMEBIASIS.

Blood, pus and mucus in, with fever, pain in abdomen, diarrhea, straining at stool, dehydration, weight loss: BACILLARY DYSENTERY.

Blood, pus and mucus in, with painful diarrhea, rectal discomfort, repeated urge to defecate: PROCTITIS.

Large, frequent, foul-smelling, in a child, with chronic cough, rapid breathing, protuberant abdomen, barrel-like chest, blueness, chronic respiratory infection: CYSTIC FIBROSIS.

Malodorous, light, greasy, tending to float, with abdominal distention, muscle wasting and weakness, vomiting, failure to thrive: CELIAC DISEASE.

Tarry, following early symptoms of profuse sweating, faintness, dizziness, weakness: PEPTIC ULCER (hemorrhage).

Change in, from few to many or from many to few, sometimes with one or more other symptoms: change in size and form of stools, blood or mucus in stools, intermittent lower abdominal cramps not necessarily succeeded by bowel movement, unexplained anemia: CANCER OF THE COLON.

## STUPOR

With chills, fever, headache, pain behind eyes, joint and muscle pain, intolerance of light, nausea, vomiting, sore throat, abdominal pain: ROCKY MOUNTAIN SPOTTED FEVER.

With chilly sensations, malaise, headache, appetite loss, nose-

bleeds, backache, diarrhea or constipation, sore throat: TYPHOID FE-
VER.

With diarrhea, dehydration, great thirst, diminished urination,
muscle cramps, weakness, wrinkling of skin: CHOLERA.


## SWALLOWING DIFFICULTY

With pain in the tonsil area during swallowing, chills, fever to 105°
or 106°, headache, malaise, swelling and tenderness of lymph nodes
at the jaw, sometimes stiff neck: TONSILLITIS (acute).

With burning, dryness, lump in throat, chills, fever, hoarseness,
swelling of neck glands: PHARYNGITIS.

With sore throat, fever, headache, nausea, prostration: DIPH-
THERIA.

With sore throat, stiff neck, arms or legs, fever: TETANUS.

With difficulty in speaking, double vision, drooping of upper eyelids, muscle weakness: BOTULISM.

Sometimes with heartburn, pain under breastbone, vomiting of
blood or darkening of stool by blood pigments: HERNIA, HIATAL.

With speaking difficulty, eyelid drooping, double vision: MYAS-
THENIA GRAVIS.

With fever, headache, sore throat, pain and stiffness in back and
neck: POLIOMYELITIS.

With hoarseness, cough, labored breathing, chest or back pain:
ANEURYSM, INTRATHORACIC.

After comfortable swallowing of the first few mouthfuls of food,
often with gurgling noises during eating or drinking, regurgitation,
cough: ESOPHAGUS, ZENKER'S DIVERTICULUM OF.

Effortful swallowing, often with regurgitation of food, pain behind
breastbone that sometimes may radiate over whole abdominal area
and to back, jaw, neck: ACHALASIA.

Intense pain on swallowing, often with heartburn, chest pain:
ESOPHAGITIS.

Boring pain on swallowing with sensation of food sticking behind
breastbone: CANCER OF THE ESOPHAGUS.


## SWEAT, URINE SMELL ON

Also on breath, with one or more other symptoms: lassitude,
fatigue, muscular cramps and twitching, nausea, vomiting, yellow-
brown skin discoloration, hiccuping, convulsions: UREMIA.

# SWEATING, ABNORMAL

In palms, soles, underarms, groin or underbreast areas: HYPERHIDROSIS.

Excessive sweating with unpleasant odor: HYPERHIDROSIS (bromhidrosis).

With one or more other symptoms: nausea, vomiting, tearing of eyes, dilation or contraction of pupils, abdominal cramps, diarrhea, thirst, dizziness, confusion, collapse, throat constriction, blood-streaked stools and vomitus, limb numbness, itching, muscle weakness, chest pain, cramps in extremities: FOOD POISONING, NONBACTERIAL.

With flushing or pallor, chilliness, numbness, hunger, trembling, headache, dizziness, weakness, palpitation, sometimes faintness, occurring several hours after meals: HYPOGLYCEMIA.

With nervousness, heat sensitivity, overactivity, restlessness, weight loss with increased appetite, tremor, palpitation, abnormal protrusion of eye, sometimes with headache, nausea, abdominal pain, diarrhea: HYPERTHYROIDISM.

Profuse, with cold, ashen damp skin, semicomatose or unconscious condition: HEAT PROSTRATION.

Night sweats, with fever, weight loss, purulent sputum, vague chest pain: TUBERCULOSIS.

With pain or discomfort over the liver in upper right part of abdomen, especially with movement, sometimes radiating to right shoulder, one or more other symptoms: fever, chills, nausea, vomiting, weakness, weight loss: AMEBIASIS (DYSENTERY).

Profuse, after chills, followed by fever, headache, nausea, body pains, exhaustion: MALARIA.

Profuse, after swelling of upper eyelids, pain in eyes, often accompanied by one or many other symptoms: sensitivity to light, fever, muscle soreness and pain, thirst, chills, hives, weakness, prostration: TRICHINOSIS.

After gland (lymph node) swelling in neck, underarms, and groin, itching, sometimes with weakness, fever, weight and appetite loss: HODGKIN'S DISEASE.

With gland (lymph node) enlargement in neck, underarms, or groin, usually on one side, fever, debility: LYMPHOSARCOMA.

With chest pain, weakness, nausea, breathing difficulty: SHOCK.

With cough, purulent sputum, malaise, appetite loss, chills, fever, sometimes chest pain: LUNG ABSCESS.

With beads on forehead, agonizing abdominal pain, shallow breathing, boardlike and tender abdomen, fever: PEPTIC ULCER (perforation).

Profuse, with faintness, weakness, dizziness, later followed by vomiting of blood, or tarry stools: PEPTIC ULCER (hemorrhage).

## THIRST, ABNORMAL

With diarrhea, dehydration, diminished urination, muscle cramps, skin wrinkling: CHOLERA.

With chills, fever, painful lymph node swelling, vomiting, generalized pain, headache: PLAGUE.

With abdominal fullness, pain over stomach area, persistent vomiting or regurgitation of large amounts of bile-stained fluid, breathing difficulty: GASTRIC DILATION, ACUTE.

With one or many other symptoms: nausea, vomiting, tearing of eyes, dilation or contraction of pupils, abdominal cramps, diarrhea, dizziness, confusion, collapse, throat constriction, blood-streaked stools and vomitus, limb numbness, itching, muscle weakness, chest pain, cramps in extremities: FOOD POISONING, NONBACTERIAL.

With swelling of upper eyelids, pain in eyes, often one or more other symptoms: sensitivity to light, fever, muscle soreness and pain, chills, profuse sweating, hives, weakness, prostration: TRICHINOSIS.

With excessive urination, appetite loss, nausea, vomiting, weakness, nervousness, itching: HYPERVITAMINOSIS D.

With excessive urination, as many as 5 to 40 quarts of liquids consumed and excreted per day: DIABETES INSIPIDUS.

With excessive urination, episodic weakness, burning or tingling sensations, transient paralysis, muscle cramps and spasms, blood pressure elevation: HYPERALDOSTERONISM.

With weakness, appetite loss, nausea, constipation, abdominal pain, excessive urination, urinary tract stones: HYPERPARATHYROIDISM.

With excessive urination, itching, hunger, weakness, weight loss, dryness of skin: DIABETES.

## THROAT, CONSTRICTION OF

With one or many other symptoms: nausea, vomiting, dilation or contraction of pupils, tearing of eyes, sweating, abdominal cramps, diarrhea, thirst, dizziness, confusion, collapse, blood-streaked stools and vomitus, numbness of limbs, itching, muscle weakness, chest pain, cramps in extremities: FOOD POISONING, NONBACTERIAL.

## THROAT, LUMP IN

Or burning or dryness, with chills, fever, swallowing difficulty, hoarseness, swelling of neck glands: PHARYNGITIS (acute).

## THROAT, RAW, TICKLING

With constant effort to clear the throat, hoarseness or loss of voice: LARYNGITIS.

## THROAT, SCRATCHY

Followed by sneezing, nasal discharge, malaise, moderate head-ache: COLD, COMMON.

## THROAT, SORE

With high fever, sometimes joint pains, small purplish-red spots and bruises on skin, bleeding from mouth, nose, bowel, kidneys, pallor, weakness: LEUKEMIA, ACUTE.

With nasal discharge, malaise, chilliness, slight fever, back and muscle pain, dry, nonproductive cough which gradually produces sputum: BRONCHITIS, ACUTE.

With pain in tonsil area especially during swallowing, chills, fever to 105° or 106°, headache, malaise, sometimes with stiff neck: TON-SILLITIS.

With pain behind eyes, chills, fever, headache, joint and muscle pain, intolerance of light, nausea, vomiting, abdominal pain: ROCKY MOUNTAIN SPOTTED FEVER.

With blisterlike, measleslike, or scarlet-feverlike rash, malaise, headache: MONONUCLEOSIS, INFECTIOUS.

With fever, headache, pain and stiffness in back and neck: POLIO-MYELITIS.

With fever, generalized aches and pains most pronounced in back and legs, headache, weakness, appetite loss, mild distress below breastbone, sometimes nasal discharge: INFLUENZA.

With bright red rash, swelling of lymph nodes of neck: SCARLET FEVER.

With slight cold, pink spots covering body and not running together: MEASLES, GERMAN.

With stiffness of jaw, neck, arms or legs, swallowing difficulty, fever: TETANUS.

## THROAT, STICKING SENSATION IN

With pain that may extend to an ear: LARYNX, CONTACT ULCER OF.

## TICS

Sudden, quick, repetitive movements without purpose including blinking of eyes, grimacing, head nodding or shaking, throat clearing, shoulder shrugging: TICS (habit or mimic spasms).

## TINGLING SENSATIONS

With episodic weakness, transient paralysis, muscle spasms and cramps, excessive urination and thirst, blood pressure elevation: HYPERALDOSTERONISM.

Sometimes also with burning sensations, lightheadedness, agitation, fainting: RESPIRATORY ALKALOSIS.

## TOES

Clubbing of, with blueness of lower half of body: PATENT DUCTUS ARTERIOSUS.

Attacks of blueness and pallor, sometimes with numbness as the attacks pass off, redness and throbbing pain: RAYNAUD'S DISEASE.

Numbness, burning, tingling, beginning in fingers and toes, often extending elsewhere: POLYNEURITIS.

Small red to violet spots that tend to bleed spontaneously or after trivial injury: TELANGIECTASIA, HEREDITARY HEMORRHAGIC.

Throbbing, crushing pain in a big toe, appearing suddenly, with swelling, warmth, redness, shininess of overlying skin: GOUT.

Prickling or burning sensations in toes, fingers, or lips, with irritability, irregular or shallow breathing, muscle cramps: METABOLIC ALKALOSIS.

## TOENAIL

Inflammation around nail, sometimes with pus: PARONYCHIAL INFECTION.

Thickening, with loss of luster, separation of nail plate, sometimes destruction of nail: RINGWORM.

## TONGUE

Small red to violet spots that may bleed spontaneously or after trivial injury: TELANGIECTASIA, HEREDITARY HEMORRHAGIC.

Reddened tip and edges, sometimes with painful ulcers or whitish patches, or smooth area, or hairy tongue, or marked tenderness with swelling, or painful burning sensation: GLOSSITIS.

Inflamed (as in GLOSSITIS, above), with yellowish greasy scaling of scalp, fissuring of lips and angles of mouth, anemia and, in infants, convulsions: VITAMIN DEFICIENCY (pyridoxine).

Bright scarlet, also bright scarlet oral membranes, sometimes with ulcerations on undersurface of tongue and skin, gastrointestinal and nervous system disturbances: VITAMIN DEFICIENCY (niacin).

Enlarged, in a child, with thick dry wrinkled skin, thickened lips, broad face, flat nose, puffy feet and hands, dullness, apathy: CRETINISM.

Sore, with burning or tingling sensations of hands and feet, often followed by weakness, shortness of breath, palpitation, appetite loss, nausea, vomiting, diarrhea, attacks of abdominal pain: ANEMIA, PERNICIOUS.

Irritated or ulcerated area on tongue that does not heal within a week: suspected CANCER OF THE MOUTH until proven otherwise.

Coated or furry tongue: in either case, not a very helpful symptom for diagnosis, since coating may be associated with mouth breathing during sleep and minor digestive upsets, whereas furriness of the tongue may occur in mouth disorders, digestive upsets, virtually all fever-producing conditions.

## TOOTHACHE

With headache, nasal and postnasal discharge, sometimes with fever to 102° or 103°, dizziness, generalized aches, puffiness about eyes: SINUSITIS.

Intermittent pain, sharp, throbbing, shooting, sometimes difficult to localize: PULPITIS.

Gnawing pain, with swelling of face near tooth: PERIAPICAL ABSCESS.

## TREMOR (TREMBLING)

Tremor is an involuntary trembling of the body or limbs. A fleeting tremor, of no significance, may occur as the result of emotional upset, fatigue, physical exertion, excessive alcohol intake, or prolonged use of some drugs such as barbiturate sleeping pills and bromides. Tremor does, however, occur as one of the symptoms of several physical disorders:

With sweating, flushing or pallor, chilliness, numbness, hunger, headache, dizziness, weakness, palpitation, sometimes faintness several hours after meals: HYPOGLYCEMIA.

With fever, headache, vomiting, stiff neck: ENCEPHALITIS, VIRAL.

With drooling, difficulty in speaking, incoordination, open-mouthedness, rigidity, sometimes behavioral changes, anemia: WILSON'S DISEASE.

With nervousness, weakness, heat sensitivity, sweating, overactivity, restlessness, weight loss with increased appetite, palpitation, protrusion of eyes, sometimes headache, nausea, abdominal pain, diarrhea: HYPERTHYROIDISM.

Of hands and nodding of head, with movements becoming slower and more difficult, loss of mobility of face, tremors increasing and sometimes involving whole body, shuffling gait, stooped position with back bent forward: PARKINSON'S DISEASE.

Of limbs, with one or many other symptoms: vision disturbances, weakness, fatigue, slowing and monotony of speech, impaired balance, unsteady walking, stiff gait, loss of bladder and bowel control: MULTIPLE SCLEROSIS.

## TWITCHING (see also TICS)

Spasmodic, with fever, joint swellings, vague pains in limbs, nosebleeds: RHEUMATIC FEVER.

Spasmodic, jerking movements, often with facial grimacing, sometimes in severe cases wild flailing arms or legs, following a strep infection (sometimes months later): SYDENHAM'S CHOREA, also known as *chorea minor, rheumatic chorea,* and *St. Vitus' dance.*

With spasticity (stiff, awkward movements and in some cases scissorslike gait), often with speaking and swallowing disturbances: CEREBRAL PALSY.

## UMBILICUS (NAVEL)

Red patches, with blisters and pustules: CANDIDIASIS.

## UNCONSCIOUSNESS (see also COMA)

Unconsciousness may be brief, as in fainting, or prolonged, as in severe brain injury. It may vary in depth from stupor or semiconsciousness from which the person can be aroused with difficulty to coma from which arousal is impossible.

Causes are almost innumerable. They include acute alcoholism, brain injury, stroke, poisoning, epilepsy, diabetic acidosis, hypoglycemic shock, infections, uremia, liver failure, hysteria, heatstroke, extreme cold, thyroid crisis. Determination of cause depends upon other symptoms.

Some aids to helping to determine the cause in a stranger: alcoholic breath, with normal or below-normal temperature, excessive blood in the face, in *acute alcoholism;* in *head injury,* evidence of a local wound, sometimes bleeding from ear, nose or throat; in *stroke,* the person is usually middle-aged or elderly, with flushed or blue face; in *diabetic acidosis,* dry skin, flushed face, fruity odor on breath; in *heat prostration,* cold, ashen, damp skin, profuse sweating; in *cardiac arrest,* no pulse, no breathing, no heart sounds.

## URINARY INCONTINENCE

Complete incontinence in some cases, urinary retention in others: BLADDER, NEUROGENIC.

With one or more other symptoms: double vision, weakness, fatigue, tremor, slowing and monotony of speech, impaired balance, unsteady walking, stiff gait, loss of bowel control: MULTIPLE SCLEROSIS.

## URINARY RETENTION

Retention in some cases, incontinence in others: BLADDER, NEUROGENIC.

## URINATION, DIMINISHED

With diarrhea, severe dehydration, great thirst, muscle cramps, weakness, skin wrinkling: CHOLERA.

With lassitude, fatigue, one or more other symptoms: muscle cramps and twitching, nausea, vomiting, appetite loss, yellow-brown skin discoloration, hiccuping, urine smell on breath and sweat, itching: UREMIA.

Marked diminution or failure to void, sometimes with low back pain or tenderness: RENAL FAILURE, ACUTE.

## URINATION, EXCESSIVE

With excessive thirst, nausea, vomiting, itching, weakness, nervousness, appetite loss: HYPERVITAMINOSIS D.

With excessive thirst, as many as 5 to 40 quarts of liquid consumed and excreted per day: DIABETES INSIPIDUS.

With excessive thirst, episodic weakness, burning or tingling sensations, transient paralysis, muscle cramps and spasms, elevation of blood pressure: HYPERALDOSTERONISM.

With weakness, appetite loss, nausea, constipation, abdominal pain, thirst, urinary stones: HYPERPARATHYROIDISM.

With thirst, itching, hunger, weakness, weight loss, dryness of skin: DIABETES.

## URINATION: FREQUENT, PAINFUL, URGENT, AND/OR DIFFICULT

Frequent, urgent, painful, with one or more other symptoms: chills, fever, headache, pain in one or both sides of lower back: PYELONEPHRITIS.

Frequent, urgent, painful, burning, often with chills, fever, nausea, vomiting, general muscle aches, lassitude: URINARY TRACT INFECTIONS.

Increasingly frequent, urgent, difficult, with excessive urination at night, hesitancy and intermittency of the stream and decreased size and force of stream: PROSTATE ENLARGEMENT.

Frequent, painful, burning, with blood and pus in urine: CANCER OF THE URINARY BLADDER.

Increasingly difficult, frequent, with diminished stream, sometimes with blood in urine: CANCER OF THE PROSTATE.

Frequent, urgent, with bleeding following coitus, sometimes with painful coitus, watery vaginal discharge, painful defecation: CANCER OF THE VAGINA.

Painful, burning, with discharge of whitish fluid or pus: GONORRHEA.

Mild pain, with watery, whitish, often slight penile discharge, sometimes with lower abdominal pain: URETHRITIS, NONGONOCOCCAL.

Frequent, with excruciating intermittent pain starting in kidney area and radiating across abdomen into genital area and inner aspects of thigh, sometimes with nausea, vomiting, chills, fever: URINARY CALCULI (STONES).

Painful, frequent, sometimes with fever: PROSTATITIS.

Frequent, urgent, in a woman, with one or more other symptoms: vaginal discharge, lower abdominal cramps, painful coitus, vaginal pain, pain on walking: PROLAPSE OF THE UTERUS.

Painful, difficult, in a woman, with one or more other symptoms: excessive menstrual bleeding, anemia, infertility, miscarriage: UTERUS, MYOMA OF.

Painful, in a woman, with vaginal discharge or bleeding: POLYPS.

Difficult or frequent, in a man, sometimes with discharge: POLYPS.

## URINE, BLOOD IN

With coughing and spitting of blood, anemia, breathing difficulty: GOODPASTURE'S SYNDROME.

With change in urine color, reduced volume of urine, water retention appearing as puffiness of face and eyelids and later extending to legs and other parts of body: GLOMERULONEPHRITIS, ACUTE.

Also with pus, recurrent attacks of pain in kidney region, sometimes fever: HYDRONEPHROSIS.

With episodic kidney pain, abdominal discomfort: POLYCYSTIC KIDNEY DISEASE.

With abdominal mass and pain, fever, appetite loss, nausea, vomiting, in a child: CANCER OF THE KIDNEY (Wilms' tumor).

With abdominal mass, fever, flank pain: CANCER OF THE KIDNEY.

With difficult, frequent urination, diminished stream: CANCER OF THE PROSTATE.

Also with pus, frequent, painful, burning urination: CANCER OF THE URINARY BLADDER.

## URINE, DARKENING OF

With fever, headache, muscle aches, yellowing of skin, prostration: YELLOW FEVER.

With fever, nausea, abdominal discomfort, drowsiness, lassitude, weakness, appetite loss, headache, sometimes jaundice: HEPATITIS.

## UTERINE BLEEDING

Abnormal uterine bleeding includes excessively prolonged menstruation (hypermenorrhea), excessive menstrual bleeding (menorrhagia), unusually frequent menstruation (polymenorrhea), bleeding between periods (metrorrhagia), and postmenopausal bleeding.

Abnormal bleeding prior to menopause has many possible causes, including malignant tumors, endometriosis (presence of uterine tissue in places other than the uterus), hormonal imbalance, chronic tubular disease, emotional trauma, and constitutional disorders such as high blood pressure, heart disease, and vitamin deficiencies. In addition to measures such as rest, nutritious diet, and agents to combat any anemia, specific treatment is directed at the cause and may include hormonal treatment, removal of cervical polyps, anticancer therapy, antibiotics.

Abnormal postmenopausal bleeding is any bleeding from the reproductive tract nine months or more after menopause and may range from slight discharge (brownish or bloody) to profuse. A common cause is vaginitis, or inflammation of the vagina. Other causes include vulvitis (inflammation of the external parts of the reproductive system surrounding the opening of the vagina), leukoplakia (white patches on mucous membranes), malignancy of vagina, vulva, or cervix, cervical or uterine polyps, and other conditions. A cardinal rule of thumb is to consider any postmenopausal bleeding to be due to malignancy until proved otherwise. Diagnosis may be aided by history, pelvic examination, diagnostic curettage, cervical biopsy, or other studies. Treatment, directed at the cause, may be removal of polyps or any malignant growth, suitable agents to control inflammation.

## UTERUS, ABNORMAL SIZE OF, IN PREGNANCY

Rapid increase in size shortly after conception, with vaginal bleeding, lack of fetal movement: HYDATIDIFORM MOLE.

## VAGINA

Painful blisters in: HERPES SIMPLEX VIRUS, TYPE 2.

Painless sore inside vagina or on the labia, appearing about three weeks after infection through sexual contact: chancre of SYPHILIS.

Bleeding from, after coitus, sometimes with painful coitus, watery discharge, urinary frequency and urgency, painful defecation: CANCER OF THE VAGINA.

Bleeding from, in pregnancy, with rapid increase in size of uterus, lack of fetal movement: HYDATIDIFORM MOLE.

Bleeding or discharge from, with painful urination: POLYPS.

Discharge from and inflammation of: CANDIDIASIS.

Discharge from, sometimes profuse, varying from clear to bloody, from mucus-laden to purulent, with or without odor, sometimes with itching: LEUKORRHEA.

Discharge of whitish fluid or pus, sometimes with painful urination, fever, nausea, vomiting, lower abdominal pain: GONORRHEA.

Discharge, slight, watery or bloody, after intercourse, often with irregular menstruation, sometimes lower back pain, vomiting, constipation: CANCER OF THE CERVIX.

Bleeding from, sometimes with odorous discharge, irregular menstruation with heavy flow sometimes followed by none: CANCER OF THE UTERUS.

## VERTIGO (see DIZZINESS)

## VISION DISTURBANCES (see also EYES)

### Blindness

Sudden: CENTRAL ARTERY OBSTRUCTION.

Transient, with one or more other symptoms: fainting attacks or epileptic seizures, arm lameness, speaking difficulty, cataracts: AORTIC ARCH SYNDROME.

### Blurring

Sometimes with blood spots in eyes, bloodshot appearance: RETINOPATHIES.

With headache, sometimes confusion, depression, agitation, inappropriate speech or dress: CRYPTOCOCCOSIS.

Or size distortion of objects, reduced central vision: CHOROIDITIS.

With one or many other symptoms: numbness and tingling of arms or fingers, weakness of arms or hands, stiff neck or shoulder, headache, "knots" in neck, shoulder or arm muscles, swelling and stiffness of fingers, loss of balance, pain in and around eyes, fainting: CERVICAL SYNDROME.

### Flashes of light

With sensation of a curtain moving across the eye: RETINAL DETACHMENT.

### Night blindness

Sometimes with abnormal dryness of surface of conjunctiva (the membrane lining eyelid and covering eyeball) and softening of cornea (the transparent front covering of eye): VITAMIN DEFICIENCY (vitamin A)

### Reduced vision

Beginning as a small area of reduced vision in the center or at the edge of one or usually both eyes, which slowly enlarges and progressively reduces acuteness of vision: TOXIC AMBLYOPIA.

Ranging from slight contraction of field of vision to blindness: OPTIC NEURITIS.

Loss of vision that may range from only moderate to blindness: OPTIC ATROPHY.

Loss of acuity, with distortions of size and shape of objects, eye discomfort: RETINITIS.

Progressive, painless loss of vision, with blurring, dimming, need for brighter light for reading, sometimes frequent changes of glasses, occasionally with double vision: CATARACT.

With one or many other symptoms: headache, muscle weakness, vomiting, loss of balance and coordination, drowsiness, lethargy, personality changes: CANCER OF THE BRAIN.

With headache, pain and tenderness of the temporal arteries in the head: TEMPORAL ARTERITIS.

### Side vision loss

With blurred or fogged vision, appearance of colored rings or halos around bright objects: GLAUCOMA.

Increasing narrowness of side vision, producing "tunnel vision": RETINITIS PIGMENTOSA.

### Spots before eyes

With one or more other symptoms: headache, ringing in ears, easy fatigability, weakness, drowsiness, pallor, heart pounding and shortness of breath on exertion: ANEMIA.

## VOICE, ABNORMAL CHANGE IN

Hoarseness or loss of voice, with throat tickling and rawness, constant effort to clear the throat: LARYNGITIS.

Drop in pitch, becoming monotone: POLYPOSIS OF THE VOCAL CORDS.

Loss of, sometimes with breathing difficulty: LARYNX, PAPILLOMA OF.

## VOMITING (see NAUSEA AND VOMITING)

## VULVA (see also VAGINA)

The vulva consists of the exterior opening of the vagina and surrounding organs: the labia majora, the labia minora, the vestibule, and the clitoris.

Reddening, with edema and swelling, burning, itching, sometimes pain severe enough to interfere with sitting and walking: VULVITIS.

Red, scaly, greasy areas on vulva, also often on ears, eyelids, with dry scaling and fissuring of lips and angles of mouth, sometimes also with tearing of eyes and sensitivity to light: VITAMIN DEFICIENCY (riboflavin).

## WALKING

Pain on walking, with weakness, intensifying until walking is impossible, disappearance of symptoms after leg rest: INTERMITTENT CLAUDICATION.

Unsteady walking, often with impaired balance, stiff gait, one or more other symptoms: vision disturbances, weakness, fatigue, tremor of limbs, slowing and monotony of speech, loss of bladder and bowel control: MULTIPLE SCLEROSIS.

## WARTS

Caused by viruses, and contagious, warts take several forms:

**Common warts.** Usually grayish, rough, firm, round or irregular in shape, occurring most often on fingers, elbows, knees, face, scalp, but may spread elsewhere.

**Moist warts.** In the anal and genital area, sometimes coalescing to form larger plaques.

**Plantar warts.** The same as the common type (above) but occurring on soles of feet where they are flattened by pressure and often become extremely tender.

**Flat warts.** Yellow-brown, smooth and flat, occurring most often on the face.

**Unusual shape warts.** Threadlike or resembling a cauliflower, most common on scalp and bearded area of face.

**Treatment of warts.** Many treatments have been developed. None is 100 percent effective in all cases. In some cases, warts reappear at the same or different sites. Physicians may apply one or another of many topical agents to warts, including caustics such as trichloroacetic acid and nitric acid. Plantar warts may be treated by peeling away some of the wart tissue, applying concentrated phenol solution followed by nitric acid, and covering with salicylic acid plaster and adhesive bandage. Other methods of treatment include freezing with liquid nitrogen, x-ray, surgical or electrosurgical removal. Anal warts have tended to be notably resistant to treatment, recurring in as many as half or more of patients after use of surgical or electrosurgical removal, freezing, drug applications. Promising early results have been reported very recently in the treatment of anal warts with a vaccine that is prepared from the wart tissue and treated with the antibiotics penicillin and streptomycin, then frozen and thawed several times.

## WEAKNESS (see also MUSCLE WEAKNESS)

### In infections

With chills, fever, severe headache, malaise, sometimes diarrhea: BRUCELLOSIS.

With chills, fever, headache, nausea, vomiting: TULAREMIA.

With diarrhea, dehydration, thirst, diminished urination, muscle cramps, wrinkling of skin: CHOLERA.

With fever, breathing difficulty and blueness, loss of appetite, weight, strength: COCCIDIOMYCOSIS.

With pain or discomfort over the liver in upper right part of abdomen, especially with movement, sometimes radiating to right shoulder, one or more other symptoms: fever, sweats, chills, nausea, vomiting, weight loss: AMEBIASIS (HEPATITIS).

With fever, headache, nausea, drowsiness, lassitude, appetite loss, sometimes jaundice: HEPATITIS.

## In parasitic disease

With swelling of upper eyelids, pain in eyes, one or more other symptoms: fever, light sensitivity, muscle soreness and pain, thirst, chills, profuse sweating, hives, prostration: TRICHINOSIS.

## In malignancies

With breastbone tenderness, vague upper abdominal distress or heaviness, appetite loss, weight loss, fatigue: LEUKEMIA, CHRONIC (myelocytic).

Increasing weakness, with fatigue, mild pallor, lymph gland (node) swellings, appetite loss: LEUKEMIA, CHRONIC (lymphocytic).

With gland (lymph node) enlargement in neck, underarms, or groin, usually on one side, fever, sweating, sometimes itching, weight and appetite loss: HODGKIN'S DISEASE.

With cough, wheezing, blood-streaked sputum, chest pains, breathing difficulty, loss of weight: CANCER OF THE LUNG.

With persistent pain in back, chest or pelvis, weight loss, recurrent bacterial infections: MYELOMA, MULTIPLE.

## In deficiency states

With vague muscle and joint aches, swollen and bleeding gums, small black and blue spots on skin, weight loss, irritability, lassitude: SCURVY.

With swelling first of legs, then becoming generalized, digestive disturbances, weight loss, lethargy, appetite loss: PROTEIN DEFI-CIENCY (chronic).

## In vitamin excess states

With sparse and coarse hair, loss of eyebrows, dry rough skin, cracked lips, headaches: HYPERVITAMINOSIS A.

With nausea, vomiting, itching, excessive urination and thirst, appetite loss, nervousness: HYPERVITAMINOSIS D.

## In other conditions

With one or more other symptoms: pallor, shortness of breath and pounding of heart on exertion, headache, ringing of ears, spots before eyes, low-grade fever, irritability, dizziness, gastrointestinal complaints: ANEMIA.

Overpowering weakness, with fatigue and, two or three days later, sudden malaise, chills, high fever, sore throat, swallowing difficulty, ulcers in mouth, extreme prostration: AGRANULOCYTOSIS.

With nausea, vomiting, malaise, appetite and weight loss, abdominal discomfort, loss of libido, absence of menstruation, nose and other bleeding tendencies: CIRRHOSIS OF THE LIVER.

With enlarged spleen, progressively severe anemia, vomiting of blood, blood in stools: BANTI'S DISEASE.

With vague ill health and weight loss, followed by repeated infections, bleeding of mucous membranes, anemia: MACROGLOBULINEMIA.

With fatigue: MITRAL INSUFFICIENCY.

With sudden fast heartbeats of 100 or more a minute, fluttering sensations in chest, faintness, sometimes nausea: PAROXYSMAL TACHYCARDIA.

With palpitation, pallor, nausea, fainting: ATRIAL FLUTTER OR FIBRILLATION.

With breathing difficulty, chest pain, sweating, nausea: SHOCK.

With dull or sharp pain in chest under breastbone or over heart and stomach, fever, chills, anxiety, sometimes with nonproductive cough, quick, shallow breathing: PERICARDITIS.

With one or more other symptoms: fatigue, nervousness, dizziness, palpitation, insomnia, headache: HYPERTENSION.

With faintness, dizziness, profuse sweating, followed by vomiting of blood or passage of tarry stools: PEPTIC ULCER (hemorrhage).

After prolonged diarrhea, appetite loss, weight loss becoming increasingly marked after weeks to months, with anemia, muscle cramps, fatigability: SPRUE, TROPICAL.

With diarrhea, appetite and weight loss, anemia, fever of 102° or 103°, joint pains and arthritis of knees, wrists and back, nonproductive cough, abdominal and chest pain: WHIPPLE'S DISEASE.

With sweating, flushing or pallor, chilliness, numbness, trembling, hunger, headache, dizziness, palpitation, sometimes faintness, several hours after meals: HYPOGLYCEMIA.

Episodic weakness, with burning or tingling sensations, transient paralysis, muscle cramps and spasms, excessive urination and thirst, blood pressure elevation: HYPERALDOSTERONISM.

With abdominal pain, appetite loss, nausea, constipation, thirst, excessive urination, urinary tract stones: HYPERPARATHYROIDISM.

With excessive urination, thirst, itching, hunger, weight loss, skin dryness: DIABETES.

With one or many other symptoms: double vision or loss of part of visual field, tremor or shaking of limbs, slowing and monotony of speech, impaired balance, unsteady walking, stiff gait, loss of bladder and bowel control: MULTIPLE SCLEROSIS.

With headache or malaise, sometimes with abdominal pain, nausea, vomiting: METABOLIC ACIDOSIS.

With nervousness, restlessness, heat sensitivity, sweating, weight loss with increased appetite, tremor, palpitation, protrusion of eyes, sometimes with headache, nausea, abdominal pain, diarrhea: HYPERTHYROIDISM.

Increasing weakness, with increased skin pigmentation, black freckles over forehead, face, neck and shoulders, bluish-black discolorations of mucous membrance of lips, mouth and other sites, weight loss, often with appetite loss, nausea, vomiting, diarrhea, decreased cold tolerance, dizziness, fainting attacks: ADDISON'S DISEASE.

## WEIGHT, FAILURE TO GAIN

With irritability, appetite loss, fever, anemia, swollen and bleeding gums, in a child: SCURVY.

## WEIGHT GAIN

With decreased appetite, one or many other symptoms: chilliness, dry, cold skin, puffiness of hands and face, slow speech, mental apathy, drowsiness, constipation, hearing loss, poor memory, excessive or absent menstruation: HYPOTHYROIDISM.

With rounded face, fat accumulation in the back (buffalo hump), muscle wasting and weakness, easy bruising, menstrual irregularities: CUSHING'S SYNDROME.

## WEIGHT LOSS

### In infections

With chills, fever, severe headache, malaise, sometimes diarrhea: BRUCELLOSIS.

With fever, abdominal pain, painful straining at stool, stools containing blood, pus, and mucus and increasing to 20 or more a day: BACILLARY DYSENTERY.

With fever, fatigue, appetite loss, listlessness, vague chest pain, purulent sputum, night sweats: TUBERCULOSIS.

With pain or discomfort over liver in upper right part of abdomen, especially with movement, sometimes radiating to right shoulder, with one or more other symptoms: fever, sweats, chills, nausea, vomiting, weakness: AMEBIASIS (HEPATITIS).

With muscular weakness, headache, diarrhea, eye inflammation: TOXOPLASMOSIS.

With mucous diarrhea, abdominal pain, especially in children: GIARDIASIS.

## In malignancies

With gland (lymph node) swellings in neck, underarms, and groin, itching, sometimes accompanied by weakness, fever, appetite loss: HODGKIN'S DISEASE.

With gland (lymph node) swellings in neck, underarms, or groin, usually on one side, fever, sweating, debility or lack of strength: LYMPHOSARCOMA.

With persistent pain in back, chest or pelvis, weakness, repeated bacterial infections: MYELOMA, MULTIPLE.

With cough, blood-streaked sputum, chest pain, breathing difficulty, wheezing, weakness: CANCER OF THE LUNG.

With firm but not tender abdominal mass, in a child, with fever, sometimes breathing difficulty: NEUROBLASTOMA.

With upper abdominal distress and pain over stomach area, usually but not necessarily intensified soon after eating, sometimes with one or more other symptoms such as appetite loss, vomiting, anemia: CANCER OF THE STOMACH.

With variable abdominal pain often extending to the back and relieved by sitting up or bending forward, with one or more other symptoms: jaundice, nausea, vomiting, appetite loss, constipation or diarrhea, vomiting of blood, darkening of stool with blood pigments: CANCER OF THE PANCREAS.

With weakness, fatigue, appetite loss, vague upper abdominal distress, breastbone tenderness: LEUKEMIA, CHRONIC (myelocytic).

## In deficiency states

With weakness, irritability, lassitude, vague muscle and joint aches, swollen and bleeding gums, black and blue spots on skin: SCURVY.

With swelling in legs, later becoming generalized, weakness, lethargy, digestive disturbances, appetite loss: PROTEIN DEFICIENCY (chronic).

## In other conditions

With fever, joint pains, sometimes also cough, breathing difficulty, hoarseness: SARCOIDOSIS.

With vague ill health, followed by repeated infections, bleeding of mucous membranes, anemia: MACROGLOBULINEMIA.

With cough, with or without a stitch in the side, slight fever, sometimes with asthma or increased severity of asthma in previous sufferers of asthma: LOEFFLER'S SYNDROME.

With abdominal pain, diarrhea: BOWEL ARTERY ATHEROSCLEROSIS.

With appetite loss, breathing difficulty, one or more other symptoms: blueness after exercise, rapid pulse, dry nonproductive cough, fever, malaise, easy fatigability: PULMONARY GRANULOMATOSES.

With progressively increasing breathing difficulty, cough, thick yellow sputum sometimes containing bits of yellow-gray material, malaise: PULMONARY ALVEOLAR PROTEINOSIS.

With chronic diarrhea (several loose, nonbloody stools a day), abdominal pain, fever: REGIONAL ENTERITIS.

Becoming increasingly marked after weeks to months, with diarrhea, appetite loss, anemia, weakness, fatigability, muscle cramps: SPRUE, TROPICAL.

With appetite loss, diarrhea, anemia, weakness, fever of 100° to 103°, joint pains and arthritis of knees, wrists and back, nonproductive cough, abdominal and chest pain: WHIPPLE'S DISEASE.

With appetite loss, nausea, vomiting, malaise, weakness, abdominal discomfort, loss of libido, nose and other bleeding tendencies, and, in a woman, absence of menstruation: CIRRHOSIS OF THE LIVER.

With one or many other symptoms: apathy, appetite loss, easy fatigue, cold intolerance, diminished libido, absence of pubic and underarm hair, scanty menstruation, failure to lactate after childbirth: HYPOPITUITARISM.

With increased appetite, nervousness, heat sensitivity, sweating, restlessness, overactivity, tremor, palpitation, abnormal eye protrusion, sometimes with headache, nausea, abdominal pain, diarrhea: HYPERTHYROIDISM.

With increasing weakness, easy fatigability, increased skin pigmentation, black freckles over forehead, face, neck, shoulders, bluish-black discolorations of mucous membranes of lips, mouth, other sites, appetite loss, nausea, vomiting, diarrhea, decreased cold tolerance, dizziness, fainting attacks: ADDISON'S DISEASE.

With excessive urination, thirst, itching, hunger, weakness, dryness of skin: DIABETES.

With fever, one or many other symptoms: severe abdominal pain, diffuse muscle pain, joint pain, bloody diarrhea, wheezing, pneumonia, skin reddening, hives: POLYARTERITIS.

## WHEEZING (see also BREATHING DIFFICULTY)

With labored breathing, sense of constriction in chest, sometimes blueness: ASTHMA.

With cough, followed by labored breathing, ability to breathe only in upright position, sometimes a sense of oppression in the chest: PULMONARY EDEMA.

With labored breathing, often on mild exertion, even talking, with chronic, spasmodic, hard, tiring cough, expectoration of thick sputum: EMPHYSEMA, PULMONARY.

With cough, with or without a stitch in the side, sometimes weight loss: LOEFFLER'S SYNDROME.

With cough, blood-streaked sputum, chest pain, weakness, weight loss: CANCER OF THE LUNG.

With fever, weight loss, one or more other symptoms: severe abdominal pain, diffuse muscle pain, joint pain, bloody diarrhea, pneumonia, skin reddening, hives: POLYARTERITIS.

## WRIST

Abnormal bending, with similar flexion of ankle joints, muscle twitchings, cramps, convulsions: TETANY.

Painless lump on back of wrist: GANGLION.

Throbbing, crushing pain, appearing suddenly, with swelling, warmth, redness, shininess of skin: GOUT.

Inflammation, pain, tenderness: ARTHRITIS.

Swelling, with pain, numbness and tingling of fingers: CARPAL TUNNEL SYNDROME.

# SECTION TWO Diseases

## ACHALASIA

A failure of the lower esophagus to relax normally and permit free passage of food into the stomach, achalasia is of unknown cause, but emotional tension can aggravate it and trigger attacks. Symptoms may include vomiting, with the possibility that some material may get into the breathing passages, pain behind the breastbone that may sometimes radiate to back, neck, and jaw. Treatment in mild cases: avoidance of very large meals, eating slowly, drinking fluids during meals. For severe cases, relief by surgery may be required to allow stretching of the esophagus.

## ACHILLES TENDON CONTRACTURE

The Achilles tendon at the back of the heel connects calf muscle to heel bone. Contracture or shortening of the tendon may be congenital, an aftermath of neurologic disease, or the result of wearing high heels. Restricted ankle movement, foot pain, and pain in the arch sometimes extending to the calf can develop. In many cases, gradual tendon-stretching exercises or manipulation help. In severe cases, lengthening of the tendon by surgery may be required.

## ACNE ROSACEA

Marked by flushing of the skin of the nose, forehead, and cheeks, followed by reddening due to dilation of tiny blood vessels, and appearance of acnelike blackheads, papules, and pustules, acne rosacea is a chronic disorder that occurs mostly in the middle-aged but sometimes in younger people. It has a familial tendency, may be intensified by heat, cold, exposure to sun and wind, emotional disturbances, gastrointestinal disorders, alcohol, some foods such as coffee, tea, chocolate, nuts, and very hot, cold or highly spiced dishes. Often, more important than various topical applications that may be prescribed is attention to avoiding the intensifying factors just noted. In severe cases, disfiguring blood vessels may be treated by electrodessication with an electrical needle.

## ACNE VULGARIS

This is the common inflammatory disease, usually occurring in adolescence, with its blackheads and pimples on the face, neck, and upper part of the body. It is associated with increased hormonal activity and production of sebum by the sebaceous glands in the skin. Severe cases require expert medical treatment, which may include use of an antibiotic such as tetracycline and topical applications such as vitamin A acid.

## ACTINOMYCOSIS

Sometimes also called "lumpy jaw," this is a fungal infection that most commonly involves the head and neck and most often affects men. A small, hard swelling, with or without pain, appears under the mucous membrane of the mouth, or skin of the neck, or around the jaw. Other parts of the head—cheek, tongue, throat, salivary glands, cranial bones—may be affected to begin with or by extension. The masses break down and discharge little granules, usually yellowish, through sinuses or channels extending through the skin. The infection progresses slowly, at first seeming not to affect general health, but if not treated successfully, it can be fatal. In some cases, the lungs are involved, with symptoms including chest pain, fever, cough. Intestinal involvement sometimes occurs, with abdominal mass and pain, fever, vomiting, diarrhea or constipation, and emaciation. Most cases respond to medical measures, including use of penicillin, but treatment is commonly prolonged, ranging upward of eight weeks.

## ACUTE ARTERIAL OCCLUSION

When a leg artery is suddenly occluded, or blocked, symptoms may include sudden coldness, numbness, tingling, followed soon by severe pain and blanching or mottling with blue patches. The blockage may be due to a blood clot arising in the artery because of atherosclerosis or to a clot (embolus) formed elsewhere and carried to the leg artery in the bloodstream. Immediate treatment may include use of anticoagulants (anticlotting agents) along with other measures such as injections of procaine and papaverine, and improvement may begin within a few hours; if not, surgery to remove the clot through incision in the artery may be required without further delay.

## ADDISON'S DISEASE

The result of underfunctioning of the adrenal glands atop the kidneys, Addison's disease, or adrenal hypofunction, may occur at any age and affects both sexes about equally. In most cases, the cortex of the adrenals atrophies or decreases in size from unknown cause; in some cases, partial destruction of the gland follows other disease such as tuberculosis or cancer. Symptoms may include increasing weakness and easy fatigability, increased skin pigmentation, black freckles over forehead, face, neck and shoulders, bluish-black discoloration of mucous membranes of lips, mouth and other sites, appetite and weight loss, nausea, vomiting, diarrhea, dizziness, decreased cold tolerance, fainting attacks. Diagnosis is aided by tests of adrenal function. Treatment includes administration—by injection at first, oral doses later—of an adrenal gland hormone or equivalent, such as hydrocortisone.

## ADENOFIBROMA (see FIBROADENOMA, BENIGN)

## ADENOID HYPERTROPHY

Hypertrophy or enlargement of the adenoid tissue in the throat area, most common in children, may cause obstruction of the outlet from the nose, leading to such symptoms as mouth breathing, halitosis, postnasal discharge, nasal speech, cough, and a facial expression that may make the child appear to be dull and apathetic. The tissue enlargement also may obstruct the eustachian tube to the ear, causing pain in the ear or a sense of pressure, and sometimes interfering with hearing. Surgery, called adenoidectomy, can be used to remove the obstructing tissue.

## AEROPHAGIA

Aerophagia, or habitual swallowing of air, can when extreme produce alarming symptoms, including abdominal distention, breathing difficulty, smothering sensations, palpitation, seeming heart pain. Unavoidably, some air is swallowed with food and drink and is of no consequence. But large, disturbing amounts may be swallowed when eating rapidly or while emotionally upset, chewing gum, smoking, drinking large amounts of carbonated beverages. Belching, to relieve discomfort, may at the same time cause additional air swallowing, especially if the mouth is kept closed. Overcoming aerophagia may require avoidance of gum, candy mints, carbonated drinks, animated mealtime conversations that may lead to food gulping, and rapid eating for any reason.

## AGRANULOCYTOSIS

An acute disease in which there is a sudden sharp drop in production of white blood cells, leaving the body defenseless against bacterial infection, agranulocytosis sometimes is of unknown cause but commonly results from sensitization to drugs or chemicals that affect the bone marrow and thus interfere with white cell formation. Symptoms often begin with several days of great fatigue and weakness, after which there may be chills, high fever, sore throat, swallowing difficulty, mouth ulcers. Laboratory tests show a greatly reduced count of white cells in the blood. Treatment is double-pronged: immediate withdrawal of the drug or chemical involved, and control of infection. In most cases, antibiotics are effective for infection control, and if the bone marrow has not been irreparably damaged, healthy white blood cell production will resume.

## AIR SWALLOWING (see AEROPHAGIA)

## ALLERGIC CONJUNCTIVITIS (see CONJUNCTIVITIS, ALLERGIC)

## ALLERGIC PURPURA (see PURPURA, ALLERGIC)

## ALLERGIC RHINITIS (see RHINITIS, ALLERGIC)

**ALLERGY, GASTROINTESTINAL** (see GASTROINTESTINAL ALLERGY)

## ALLERGY, PHYSICAL (HEAT OR COLD)

Of unknown cause, heat or cold allergy produces hives, or sudden outbreaks of itching and burning swellings on the skin. The outbreaks occur on exposed areas and may, after swimming or bathing, affect virtually the whole body. Cold sensitivity sometimes can be reduced by daily showers at gradually colder water temperatures. For relief of itching, an oral antihistamine such as diphenhydramine or cyproheptadine may be prescribed.

## AMBLYOPIA, TOXIC (see TOXIC AMBLYOPIA)

## AMEBIASIS

An infectious disease caused by a protozoan organism, *Entamoeba histolytica*, amebiasis, according to various surveys, affects from 1 to 10 percent of Americans. The infection is transmitted through feces-contaminated food or drink, with carriers of the disease, especially food handlers, themselves having no disturbing symptoms, being merely the principal source. The parasites reach the intestine and multiply.

**Amebic dysentery.** Amebiasis may cause amebic dysentery in some cases and is more likely to do so in tropical regions than in the United States. It is marked by diarrhea, with stools containing blood and mucus, slight fever, recurrent cramps, anemia, emaciation.

**Amebiasis in the United States.** Symptoms often include slight fever, fatigue, vague aches and pains, diarrhea, constipation, with abdominal pain that may be generalized or limited to the right lower abdomen.

**Amebic hepatitis.** In some cases, amebiasis leads to involvement of the liver, with pain or discomfort over the liver area (on the right side of the abdomen, just under the diaphragm) which may radiate to the right shoulder. Intermittent fever, sweats, chills, nausea, vomiting, weakness, and weight loss may occur.

Diagnosis of amebic infection can be established definitively by recovery of the parasite in the stool.

Treatment for patients with mild symptoms and for carriers consists of either diiodohydroxyquine for 20 days, tetracycline for 10 days, or paromomycin for 7 days, all by mouth. For severe infections, bed rest is needed and blood transfusion may be required. For acute amebic dysentery, emetine may be administered by injection for 4 to 6 days, followed by tetracycline by mouth for 5 days and diiodohydroxyquine by mouth for 20 days. In resistant cases, other agents such as penicillin, paromomycin, and succinylsulfathiazole may be used. Amebic hepatitis often responds well to chloroquine, emetine, or metronidazole.

## AMENORRHEA (ABSENCE OF MENSTRUATION)

Called *primary* when menstruation fails to begin at puberty and *secondary* when flow stops in women who have previously menstruated, amenorrhea has many possible causes, including mechanical obstruction, ovarian disorders, other glandular disturbances, central nervous system disorders, emotional stress, and great weight changes. Treatment must be directed at the underlying cause.

## AMYOTROPHIC LATERAL SCLEROSIS

A grave disease of unknown cause, amyotrophic lateral sclerosis is marked by degenerative changes in the nervous system. It usually occurs after the age of 40, affecting men more frequently than women. Symptoms include weakness and wasting of hand muscles and then of muscles of forearms and shoulders, weakness and spasticity of the legs, difficulty in swallowing. No specific treatment is known. Physical therapy may help to relieve spasticity and keep muscles functioning.

## ANAPHYLAXIS

This is an extremely acute, severe reaction in a person who has become sensitized to a drug, serum, or insect sting. Commonly, within 15 minutes after reexposure to the material or sting, the patient becomes flushed and agitated. Other symptoms—breathing difficulty, itching, throbbing in the ears, coughing, sneezing—follow. SHOCK may develop and involves dangerous reduction of blood pressure. With shock, the patient may become lethargic and comatose and may die without treatment. *Shock is an emergency, requiring immediate treatment.* Drugs to elevate blood pressure may be required and, depending upon the patient's condition, other measures, including artificial respiration, may be required.

## ANEMIA

The red cells in blood contain hemoglobin, the pigment that transports oxygen from the lungs to body tissues. Anemia is present when either the number of red cells or the amount of pigment in them is reduced below normal values.

There are many types of anemia but some symptoms are common to all. With mild anemia, there is lack of energy and easy fatigability. With somewhat more severe anemia, there may be shortness of breath on exertion, pounding of the heart, a more rapid pulse than usual. With very severe anemia, there may be weakness, dizziness, headache, ringing of the ears, spots before the eyes, drowsiness, irritability, euphoria, psychotic behavior, failure of menses, loss of libido, low-grade fever, varied gastrointestinal complaints.

Even mild anemia can be detected by determination of red cell count and hemoglobin in blood.

Iron-deficiency anemia. Iron is required for hemoglobin and iron-deficiency anemia is common. Often it results from chronic loss of blood—through excessive menstrual flow, slow bleeding from a peptic ulcer, hemorrhoids, sometimes stomach disturbances caused by aspirin or other drugs, stomach or intestinal tumors, hookworm infestation. Failure to get enough iron in a limited diet may be a cause. Treatment may include use of an iron preparation and diet changes. If blood loss is involved, it's vital not only that the anemia be corrected but that the underlying cause be found and treated.

Pernicious anemia. For red blood cell production in the bone marrow, vitamin $B_{12}$ is required. The vitamin is present in adequate amounts in any well-balanced diet. But for absorption by the body, $B_{12}$ requires the presence in the stomach of a substance called *intrinsic factor.* In pernicious anemia, intrinsic factor is lacking or inadequate. In addition to the common symptoms (above) of anemias, pernicious anemia manifests itself in a red, sore tongue, difficulty in swallowing, pale lemon skin color and, in some cases, numbness and tingling of the legs and fingers, unsteady gait, impaired memory. Blood, bone marrow, and stomach tests can be used for diagnosis. Treatment with injections of vitamin $B_{12}$, especially when started early, may completely eliminate symptoms.

**Aplastic anemia.** Since blood cells are made in the bone marrow, anemia may result when the bone marrow is damaged and fails to function adequately or at all. In this type of anemia, not only are red blood cells reduced in numbers, so, too, are the white cells which help to combat infections. The general symptoms common to all anemias are usually severe in aplastic anemia. In addition, there may be brown skin pigmentation, blood seepage into the skin and mucous membranes, severe sore throat, lowered resistance to infections. Some cases of aplastic anemia, especially in adolescents and young adults, are of unknown cause. In other cases, the anemia results from exposure to some drugs or chemicals such as benzene, methotrexate, nitrogen mustard, quinacrine, phenylbutazone, chloramphenicol, gold compounds, some sulfa drugs, insecticides. Treatment requires blood transfusion until the marrow can resume functioning, control of infection with antibiotics, avoidance of any materials that might be involved in depressing marrow function, and sometimes use of drugs such as cortisonelike agents and compounds related to the male sex hormone, testosterone.

**Hemolytic anemia.** In this type of anemia, red blood cells are destroyed faster than they can be replaced. In addition to symptoms (above) common to other anemias, hemolytic anemia usually produces some degree of jaundice because the hemoglobin released by the destroyed red cells is converted into jaundice pigments. Hemolytic anemia may be congenital or acquired, acute or chronic. An acute form may appear suddenly, with chills, fever, nausea, vomiting, abdominal pain. The cause may be a drug to which the patient is sensitive, infection, cancer, or Hodgkin's disease. If the cause can be removed (an offending medicine) or cured (an infection), the outlook is good. Usually, prompt hospitalization is required so that fluids can be injected and transfusions of packed red cells and cortisonelike medications can be given. Chronic hemolytic anemias may last for years and, if neglected, may lead to gallstones, sometimes leg ulcers and spleen enlargement. It is in the spleen that red cells are destroyed, and, in some cases, surgical removal of the spleen may be required and produces great benefit as the excessive destruction is stopped.

**Sickle cell anemia.** This is a form of hemolytic anemia that affects mainly blacks. It is called *sickle cell* because the ordinarily round red blood cells become sickle-shaped, making them more fragile and easily destroyed. The cells, because of their distorted shape, may also sometimes block small blood vessels. The anemia is usually severe, with jaundice. There may be episodes of joint pain and fever, severe abdominal pain with vomiting. Hospitalization may be needed for severe pain attacks.

**Other anemias.** Other hemolytic anemias may sometimes result from mismatched blood transfusions, industrial poisons (such as benzol and aniline), and other substances such as sulfa drugs, quinine, lead, or fava beans; and the outcome will depend upon how quickly the cause can be found and withdrawn as well as on prompt treatment with fluids, transfusions, and other measures.

Another severe type of anemia is hereditary: *thalassemia major,* also called *Cooley's* and *Mediterranean anemia.* It occurs most often in people with ancestry tracing to northern Africa, southern Europe, and such Asian areas as Iran, Iraq, Indonesia, Thailand, and southern China. In addition to general symptoms of anemia plus jaundice, the liver and spleen enlarge, and leg ulcers, gallstones, and heart failure may develop. Treatment is by transfusion, which prolongs life to some extent.

Still other anemias are associated with various diseases. For example, the anemia associated with low thyroid function yields to thyroid treatment; anemia associated with intestinal parasites yields when the parasites are eliminated by suitable treatment; anemia associated with lead poisoning yields when the poisoning is treated effectively; anemia accompanying chronic infection clears when the infection is cured.

## ANEURYSMS

An aneurysm is a dilation or ballooning out of a part of a blood vessel, usually an artery, and most often of the aorta, the trunkline artery emerging from the heart. Shortly after it emerges upward from the heart, the aorta makes a 180-degree turn, much like the head of a cane, and runs downward from the chest or thoracic area to the abdomen, where it divides into the main leg arteries. Some aneurysms (intrathoracic) occur at the turn of the aorta in the chest; others (abdominal) occur lower down within the abdomen. At first, an aneurysm may be small, but in time it tends to increase in size until finally it may rupture, spilling blood and producing excruciating pain. To avoid this, preventive surgery in advance of rupture is advisable when a still-intact aneurysm producing no symptoms is seen on a routine x-ray or felt during a routine physical examination. Replacing a diseased ballooning-out portion of the aorta with a prosthetic graft is often successful.

**Abdominal aortic aneurysm.** The chief symptom is excruciating, boring pain, usually in the abdomen, but sometimes in the back.

**Intrathoracic aneurysm.** Symptoms are chest or back pain, with cough, labored breathing, difficulty in swallowing.

**Dissecting aortic aneurysm.** In a dissecting aneurysm, in addition to the ballooning out, the inner coat of the artery ruptures, permitting blood to escape between layers of the artery wall, splitting or dissecting the wall. Severe chest pain, much like that of a heart attack, occurs. Often medical treatment, which may include the drug propranolol or antihypertensive agents to bring down blood pressure, can be used. When medical therapy is inadequate in very severe cases, surgery may be performed.

## ANKYLOSING SPONDYLITIS

A chronic, progressive disease of the small joints of the spine, ankylosing spondylitis produces stiffening of the joints, making movement increasingly difficult and painful. The stiffening may extend to the ribs, impairing breathing. Although no curative treatment is known, aspirin is often helpful and, in other cases, either phenylbutazone or indomethacin may be useful. Posture-maintaining exercises are important, and braces may be used in some cases; as long as good posture can be maintained, a useful life can be expected.

## ANORECTAL ABSCESS

A painful red swelling, often producing pain on walking, sitting, or defecation, an anorectal abscess may start as an infection of glands in the anus or rectum or may be associated with FISSURE-IN-ANO, ulcerative COLITIS, REGIONAL ENTERITIS, or TUBERCULOSIS. Treatment involves incision and drainage, with antibiotics used if the infection is widespread.

## ANOREXIA NERVOSA

Occurring most often in young, single women, anorexia nervosa is a loss of appetite and a food aversion due to emotional and mental disorders ranging from a neurotic anxiety over becoming obese to delusions of a schizophrenic nature. Victims may weigh as little as 65 pounds and commonly experience constipation and other gastrointestinal complaints, dry hair and skin, pallor, sometimes puffiness of the ankles. Hospitalization and psychiatric help are often required.

## ANTHRAX

An infectious disease of cattle, horses, mules, sheep, and goats, anthrax rarely may be transmitted to humans through contact with infected animals or their by-products, such as skins. After an incubation period, usually of three to five days, the common skin form begins as a red-brown skin elevation that enlarges, reddens, and blisters. Other symptoms may include swelling of nearby lymph glands (nodes), fever, headache, muscle aches, nausea, vomiting, malaise. Treatment with penicillin or a tetracycline antibiotic is effective. Less common forms of anthrax may involve the lungs, causing lung congestion, or the nervous system, causing breathing difficulty, blueness, shock, and coma. In addition to an antibiotic, treatment may include a cortisonelike drug.

## AORTIC ARCH SYNDROME

This is a condition in which one or more arteries branching off from the main artery, the aorta, become narrowed by atherosclerosis or inflamed. Symptoms, which depend upon the arteries involved and stem from reduced blood flow, may include transient blindness, fainting attacks or epileptic seizures, arm lameness, disturbances of ability to understand or express speech concepts (aphasia), cataracts, wasting of the iris and retina of the eye. Once almost uniformly fatal, aortic arch syndrome now can be treated effectively with surgery to bypass diseased artery sections with Dacron grafts.

## AORTIC INSUFFICIENCY

Aortic insufficiency is an aftermath of rheumatic fever when the latter disease affects the aortic valve, which controls blood flow from the left ventricle, or pumping chamber, of the heart into the aorta, or main body artery. Because the valve fails to close completely, blood leaks backward, forcing the left ventricle to pump harder, enlarge, and, after many years, lose ability to pump effectively. This leads to heart failure, with pumping efficiency diminished to the point that labored breathing and fluid accumulations in the lungs, abdomen, and ankles develop. The heart failure usually responds to medical treatment. In some cases, surgery to replace the defective valve with an artificial valve may be required.

## AORTIC STENOSIS

Either present at birth or resulting from rheumatic fever, aortic stenosis is a narrowing of the aortic valve, which regulates the flow of fresh blood from the left ventricle of the heart into the main artery, the aorta. Many children tolerate the defect well in early years, without symptoms and with normal development. In time, however, obstruction to blood flow through the valve may increase, leading to fatigability, chest pain, labored breathing on exertion, fainting. Medical treatment with a drug such as propranolol sometimes decreases the degree of stenosis or narrowing, lightening the burden on the heart. When medical treatment is inadequate, surgery may be used to cut apart abnormally fused portions of the valve or, when necessary, to replace it with a plastic substitute.

## APPENDICITIS

The appendix is a hollow, 2½- to 3-inch structure located where the large and small intestines join. In appendicitis, the appendix becomes inflamed, sometimes as the result of obstruction by worms, more commonly by fecal material. Once inflamed, the appendix can cause serious trouble if it ruptures and spreads pus through the abdomen (PERITONITIS). Symptoms of appendicitis usually are nausea, abdominal pain, loss of appetite, sometimes fever, constipation or diarrhea. Typically, the pain may begin in the navel area and then shift to the right lower quadrant of the abdomen, and may be accentuated by coughing, sneezing, and movement. Since the appendix in some individuals may be located in an unusual position, pain may localize elsewhere. Expert history-taking and physical examination are important in diagnosis. Other clues include increased white blood cell count, fever, and failure of symptoms to subside. Treatment is surgical removal. Since the risk in surgery is virtually zero, while problems after an appendix ruptures can be formidable, appendectomy may be advisable when appendicitis is suspected but cannot be definitively diagnosed.

## ARTERIAL OCCLUSION, ACUTE (see ACUTE ARTERIAL OCCLUSION)

**ARTERITIS** (see TEMPORAL ARTERITIS)


**ARTHRITIS**

Arthritis, which means inflammation of a joint, is a term that covers many different types of joint diseases, some rare. The most common are *rheumatoid arthritis* and *osteoarthritis,* the latter also known as degenerative joint disease. In *psoriatic arthritis,* both skin and joint disease are present. *Gonococcal arthritis* arises from the venereal disease.

**Gonococcal arthritis.** Caused by invasion of joints by the gonococcus organism, gonococcal arthritis most commonly affects the knee, wrist and ankle, making them hot, red, extremely tender and painful when moved. Fluid accumulations are usually present in the joints. Often gonorrheal infection can be detected in urethral discharges. Penicillin is highly effective for gonococcal arthritis.

**Osteoarthritis.** Rarely occurring before middle age except when a joint has been injured or put to excessive use, osteoarthritis is not as severe a disease as rheumatoid arthritis and is unlike the latter in producing no fever or other constitutional symptoms. Its cause is not clear, although aging, obesity, and joint injury apparently tend to predispose to it. The joints usually affected are the weight-bearing ones such as hips, spine, knees, and ankles. Often, swellings of small finger joints are seen. Affected joints may "creak" and grate on movement. Although, typically, osteoarthritic pain is increased by vigorous exercise and relieved by rest, moderate activity may be needed to avoid joint stiffness. Treatment includes weight reduction where necessary, use of aspirin and other drugs to relieve pain and improve mobility, and applications of heat. In very severe cases, joint replacement—in knee, hip, and elsewhere—may be used.

**Psoriatic arthritis.** This condition is similar to rheumatoid arthritis in many ways except that the joint flare-ups tend to coincide with flare-ups of psoriasis. Treatment measures are similar to those for rheumatoid arthritis (below).

**Rheumatoid arthritis (RA).** Its cause unknown, RA is really a systemic illness that manifests itself primarily by joint pain and inflammation, often leading to deformities. In some cases, other organs, such as the lung, may be affected. Often, RA may begin with nonspecific symptoms such as fever, chills, poor appetite, and general run-down feeling. Later, the joints become stiff, sore, and painful. Usually, the disease begins between ages 20 and 40, most frequently affecting finger joints, wrists, knees, ankles and toes, individually or in combination, although in some cases all joints may be involved. One hallmark of RA is that commonly both sides of the body are affected. Although there is no cure, early treatment often can help prevent crippling deformities. Aspirin is a mainstay of treatment because of its antiinflammatory as well as fever-reducing and pain-relieving activity. When aspirin is inadequate, gold salts or other agents such as prednisone, a cortisonelike drug, may be used. Exercise is important to prevent joint stiffening, and local heat helps relieve muscle spasm and pain. Surgery may be used to remove overgrown tissue in a joint, to loosen any tendons or ligaments that may be distorting a joint, or to replace a severely diseased joint with a prosthesis or artificial joint.

*Juvenile rheumatoid arthritis* is similar in most respects to adult RA. Often, fever may precede joint paint. Spleen and lymph node enlargement may occur. Treatment is similar to that for adult RA, and the outlook for juvenile RA is more favorable, with as many as 80 percent of children experiencing complete remissions.

## ASBESTOSIS

A lung disease resulting from prolonged inhalation of asbestos dust, which mechanically irritates lung tissue, asbestosis produces labored breathing, dry cough, blueness on exercise. Once exposure is stopped, there is little or no further progression of the disease. Long-continued exposure may increase risk of lung cancer. When necessary in severe cases, bronchodilating medication may be used to help breathing. Good nutrition and a program of graded exercise are valuable.

## ASTHMA

A chronic disease, asthma involves obstruction of air flow in the smaller air passages. It usually occurs in people with an inherited allergic constitution. In half or more, allergy to molds, pollens, animal danders, lint, insecticides, or foods or drugs may be present. In other cases, there is often sensitivity to the bacteria causing respiratory infections. In still others, however, nervous tension appears to be largely responsible, and the asthma may improve when emotional difficulties are overcome. Episodes of the disease occur periodically rather than constantly, with attacks varying greatly in frequency, duration, and intensity. Typically, an attack is characterized by breathing difficulty and wheezing, with the patient often sitting upright and leaning forward in order to use all the breathing muscles. Blueness is rare, occurring only in extremely severe attacks. Treatment may begin with efforts to detect the cause or causes of allergy so they may be avoided if possible. Drugs for relief of symptoms include bronchodilators such as epinephrine and aminophylline which enlarge air passages. Other drugs that thin secretions and help in coughing up obstructing mucus may be prescribed. Acute flare-ups of infective asthma are treated with antibiotics.

## ATELECTASIS

Atelectasis is a shrunken, airless state of all or part of a lung, often with infection. It may develop slowly, producing increasing breathing difficulty and weakness. With rapid development, especially with infection, it may cause sudden breathing difficulty, blueness, fever, drop in blood pressure, chest pain on the affected lung side. The major factor producing atelectasis is airway obstruction. In atelectasis of the newborn, the lungs fail to expand normally at birth because of excessive or excessively sticky lung secretions, with other factors such as prematurity and diminished nerve stimulation for breathing and crying sometimes entering in. Treatment of newborn atelectasis includes suctioning the windpipe to establish an open airway, administration of oxygen, and measures to stimulate breathing and crying. In other types of atelectasis, which may be acute or chronic, airway obstruction may be caused by sticky secretions, foreign bodies, tumors or lymph nodes that press on the air passages. Atelectatic lung collapse sometimes is a postoperative complication contributed to by accumulated secretions and inadequate coughing. Acute atelectasis is treated by eliminating the cause whenever possible, stimulating coughing (sometimes with a cough-inducing machine), suctioning, use of detergent aerosols, and antibiotics to combat infection. Chronic atelectasis often can be treated successfully by surgical removal of the affected segment or lobe of the lung.

## ATOPIC DERMATITIS (see DERMATITIS, ATOPIC)

## ATRIAL FLUTTER OR FIBRILLATION

Producing pallor, palpitation, nausea, weakness, and fainting, atrial flutter and atrial fibrillation are abnormally rapid rhythms of the atria, the two upper, blood-receiving chambers of the heart. With flutter, atrial contractions may range between 200 and 400 times a minute; with fibrillation, the range is even higher, 400 to 600, sometimes going to 1,000 a minute. The abnormal rhythms may occur in coronary heart disease, heart attack, rheumatic heart disease, hyperthyroidism, cancer invasion of the atria, and following operations within the chest. In some cases, they may occur without known cause. Digitalis, a long-used heart drug, often can turn flutter into normal rhythm. Quinidine may also do this. Quinidine or procainamide also can be used for atrial fibrillation. Once return to normal rhythm is achieved, drug treatment may be continued for several weeks.

## ATRIAL SEPTAL DEFECT

A congenital abnormality, an atrial septal defect is an abnormal opening in the septum, or wall, separating the two atria, or upper chambers of the heart. Symptoms may include easy fatigability, shortness of breath, reduced resistance to respiratory infections, some degree of growth failure. The septal defect allows blood returning fresh from the lungs to the left atrium, ready to be pumped out to the body, to move instead into the right atrium for needless return again to the lungs. Diagnosis can be made on the basis of a distinctive heart murmur, x-ray study of the heart, and changes in the electrocardiogram. The defect can be repaired by surgery carried out with the aid of the heart-lung machine.

## ATRIOVENTRICULAR BLOCK

This is a disturbance in the electrical conduction system of the heart which may lead to one or more dropped heartbeats or in some cases independent beating of the upper and lower heart chambers. Depending upon the degree of block, symptoms vary. In most cases, the symptoms are palpitation and a sensation of "shock in the chest" or "something turning over in the chest." In other cases, there may be faintness and dizziness. In a more severe type of block, called *Adams-Stokes syndrome,* there may be episodes of giddiness, loss of consciousness, and convulsions. The causes of atrioventricular (AV) block include coronary heart disease, rheumatic heart disease, heart attack, diphtheria, syphilis, sometimes drugs such as digitalis, quinidine, procainamide, rauwolfia, and propranolol. When the block is due to heart attack, acute rheumatic heart disease or diphtheria, it often becomes less severe or may even disappear once the acute episode of underlying illness is over. In other cases, drug treatment (phenobarbital, ephedrine, or others) may be helpful. In some cases, installation of an electrical pacemaker may be required.

## BACILLARY DYSENTERY

Also known as *shigellosis,* this is an acute bowel infection caused by *Shigella* bacteria spread through fecal contamination of food or drink by carriers of the disease. After a one- to four-day incubation period, the infection manifests itself. In children, it often begins suddenly with fever, drowsiness or irritability, abdominal pain, and painful straining at stool. Within 72 hours, blood, pus, and mucus appear in the stools, which increase to 20 or more a day. Dehydration and severe weight loss may occur. In most cases in adults, fever does not occur, diarrhea is nonbloody and free of mucus, and there is little or no straining at stool. In some adults, however, the disease begins with griping abdominal pain and urgency to defecate, with pain relief following passage of a formed stool. But such episodes occur more and more often, with diarrhea becoming severe and stools containing mucus, pus, and often blood. Bacillary dysentery is usually over after a few weeks, although an attack in a child may be more serious and last longer. Of major importance in treatment is replacement of fluids, sometimes by intravenous administration. Antibiotics may be used.

## BACK PAIN, LOW (see also SCIATICA)

*Acute* low back pain may be produced by a fall, blow, heavy lifting, snow shoveling, or there may appear to be no cause. Pain is usually severe, with difficulty in walking and standing. Commonly, acute attacks improve after several days of rest in bed on a firm mattress, preferably with a bed board under it. Aspirin or a stronger pain reliever may be used when necessary. Muscle spasm, a major factor in the pain, will be helped by warm, moist packs changed frequently to maintain warmth.

*Chronic* low back pain may result from protracted poor posture, obesity, sedentary living which allows deterioration of abdominal muscles that adds to the burden on back muscles. Treatment may require weight reduction, exercises, efforts to improve posture, sometimes a corset. If a difference in length of the legs is involved, an extra heel or a shoe lift may be helpful. In some cases, spinal tuberculosis or other infection may be involved and require appropriate treatment. Spinal osteoarthritis may be a factor and may be treated with rest on a firm bed, local heat, massage with chloroform liniment, aspirin and, if necessary, other medication.

Spinal disk degeneration, of course, can be a factor in backache. In the acute phase, treatment is the same as for other acute back pain (above). Later, conservative medical management, including a program of exercises, may be effective in preventing recurrences. If not, disk surgery may be performed.

## BACTERIAL ENDOCARDITIS (see ENDOCARDITIS, BACTERIAL)

## BAGASSOSIS (see FARMER'S LUNG AND BAGASSOSIS)

## BALANOPOSTHITIS

An inflammation of the foreskin and the glans penis (the cone-shaped body at the end of the penis), balanoposthitis results from a bacterial infection beneath the foreskin and, unless it can be controlled, may lead to interference with urinary flow.

## BANTI'S DISEASE

Occurring along with cirrhosis of the liver, Banti's disease may cause fatigue, spleen enlargement, progressively more severe anemia, vomiting of blood, blood in stools. The disorder may be the result of cirrhosis or of clotting in or narrowing of splenic or other veins. Spleen removal may partially or completely correct the anemia. The cirrhosis of the liver requires separate treatment.

## BED-WETTING

The inability to control urination, especially at night during sleep, also called *enuresis*, occurs often in children who are sound sleepers or have small bladder capacity. If it persists beyond the age of 5 or 6 years, it may be an indication of physical or emotional disorder.

Physical causes include obstructions, strictures, and infections, which can be treated with suitable medical or surgical measures. When physical causes are absent, bladder training may be used. In children with small capacity, the capacity may be increased by deliberate restriction of urination during the day. For sound sleepers, a drug such as ephedrine or dextroamphetamine may be prescribed. Recently reported useful is an antidepressant drug, imipramine.

## BELL'S PALSY

Bell's palsy is a *neuritis*, an inflammation of a nerve, in this case a facial nerve that controls expression. The inflammation results in paralysis of muscles on one side of the face, leading to inability to close the mouth and sometimes to close the eye on the affected side, producing a distortion of the face. Although often of unknown cause, Bell's palsy may involve injury to or pressure on a nerve. Often the palsy is temporary and may last a few days or weeks. When a cause such as injury can be established, its treatment may speed relief.

## BENIGN INTRADUCTAL PAPILLOMA (see PAPILLOMA, BENIGN INTRADUCTAL)

## BERYLLIOSIS

A disease affecting the lungs and other tissues, berylliosis is associated with inhalation of fumes or dust containing beryllium compounds and occurs mainly in jobs involving extraction of beryllium from its ore and in manufacture of corrosion-resistant alloys. It may take as long as five years of exposure before berylliosis in chronic form develops and leads to labored breathing, with blueness and cough. Promising results have been obtained with a corticosteroid drug such as prednisone, especially in cases treated relatively early, with disappearance of symptoms and improvement maintained for many years.

## BILIARY CIRRHOSIS (see CIRRHOSIS, BILIARY)

## BLADDER CANCER (see CANCER OF THE URINARY BLADDER)

## BLADDER, NEUROGENIC

Involving loss of normal nerve control of bladder function, neurogenic bladder may manifest itself as urinary retention or urinary incontinence. As a result of incomplete bladder emptying, urinary infection may occur. Urinary stones also may develop. The condition of neurogenic bladder may result from congenital abnormality, spinal cord injury, or disease such as syphilis, diabetes, or multiple sclerosis. Catheter or other drainage may be required, sometimes continuously. In some cases, one of several different types of surgery may be done for urinary diversion.

## BLASTOMYCOSIS

An infectious disease caused by a fungus, *Blastomyces dermatitidis*, blastomycosis occurs mainly in the southeastern United States and Mississippi Valley, most frequently in adults in the 20-to-40-year age group, at least six times more often among men than women. One type, which affects the lungs, produces dry hacking cough, chest pain, fever, chills, drenching sweats, and breathing difficulty. A systemic form, spread through the bloodstream, may affect skin, prostate, bone, mouth, and nose. On the skin, papules or small firm elevations appear and spread slowly. Pus-laden abscesses develop. In bone, swelling, heat, and tenderness occur. In the prostate and the genital tract, the disease produces painful swellings. Diagnosis is made by recovery of the causative fungus. A drug, hydroxystilbamidine, administered by injection, often is effective against blastomycosis, with relief of symptoms beginning after about two weeks of treatment. Amphotericin B, another drug, also can be used and often is effective when hydroxystilbamidine fails.

## BLEPHARITIS

An inflammation of the eyelid margins that may result from infection or allergy, blepharitis causes itching, burning and redness of the lid margins, swelling of the lids, loss of eyelashes, irritation of the conjunctiva, excess tearing of the eyes, and sensitivity to light. Treatment is with antibiotic ointments or solutions or with combinations of antibiotics and corticosteroids.

## BODY ODOR (see HYPERHIDROSIS)

**BOIL** (see FURUNCLE)

**BONE CANCER** (see CANCER OF BONE)

## BOTULISM

An acute intoxication affecting nerves and muscles, botulism results from eating food contaminated by a toxin produced by the organism *Clostridium botulinum*. Almost always, the disease comes from improperly preserved food, usually home-canned. A grave disease, with mortality as high as 65 percent, botulism develops abruptly, with symptoms that may include double vision, loss of visual acuity, drooping of upper eyelids, loss of visual accommodation, followed by difficulty in swallowing and speaking, muscle weakness. Fever usually is not present unless another infection is superimposed. In only about one third of cases do vomiting and diarrhea occur. Hospitalization is required. Treatment may include use of antiserum, intravenous feeding, sedation, administration of oxygen, and use of a respirator. Recovery occurs slowly, with eye muscle weakness often persisting for months, but in those who recover there are no permanent aftereffects.

## BOWEL ARTERY ATHEROSCLEROSIS

Atherosclerosis, a disease process in which deposits form on the inner walls of arteries and interfere with blood circulation, most often affects the coronary arteries feeding the heart and other arteries feeding the brain and limbs. But it may sometimes affect other vessels, including arteries supplying the gastrointestinal tract. In the latter case, there may be abdominal pain, diarrhea, and weight loss. Atherosclerosis and its further development are believed to be associated with such factors as cigarette smoking, lack of exercise, high blood pressure, obesity, and diet that tends to raise blood fat levels. For treatment as well as prevention, cessation of smoking, correction of high blood pressure and diet, and a program of graduated exercises may be used.

## BRAIN CANCER (see CANCER OF THE BRAIN)

**BROMHIDROSIS** (see HYPERHIDROSIS)

## BRONCHI, FOREIGN BODY IN

When a foreign body—a particle of food, loose dental filling, nail, or other object—is inhaled, it may, depending upon its size, cause asphyxiation or choking, gagging, and blueness. There is risk, too, that if it remains lodged in an airway, it may cause infection and, sometimes, lung abscess or bronchiectasis. Although sometimes expelled by coughing, more often it is not and constitutes an emergency, calling for its location and removal by means of a long, metal, tubelike instrument, the bronchoscope.

## BRONCHIECTASIS

Bronchiectasis is a chronic dilation of air passages (bronchi or bronchioles) which can be congenital but is more likely to be secondary to other conditions such as chronic sinusitis, allergy, whooping cough, emphysema, pneumonia, silicosis, tuberculosis, lung abscess or tumor. Its seriousness derives from the general lowering of resistance it produces and the bouts of pneumonia and bronchitis to which it may make the victim prone. Commonly, it begins with a dry or slightly productive cough that gradually becomes more productive. Typical of the disease, coughing follows a regular pattern, occurring in the morning, late in the afternoon, and on retiring, often with relative freedom from coughing in between. Coughing of blood is frequent. In severe cases, there is breathing difficulty on exertion. Repeated attacks of respiratory infection are common. Treatment may include special attention to good diet and adequate rest, elimination of cigarette smoking, use of an expectorant cough medication, postural drainage, and antibiotics to combat infections. If the dilation is well localized, surgery may be performed to remove the diseased area.

## BRONCHITIS, ACUTE

An acute inflammation of the air passages, acute bronchitis may follow a cold or other upper respiratory infection and occurs most frequently in winter. Symptoms include sore throat, nasal discharge, malaise, chilliness, slight fever, back and muscle pain, followed by a cough that is dry at first but after a day or two begins to produce increasing amounts of sputum. Treatment may include rest, fluids, a fever-reducing analgesic such as aspirin, steam inhalation, a cough mixture if the cough is very troublesome and, if high fever occurs and persists, an antibiotic. Usually, there is complete recovery.

## BRONCHITIS, CHRONIC

Major causes of chronic bronchitis, which involves chronic inflammation of the airways, are believed to be cigarette smoking and air pollution. The condition in mild form may be present for years with slight cough that is intensified with upper respiratory infections. As the disease progresses, degenerative changes disturb the normal action of the cilia, the tiny hairlike processes in the airways, which normally wave up bacteria and foreign matter for elimination. At the same time, inflammation leads to increased sputum production and there is a tendency, with cilia action inadequate, for matter to be retained except when it can be coughed up. With disease progression, other symptoms appear: breathing difficulty, wheezing, blueness, sometimes paroxysms of coughing that may be incapacitating. Treatment includes strict attention to general good health and nutrition, avoidance of exposure to irritants and to sources of acute respiratory infections, prompt treatment of any acute infections that may develop, elimination of smoking, use of expectorants, steam and other inhalations to raise sputum and help clear air passages, use of aerosols that dilate the airways when there is increasing breathlessness on exertion. Postural drainage may be prescribed and mild regular exercise encouraged.

## BRUCELLOSIS

Also known as *undulant fever* or *Malta, Mediterranean,* and *Gibraltar fever,* brucellosis is an infectious disease transmitted to humans from domestic animals such as pigs, goats, and cattle, especially through infected milk or contact with an infected carcass. The disease is most frequent in rural areas and among farmers, livestock producers, veterinarians, and others who work with animals. The incubation period ranges from five days to several months. The disease may begin suddenly and acutely, with chills, fever, severe headache, malaise, and occasionally diarrhea. But it can also begin insidiously with mild malaise, muscular pain, headache, pain in the back, and a rise in evening temperature. As the disease progresses, temperature may reach 104° or 105° in the evening and come down to normal or near normal in the morning when profuse sweating occurs. The intermittent fever may last one to five weeks, and all symptoms may disappear, only for the fever and other symptoms to return after a few days to a few weeks, often in repeated episodes over a period of months or years. When the disease becomes chronic, other symptoms often develop: appetite and weight loss, abdominal and joint pain, headache, backache, weakness, irritability, mental depression, emotional instability, insomnia. Most patients respond well to treatment with a tetracycline antibiotic or, in more serious cases, to a combination of tetracycline and streptomycin.

## BUERGER'S DISEASE

Also known as *thromboangiitis obliterans*, Buerger's disease is an inflammatory condition that affects veins and arteries, particularly those in the legs, roughening the inner walls and sometimes leading to clot formation. When severe, the disease can obliterate or destroy vessels, causing gangrene. It occurs almost entirely in men between the ages of 20 and 45 and the cause is still in question, although excessive use of tobacco over an extended period is believed to be involved. Coldness of an involved leg is typical. There may also be numbness, tingling, burning. Pain on walking may occur. To treat the disease, a first essential step is elimination of tobacco in any form. Other measures include avoidance of exposure to extremes of temperature and injury from ill-fitting shoes. Special exercises are prescribed to stimulate circulation.

## BUNION

Also called *hallux valgus*, a bunion is a swelling of the bursa of the first joint below the base of the great toe, producing pain. Commonly, it results from the pressure of tight shoes. In mild cases, heat may relieve pain and the condition may clear by itself after properly fitting shoes are worn for some time. In more severe cases, special corrective "bunion last" shoes may be prescribed or a simple surgical procedure, bunionectomy, may be done to correct the condition.

## BURSITIS

A bursa is a small, fluid-filled sac that allows one part of a joint to move easily over another part or over other structures. Bursae are found throughout the body but the most important are those in the shoulder, elbow, knee, and hip. In bursitis, a bursa becomes inflamed, as the result of injury, infection, excessive use, or chilling. Acute bursitis appears suddenly; severe pain and limitation of movement of the affected joint are the principal symptoms. Resting the joint in a sling or splint until pain diminishes enough to permit motion, with applications of moist heat and use of aspirin or another analgesic, may be sufficient treatment. If necessary, other measures may be used. Injection into the affected bursa of either procaine or a corticosteroid such as hydrocortisone, or use of phenylbutazone, an antiinflammatory drug, by mouth, often is effective.

*Chronic* bursitis may follow an acute attack, especially if there is infection or repeated injury. There may be pain, swelling, tenderness, muscle weakness, and limitation of motion. X-ray examination often will show deposit of calcium salts. Hot packs or baths, or diathermy, and massage may provide temporary relief. An often-effective measure is injection of hydrocortisone or prednisolone with procaine into the affected bursa while the calcium deposits are needled to break them up.

*Tennis elbow,* also known as *epicondylitis* and *radiohumeral bursitis,* may occur not only after tennis playing but also after an activity such as screwdriving. Its exact nature is still not clear. Pain may radiate from the elbow to the outer side of the arm and forearm. In mild cases, avoidance of movements causing pain may produce gradual improvement. In other cases, one or more injections of hydrocortisone or prednisolone may bring relief. Uncommonly, if medical measures fail, surgery may be done and may consist of manipulation under local anesthesia or, rarely, removal of an inflamed bursa.

## CANCER

A *neoplasm* is a mass of new, abnormal tissue, a new growth or tumor. Not all tumors are malignant or cancerous. The nonmalignant are called *benign* tumors. They vary in size and may be no bigger than, for example, a wart, which is a benign tumor. On the other hand, they may grow so big that they obstruct organs or cause ulceration and bleeding. But benign tumors are encapsulated; they do not metastasize (or spread) to other areas; and usually they can be surgically removed without difficulty.

*Malignant* tumors, or cancers, grow in disorganized fashion, interrupt body functions and may spread to other areas of the body.

Cancer is not one disease but many. Cancers are classified into two large groups: *sarcomas* which affect such tissues as bones and muscles; and *carcinomas* which include most gland cancers and cancers of breast, stomach, uterus, skin, and tongue.

Some changes in body tissues are known as *precancerous* because they have a tendency to become malignant. They include thickened white patches (leukoplakia) in the mouth and on the vulva, some moles, chronically irritated areas in the mouth or on the tongue or the skin, and some polyps.

HODGKIN'S DISEASE, which affects lymph nodes, is considered a cancer. So are the LEUKEMIAS.

*Seven early warning signs* of cancer should be remembered:

1. A lump or thickening anywhere, especially in the breast or on the lip or tongue.
2. Any sore that does not heal, especially around the mouth, lips or tongue or on the skin.
3. Persistent loss of appetite or indigestion.
4. A change in color or size of a wart, mole, or birthmark.
5. Persistent change in bowel or bladder habits (either more or less frequent).
6. Persistent hoarseness, cough, or swallowing difficulty.
7. Any unexplained bleeding—blood in urine or stools, blood or bloody discharge from nipple or any body opening, unexplained vaginal bleeding or discharge, or any postmenopausal bleeding.

These signs do not always, by any means, indicate malignancy but do call for medical examination.

Pain may occur in some malignancies but it is not commonly one of the earliest warnings.

Various particular symptoms depend upon the site and type of cancer.

## CANCER OF BONE

Persistent pain followed later by swelling occurs in bone cancers. Malignant tumors can spread to bone from other sites—most commonly from breast, lung, prostate, kidney, and thyroid—and any bone pain in a person who has had cancer should call for x-ray or biopsy of the bone, or both. Malignant tumors also may arise originally in bone and do so most often in young people. The most frequent sites are in the knee, thigh, upper arm, pelvis, and ribs. Surgery often must be performed to excise the cancerous bone, and in some cases this may involve amputation. In some cases, radiation and drug treatment may be used.

## CANCER OF THE BRAIN

Although possible at any age, brain tumors most commonly occur in early adult and middle life. Symptoms are produced by pressure of a growth and depend upon where in the brain the pressure is exerted. Any or many of the following may be present: headache, nausea and vomiting, convulsive seizures, drowsiness, lethargy, personality changes, impaired mental processes, muscle weakness, failing vision, loss of balance and coordination, psychotic episodes, impairment of skin sensation, tremors, paralysis, ringing in an ear, hearing impairment in one ear. Diagnosis requires thorough neurologic study, with vision and hearing tests, skull x-rays, electroencephalograms, and other tests. Treatment is surgery, radiation, or both, sometimes with drug therapy.

## CANCER OF THE BREAST

The most common malignancy among women, breast cancer is rare before the age of 30, and its incidence climbs high after menopause, so that, for safety, any breast mass occurring postmenopausally has to be considered malignant until proved otherwise. The cancer is not inherited, although there is some tendency for it to run in families. In most cases, breast cancer manifests itself as a slowly growing painless mass. Other indications may include elevated or retracted nipple, some distortion of breast contour, dimpling of breast skin over the growth, and pitting of the breast skin that may give it an orange-skin appearance. In advanced disease, underarm and other glands (lymph nodes) enlarge. Diagnosis requires microscopic examination of tissue removed by biopsy. Treatment is usually surgical. Depending upon the extent of the cancer, simple mastectomy or radical mastectomy (with removal of breast and other tissue including underlying muscles) may be performed. Radiation treatment is often employed after surgery. Radiation may be used alone to slow advance of the disease when it has spread. Hormone treatment also is useful in delaying advance of the disease. Drug therapy, which has been used for palliation in advanced disease, shows promise when used with less radical surgery in early disease. Especially in early cancer, outlook is good, with five-year cures ranging up to 80 percent.

## CANCER OF THE CERVIX

The cervix, or neck of the uterus, is a relatively common site for a slow-growing malignancy in women. Vaginal discharge, often slight, either watery or containing blood, is commonly an early symptom, frequently occurring after coitus. Vaginal bleeding or spotting and irregular menstruation may be present. As the disease progresses, other symptoms—constipation, vomiting, lower back pain, weight loss, urinary disturbances—may develop. Diagnosed and treated early, cervical cancer has a high cure rate. Surgery is done and in early cases often may be limited, especially in younger women of child-bearing age; in others, hysterectomy (or removal of the uterus) may be indicated; in some cases, surgery may have to be more extensive. Radiation also may be used.

## CANCER OF THE COLON

The colon, or large intestine, is a common site for malignancy. A tumor may manifest itself by blood in the stool, by a change in bowel habits from few movements to many or from many to few, by cramps, and in some cases by anemia, weakness, and weight loss. A large proportion of colonic tumors can be seen with a sigmoidoscope, an instrument which is inserted through the rectum for a distance of ten or more inches. A new aid to diagnosis is the colonoscope, a slender, flexible instrument which, when inserted through the rectum, permits examination of the whole length of the colon. Also helpful in diagnosis: x-ray films taken after a barium enema. Surgery is the only definitive treatment for colon cancer. The growth and the section of colon containing it, plus a segment on each side, must be removed. Depending upon the extent of the growth and the site in the colon, it may be possible sometimes for the two remaining ends of the colon to be joined together. In other cases, the end of the remaining healthy colon may have to be brought up to an opening in the abdomen (a colostomy). Most colonic cancers are curable when found in early stages and some are curable at later stages.

## CANCER OF THE ESOPHAGUS

About 1 percent of all cancers occur in the esophagus, most often in men after the age of 50. Because malignant tumors of the esophagus tend to start in the lining membrane, an early symptom may be the sensation of food, particularly meat and soft bread, sticking somewhere behind the breastbone. Boring pain may occur with swallowing or may be persistent. A cancer of the esophagus usually shows up on x-ray films. It can also be viewed directly through a tubelike instrument, and a piece of it can be removed for microscopic examination (biopsy). Surgery is required. Improved surgical techniques have made it possible to remove the entire cancerous area in more and more cases. Sometimes, enough healthy esophagus remains so it can be connected to the stomach. For this, the diaphragm may be cut through and the stomach brought into the chest. In other cases, a portion of intestine may be taken and used to replace the diseased chest part of the esophagus. In some cases, a plastic tube may be used as a replacement.

## CANCER OF THE KIDNEY

Kidney malignancy accounts for 1 to 2 percent of adult cancers and occurs in children (Wilms' tumor). In adults, about two thirds of cases are in men.

In adults, the symptom most commonly noticed first is blood in the urine. Pain in the flank (the side of the body between ribs and hip), an abdominal mass, and fever are other symptoms. X-ray studies, including *pyelography*, in which the x-ray is taken after injection into a vein of a contrast medium, are important in diagnosis. Surgery to remove the affected kidney, often coupled with radiation and chemotherapy, offers the only cure. The five-year cure rate, overall, is about 45 percent and increasing, and is greater with early detection and treatment.

**Wilms' tumor.** This cancer, which begins in the fetus, lies dormant for a time even after birth. It usually manifests itself before the fifth year. Commonly, the first indication is an abdominal mass discovered by a parent or a physician. Pain, fever, appetite loss, nausea, vomiting, and blood in the urine follow. A major aid to diagnosis is pyelography (see preceding paragraph) revealing a mass within a kidney. Prompt surgery is needed and may be combined with drug and radiation therapy. Five-year cure rates of well over 50 percent, and increasing, are being reported.

## CANCER OF THE LARYNX

Usually originating on the front of a vocal cord, cancer of the larynx causes persistent, painless hoarseness—and that symptom, especially in anyone over the age of 40, calls for expert diagnosis. In some cases, difficulty in swallowing and breathing and, occasionally, cough may occur. Most patients with early laryngeal cancer can be cured by x-ray and other conservative treatment. More advanced malignancy may require surgical removal of the larynx.

## CANCER OF THE LIP

Most common in older people and more common in men than in women, lip cancer often begins as a blister or sore, usually on the lower lip, that fails to heal and tends to bleed easily. Radiation or surgery or a combination of both may be used, with total cure likely.

## CANCER OF THE LIVER

Primary cancer of the liver, a malignancy originating in the liver itself, is relatively uncommon in the United States although prevalent in Africa and the Orient, and in this country half or more of cases that do occur are associated with cirrhosis of the liver. The liver, however, is a site to which cancer originating elsewhere—in the gastrointestinal tract, pancreas, gallbladder, lung, or breast—may spread. The liver often becomes tender when affected by malignancy and enlarges rapidly; it may occupy much of the right side of the abdomen. Other symptoms may include fluid accumulation in the abdomen, backache, fever, jaundice. Diagnosis is by needle biopsy—insertion of a hollow needle through the body wall into the liver to obtain tissue for microscopic examination. For primary cancer of the liver detected at early stages, surgical removal of the tumor is sometimes effective. In other cases of primary cancer and of cancer spread to the liver from elsewhere, palliative treatment with drugs is used.

## CANCER OF THE LUNG

The most common cancer in men, lung cancer has been increasing steadily in women as well. Most cases occur after the age of 40. There are several types of lung cancer which spread by different routes. Depending upon the site of the cancer, early symptoms vary. Often, a new cough or a change in the character or severity of a chronic cough is an early symptom. Wheezing or other noises in the chest may develop. Coughing up of blood or bloody sputum may occur. There may also be chest ache or pain and shortness of breath not caused by obvious exertion. In advanced disease, symptoms may include weight loss, loss of appetite, weakness, hoarseness. In some cases, there may be clubbing of fingers and toes, joint pains, and other symptoms that may resemble those of CUSHING'S SYNDROME, POLYCYTHEMIA VERA, or MYASTHENIA GRAVIS. Diagnosis makes use of careful physical examination and chest x-ray. If a suspicious density appears on the x-ray film, sputum samples are examined microscopically for presence of malignant cells. Bronchoscopy—inspection of the breathing passages with an instrument through which a specimen of tissue also may be obtained for miscroscopic study—may be used.

Prompt treatment is essential. When surgical treatment is possible because the cancer is still confined to the lung area, a whole lung or a lobe of a lung may be removed. Radiation therapy may be used before or after surgery or when surgery is not possible. Drug treatment also can be employed for temporary improvement, and there is some hope that new drugs, new combinations of drugs, and new methods of administering drugs may before long offer more than palliation.

## CANCER OF THE MOUTH

Although possible at any age, malignancy in the mouth—on the gum, palate, tongue, cheek, floor of mouth, or other site—primarily affects older people, men more often than women. Smoking and high alcohol intake are suspected factors. Although there can be other, nonmalignant causes, including LEUKOPLAKIA and even vitamin deficiency, any sore that does not heal in two weeks or any white patch taking the place of the normal pink color of the tongue or inside of the mouth should, for safety, be considered cancerous until proved otherwise. Diagnosis requires biopsy—microscopic examination of a small sample of tissue. With early treatment by radiation or surgery, the cure rate is high.

## CANCER OF THE OVARY

This cancer has its peak incidence in women in their 50s. It is difficult to detect in the very earliest stages, since it develops silently until it reaches a size to produce symptoms. Earliest symptoms are vague lower abdominal discomfort and mild digestive disturbances. Abnormal vaginal bleeding is not common. Such symptoms as abdominal swelling, pelvic pain, anemia, and emaciation appear late in the course of the disease. Treatment depends upon the size of the tumor and whether it has extended beyond the ovary and may involve removal of the ovary and radiotherapy of the area, or more extensive surgery to remove uterus and tubes as well. Drug treatment also is employed. The overall five-year survival rate ranges up to 60 percent or more for some types of ovarian cancer, less for others.

## CANCER OF THE PANCREAS

When malignancy affects the pancreas, a prime symptom is abdominal pain that often radiates to the back and may be relieved by sitting up or bending forward. Jaundice is common, as are weight and appetite loss, nausea, vomiting (sometimes with blood in the vomitus), and constipation or diarrhea (with stools sometimes darkened by blood pigments). Various laboratory procedures, including blood and urine tests, tests for blood in the stool, and x-rays may suggest cancer. When cancer is confined to the tail of the pancreas, cure sometimes may be achieved by removal of the affected area. More commonly, however, the malignancy affects the head of the pancreas. There, it may press upon the bile duct, producing jaundice. When the cancer has advanced to the point where it cannot be removed entirely, a short-circuit operation—connecting gallbladder to small intestine or stomach so bile can bypass the obstructed bile duct, relieving the jaundice and severe itching that may accompany it—may be performed. If the cancer has affected most of the pancreas but has not spread elsewhere, and if the condition of the patient permits, an extensive surgical procedure may be carried out. All of the affected portion of the gland, and sometimes the whole of it, is removed, along with all of the duodenum to which the cancerous pancreas has become adherent. The stomach is attached to the small intestine in the area beyond the duodenum, and the common bile duct is attached to the small intestine.

## CANCER OF THE PROSTATE

Prostate cancer is the number-one malignancy in men over 65 but may occur at younger ages. It is a slowly progressive disease. Its urinary symptoms—increasing difficulty and frequency of urination, with diminished stream, sometimes with blood in the urine—are similar to those of benign PROSTATE ENLARGEMENT or hypertrophy. When the cancer seeds or spreads to the pelvis and lower spine, it may cause bone pain. Diagnosis is made by digital rectal examination, by needle biopsy to obtain a tissue specimen for microscopic study, and by blood and bone marrow tests. In localized prostate cancer, surgical removal is the treatment and ten-year cure rates of almost 65 percent are obtained. In other cases, hormone treatment or removal of the testes may extend life for many years. Radiation often provides dramatic relief of pain when the cancer has spread to bone.

## CANCER OF THE SKIN

The most common malignancy—and the most readily curable—skin cancer has to be suspected when any sore or ulcer fails to heal promptly or when there is any sudden change in the color, size, and texture of a mole. By far, the two most common forms of skin cancer are basal cell carcinoma and squamous cell carcinoma, with basal cell alone accounting for three of every four skin cancers.

Basal cell carcinoma does not metastasize or spread to other sites in the body although it may invade underlying tissue. Most common after the age of 40, it usually occurs on exposed skin sites, beginning as a small papule or solid elevation which slowly enlarges and after some months shows a central ulcer. Treatment by a specialist may involve electrocoagulation or surgical removal, with radiation sometimes used.

Squamous cell carcinoma, which tends to spread, appears as a small reddish papule or patch. After a period of months or years, it starts to grow and form a crusted ulcer with hard edges, and may then spread rapidly to mouth, nose, or vulva as well as on the skin. Treatment, by a specialist, is by surgical excision or radiation.

Malignant melanoma. This is the most dangerous skin malignancy, although fortunately it is rare. Most malignant melanomas develop from pigmented moles, especially those on the lower legs and on mucous membranes. There is some evidence that moles exposed to repeated irritation or injury may be more likely than others to become malignant. The development of malignancy in a mole is indicated by sudden increased growth and darkening, ulceration and bleeding. *Immediate* medical attention is essential, followed by surgery to remove the mole and surrounding area. When melanoma has spread, new drug therapy techniques may be used and may be helpful.

## CANCER OF THE SMALL INTESTINE

For unknown reasons, cancer, although common in the large intestine, is rare in the small. Symptoms may include intermittent, crampy, midabdominal pain, stools darkened by blood pigments, and anemia. Diagnosis is aided by small intestine x-ray study. Surgery is the only definitive treatment.

## CANCER OF THE STOMACH

Declining in incidence in the United States in recent years, stomach cancer is largely concentrated at ages over 60 and affects men twice as often as women. Symptoms include upper abdominal discomfort, which sometimes but not always is worse after eating; pain, sometimes irregular, over the pit of the stomach; appetite loss; weight loss; vomiting; anemia. The symptoms may occur singly or in various combinations. Diagnosis is aided by x-ray films of the stomach. Another important aid is gastroscopy in which, under local anesthesia, a lighted tube is passed via the mouth into the stomach for examination of a growth and removal of a small piece for microscopic examination (biopsy). Immediate surgery is essential when stomach cancer is diagnosed. Overall, the five-year survival rate after stomach cancer surgery has been 11 percent for men, 14 percent for women. However, when surgery is done early, with the cancer still confined to the stomach, the rate has been 37 percent for men and 43 percent for women. There is increasing hope that with earlier recognition and treatment survival rates may be improved.

## CANCER OF THE TESTIS

This cancer accounts for a significant number of malignancies in men under 30. The cause is unknown. The usual symptom is a scrotal mass that increases in size, with or without pain. The mass, which may be soft or hard, can be felt in the scrotum. Treatment is surgical removal of the testis. Radiation may be used and drug therapy often may be valuable when spread of the cancer has occurred. Depending upon the type of malignancy and the extent, five-year survival rates range up to 80 percent.

## CANCER OF THE THYROID

More common in women than in men, thyroid cancer is often slow-growing. The first indication is a mass in the neck, commonly without pain or tenderness. When the mass is soft, mobile, made up of many nodules, it is likely to be a benign tumor. When it is hard, irregular, and fixed, it may be malignant. Various tests are used in diagnosis. In one, doses of radioiodine are administered and followed with a scanner device to determine how the thyroid picks up the material. Usually, "cold nodules" (which collect less radioactivity) are more likely to be malignant. Surgical removal of the gland may be required, followed by regular doses of thyroid hormone for a lifetime.

## CANCER OF THE URINARY BLADDER

Bladder cancer affects men about twice as often as women. Known causes include aniline dyes and, possibly, the products of nicotine tars that are excreted in the urine. The most common first symptoms are urinary frequency, pain and burning, with blood and pus present in the urine. A definitive diagnosis of cancer can be made by examination of the bladder through an instrument, the cystoscope, and removal of a small amount of tissue for microscopic examination. Early, superficial malignancy may be removed surgically. When the cancer has invaded the wall of the bladder, part or all of the bladder may have to be removed. Radiation treatment prior to surgery may slow tumor growth, and some growths may be retarded by repeated instillations into the bladder of a drug such as thio-TEPA.

## CANCER OF THE UTERUS

Uterine cancer may occur at any age but most often affects older women after menopause. Commonly, the disease produces vaginal bleeding and odorous discharge. Subsequently, constipation, lower back or abdominal pain, and urinary irregularities may appear. When the malignancy affects women prior to menopause, it may produce menstrual irregularities, often with several heavy flows followed by none, then return of menstruation. In treatment, the uterus is removed if the malignancy has not spread beyond the uterus. In the latter case, radiation may be used, often with good results.

## CANCER OF THE VAGINA

The peak incidence of vaginal cancer is from age 45 to 65. Patients experience bleeding following intercourse. Ulceration of the tumor may produce bleeding at other times. Watery discharge, urinary frequency and urgency, and painful intercourse may occur when the bladder as well as the vagina is involved, and defecation may be painful when the rectum is involved. A Pap smear test may disclose cancer cells. Depending upon where the cancer is located, treatment may be by surgery, radiotherapy or radium.

## CANDIDIASIS

An infection caused by a fungus, *Candida albicans,* candidiasis often affects the mouth (thrush), producing slightly raised, milk-curd-like patches, usually beginning on the tongue and inside the cheeks. The infection may spread to palate, gums, tonsils, throat, and larynx. The mouth usually appears dry. Thrush usually responds to an anti-fungal drug, nystatin. Candidiasis may also affect the fingernails (inflaming the nailbed and surrounding tissue, producing painful red swellings), the underarm areas, underbreast areas, navel and groin, producing red patches of various sizes and shapes, sometimes rimmed by blisters and small pustules. It may affect the area about the anus, producing itching, and the vaginal area, producing inflammation and discharge. Frequent soaking of the skin in soapy water by housewives and others whose work requires it, excessive sweating, pregnancy, and diabetes are factors tending to favor development of candidiasis. The infection also may follow use of antibiotics for other infections. Treatment is with nystatin or when necessary with another potent antifungal agent, amphotericin B.

## CARBUNCLE (see FURUNCLE)

## CARCINOID SYNDROME

This disorder involves the release of excessive amounts of chemicals such as serotonin, a potent blood vessel constrictor, by tumors that usually arise in the small intestine but may originate elsewhere in the gastrointestinal tract, in an ovary, or in an air passageway. Commonly, the earliest symptom is flushing of the skin triggered by emotion, food, or alcohol. Abdominal discomfort and repeated episodes of diarrhea follow. In some cases, flushing may be accompanied by asthmatic wheezing. Diagnosis is made with the help of a urine test showing excretion of certain materials. Treatment may include surgery and the use of various drugs to control symptoms, including prochlorperazine or chlorpromazine or in some cases prednisone for flushing, cyproheptadine or other agents for diarrhea.

# CARDIAC ARREST

When the heart stops beating—evident from lack of pulse, breathing, or heart sounds—treatment must begin at once. A delay of more than three to five minutes may lead to irreversible brain damage.

The victim's airway must be open. An effective technique to assure this, called the *chin lift,* calls for placing the fingers of one of your hands under the lower jaw at the chin, lifting, bringing the chin forward while supporting the jaw and tilting the head back. Press the other hand on the forehead, tilting the head backward. Use the thumb of the hand under the chin to lightly depress the lower lip. The chin should be lifted gently.

Immediately begin mouth-to-mouth breathing, closing the nostrils with the thumb and forefinger of the hand on the forehead. If someone else is not present to help, stop the mouth-to-mouth breathing after five respirations and start external heart compression at a rate of 80 times a minute. This involves placing both hands, one over the other, at the lower end of the breastbone in the middle of the chest, and exerting brief strong (but never violent) pressure downward with the heel of the underhand. Interrupt the compression every 15 seconds to give two quick mouth-to-mouth resuscitations. If someone is present to help, the mouth-to-mouth resuscitation and heart compression can be carried out simultaneously. Carried out successfully, the compression and resuscitation can maintain a flow of air even if they do not restore normal heart action and breathing. Subsequent treatment can be carried out by a physician and may include oxygen administration, electrical countershock, intravenous infusions, and other measures.

# CARPAL TUNNEL SYNDROME

Caused by compression of a nerve where it passes under a ligament of the wrist, the carpal tunnel syndrome produces pain, numbness, and tingling of the fingers. It occurs most often in middle-aged women. Causes include excessive wrist movement, arthritis, swelling of the wrist. Treatment may be by splinting the wrist for several weeks to immobilize it and give the nerve irritation time to heal. In severe cases, surgical removal of the ligament is helpful.

# CATARACT

An opacification or clouding of the lens of the eye, cataract may result from injuries to the eye or exposure to heat or radiation, but in most cases occurs with aging. Blurring and dimming of vision are commonly the first symptoms. The vision disturbance is gradual, progressive. Commonly, there is need for brighter light for reading; sometimes, there are frequent changes of eyeglasses. Double vision may sometimes occur. These symptoms do not always mean cataract, but any of them calls for examination by an ophthalmologist. Treatment requires surgery to remove the clouded lens, which is compensated for by special eyeglasses or a contact lens. Cataract removal, which can be carried out when needed, without waiting for "ripening" of the cataract as once supposed, is better than 95 percent successful in restoring sight.

## CAT-SCRATCH DISEASE

Although no causative agent has ever been recovered from cats, this disease is believed to result from transmission of a virus or other agent present between the claws of cats and kittens. Symptoms begin with a bump or sore at the site of and within a few days after a minor cat scratch. Within two weeks, glands (lymph nodes) near the site of the scratch swell, and fever, malaise, headache, and appetite loss develop. The disease is usually mild and disappears within two to four weeks. Some reports suggest that an antibiotic, tetracycline, may shorten the course of the disease. In severe cases, surgical incision and drainage of glands (lymph nodes) may be needed.

## CAVERNOUS SINUS THROMBOSIS

Caused by spread of infection to an area of the brain from the eye, face, or elsewhere, this grave disease leads to abnormal protrusion of one eye and eventually of the second, fever, headache, convulsions. Intensive treatment with antibiotics coupled with expert supportive care is required for best chance of cure.

## CELIAC DISEASE

A relatively uncommon disorder of the digestive system which may, it is thought, be associated with hereditary factors, celiac disease involves an intolerance of *gluten*, the protein of wheat and rye. The intolerance leads to abnormal changes in the lining of the small intestine and impaired absorption of nutrients. The disease typically begins in a child after about the age of 6 months, although it may sometimes begin or reappear from age 20 to 50. Symptoms may include flatulence and large, foul-smelling, bulky, frothy and pale-colored stools containing much fat. Other symptoms are abdominal distention, muscle wasting and weakness, vomiting attacks, failure to thrive. Treatment relies on a well-balanced diet, high in calories and proteins and normal in fat, but excluding all cereal grains except rice and corn. The diet, supplemented by iron, calcium, and B and other vitamins as needed to correct any deficiencies, is usually effective in eliminating symptoms. In rare cases where diet is not enough, a corticosteroid drug such as hydrocortisone, prednisone, or prednisolone is often effective.

The adult form of celiac disease is known as *nontropical sprue.*

## CENTRAL ARTERY OBSTRUCTION

A painless blockage of the central retinal artery due to a blood clot or artery spasm, this condition causes sudden blindness. Quick treatment to overcome the obstruction is needed to prevent permanent sight loss. Treatment may include surgical puncture and drainage of the front chamber of the eye as an aid in dislodging a clot, along with inhalation of amyl nitrate and oxygen and administration of nitroglycerin and sodium nitrite.

## CEREBRAL PALSY

A disorder with partial paralysis and lack of muscle coordination, cerebral palsy results from a defect, injury, or disease of nerve tissue in the brain believed to be caused at or near the time of birth by lack of oxygen, premature delivery, head injury, or infection. One or more brain areas may be affected, producing varied muscular disorders. There are three major forms of cerebral palsy: *spastic,* with muscle spasm, exaggerated stretch reflexes, and increased deep tendon reflexes; *athetoid,* with muscle tension and uncontrollable, purposeless movements; and *atactic,* with poor balance and coordination and staggering gait. Visual, hearing, and speech defects also may develop. In severely affected infants, vomiting, irritability, and difficulty in nursing may be present from birth. In milder cases, diagnosis may not be made until the second or third year when a child fails to develop normal motor skills, such as sitting up, crawling, or walking. Treatment necessarily may vary with the individual child. It may include one or many measures such as administration of muscle relaxants, orthopedic surgery, casts, braces, traction, special exercises, and muscle training.

**CEREBROVASCULAR ACCIDENT** (see STROKE)


**CERVICAL CANCER** (see CANCER OF THE CERVIX)


## CERVICAL SYNDROME

Resulting from irritation of nerve roots in the cervical (or neck) area of the spine, the cervical syndrome may produce such symptoms as numbness and tingling of arms or fingers, weakness of arms or hands, stiff neck and pain with movement, stiff shoulder, headache, "knots" in muscles of neck, shoulders or arms, finger swelling and stiffness, vision blurring, loss of balance, pain in or around the eyes, fainting. Most often, the cause of nerve root irritation is injury, sometimes well in the past, from sudden forceful movement of the neck sustained in automobile accidents, sports, falls. Rarely, infections, malignancy, or other disorder may be involved. Depending upon response, one or more treatment measures may be used, including moist heat, diathermy or ultrasound to relieve pain and spasm, a collar to hold the neck straight for a month or more, a special cervical contour pillow to position the neck properly during sleep, traction, exercises, analgesics, muscle-relaxant drugs, injection of a local anesthetic into persistently painful areas.


## CERVICITIS

An inflammation of the cervix, the narrow lower end of the uterus extending into the vagina and serving as a passageway between the two organs, cervicitis may produce discharge, bleeding, heavy menstrual flow, and pain or discomfort after coitus. Cauterization may be used in treatment, or in some cases dilatation and curettage may be used to remove infected tissues.


**CHAFING** (see INTERTRIGO)


## CHALAZION

This is a painless, slow-growing cyst or tumor on the eyelid resulting from an infection of a sebaceous, or oil, gland. In some cases, application of hot compresses may be adequate treatment, but in others incision and drainage by a physician may be required.

## CHANCROID

A localized venereal disease, chancroid begins within three to five days after sexual contact with one or more small soft sores on or near the external genitalia. The sores soon develop into ulcers, surrounding areas become red and swollen, and infection sometimes may spread to the lymph nodes of the groin, producing swelling and tenderness. A sulfa drug such as sulfadiazine or sulfisoxazole is usually effective. If not, an antibiotic, tetracycline, may be used.

## CHEILOSIS

A dry scaling and fissuring condition of the lips and angles of the mouth, cheilosis may sometimes be the result of fungal infection, which then must be treated. Most often, however, it results from deficiency of B vitamins, particularly riboflavin and pyridoxine, and responds to high doses of vitamin B complex.

## CHICKENPOX

Also known as *varicella*, chickenpox is a common acute communicable disease of childhood caused by a virus. One attack usually provides immunity. The incubation period is two to three weeks and the period of contagion extends about two weeks, beginning two days before the appearance of the rash. The disease may begin with a slight fever, headache, backache, and appetite loss. At about the same time, sometimes a day or two later, small red spots appear, usually first on the back and chest. After several hours the spots enlarge, and each develops a blister in the center filled with clear fluid which turns yellow after a day or two. A crust or scab then forms and peels off in from five to twenty days, during which time severe itching is experienced. Most cases of chickenpox are mild, and no special treatment is needed other than bed rest and forcing of fluids during the fever stage. For severe itching, calamine lotion or other applications provide some relief. A child with chickenpox should be isolated during the communicable period, or until about twelve days after the blisters first appear.

## CHOKING ON AN OBSTRUCTION

Choking on an obstruction may occur during eating. Often the obstructing object is a piece of meat. The victim often is incapable of speaking or breathing. To rule out the possibility of a heart attack, ask the victim if he can talk. If he cannot, he very probably is choking and immediate action is needed.

A recently developed technique called the *Heimlich Maneuver* is highly effective for removing an obstruction that causes choking.

If the victim is standing, stand behind him and wrap your arms around his waist. Make a fist of one hand and place it, thumb side in, against the victim's abdomen, below the rib cage and slightly above the navel. With the other hand, grasp your fist, and press into the victim's abdomen with a quick upward thrust. Repeat several times if necessary.

If the victim is sitting, stand behind his chair and carry out the maneuver in the same way.

If the victim has collapsed and you cannot lift him, turn him on his back. Face him and kneel astride his hips. Place one hand on top of the other, with the heel of the bottom hand on the abdomen below the rib cage and slightly above the navel. Press into the abdomen with a quick upward thrust. Repeat several times if necessary.

If *you* should be the victim and are alone, you can administer the maneuver to yourself. Press a fist, thumb side in, against your abdomen, below the rib cage and slightly above the navel. Then, either press your fist into the area, or drop hard on your fist against the edge of a chair or a sink.

## CHOLANGITIS, ASCENDING

An acute illness producing fever, chills, abdominal pain and jaundice, ascending cholangitis is an inflammation of a bile duct. The inflammation develops as the result of infection and partial obstruction of the duct, with the obstruction most often caused by a stone but sometimes a stricture or tumor. Surgery to reestablish a free flow of bile is needed but usually must be preceded by drug treatment for infection.

## CHOLECYSTITIS, ACUTE (see also GALLSTONES)

An inflammation of the gallbladder, acute cholecystitis is almost always caused by the lodging of a gallstone in the neck of the gallbladder or in the cystic duct. Once obstructed, the gallbladder distends and becomes inflamed by the toxic effect of the retained bile salts. The outstanding symptom is pain in the area about the stomach or right upper quadrant of the abdomen, extending into the right shoulder, severe and remaining steadily severe for hours. Fever, chills, nausea, abdominal distention, and jaundice also may develop. Diagnosis can be made by x-ray study. Treatment includes bed rest, pain relief with analgesic and antispasmodic medication, antibiotics, and sometimes stomach suction. Surgery for removal of the gallbladder is the preferred method of treatment and is carried out within 48 to 72 hours or some weeks later, depending upon the condition of the patient.

## CHOLELITHIASIS (see GALLSTONES)

## CHOLERA

This acute infection caused by a bacterium, *Vibrio cholerae,* is transmitted by contaminated food and water. It usually occurs in explosive outbreaks, is rare in the United States and Europe but still a danger in many other parts of the world, particularly in the tropics and India. The disease usually has an incubation period of one to six days and begins abruptly with painless diarrhea of such frequency that dehydration occurs quickly. The severe dehydration and loss of body minerals lead to great thirst, diminished urination, muscle cramps, weakness. The skin becomes wrinkled, the eyes swollen. Blueness and stupor may occur. Administration of fluids intravenously as well as by mouth is essential. The antibiotic tetracycline is valuable in eliminating the microorganisms and may reduce diarrhea dramatically.

## CHOROIDITIS

Its cause commonly obscure, choroiditis is an inflammation of the choroid, the middle vascular coat of the eye, and often of the retina as well. It produces visual disturbances—in some cases distortion of size of objects, in others blurring, in still others reduced central vision. In treatment, corticosteroid drugs are used to suppress the inflammation until the cause of the choroiditis disappears on its own or can be eliminated. The latter can be achieved when a cause such as toxoplasmosis, histoplasmosis, or amebiasis can be found.

**CHRONIC CYSTIC MASTITIS** (see MASTITIS, CHRONIC CYSTIC)

## CHRONIC PASSIVE CONGESTION

In this condition, blood vessels in the liver become engorged, commonly as the result of congestive heart failure, in which the heart is unable to pump blood effectively. Dull, aching, upper right abdominal pain is a usual symptom. Distention of the abdomen with fluid, spleen enlargement, and jaundice may sometimes occur. Treatment is for congestive heart failure.

## CIRRHOSIS, BILIARY

An uncommon disease, biliary cirrhosis takes two forms. In one, *primary* biliary cirrhosis, which mostly affects women aged 35 to 55, the cause is unknown. Bile ducts become inflamed, after which the liver is affected. Gradually over a period of months, jaundice, itching, excess fat in the stools from malabsorption, deposits of fatty substances in the skin and eyelids, bone softening, and liver enlargement develop. Although no specific treatment is known, the disease is only slowly progressive and survival can be prolonged. Cholestyramine may be used to control itching, and other measures, including administration of calcium and vitamins A, D and K, to prevent deficiencies, are employed.

The second form, *obstructive* biliary cirrhosis, is caused by blocking of bile ducts by stone, scar, tumor, or a congenital absence of a normal opening. Jaundice, in some cases chronic and in others intermittent, develops over a period of months to years, and fatty deposits may appear in the skin. Treatment is similar to that for primary biliary cirrhosis.

## CIRRHOSIS OF THE LIVER

A chronic disease in which liver cells degenerate and surrounding tissue thickens, cirrhosis is most likely to affect a middle-aged man with a history of chronic alcoholism. The cirrhosis may result from the severe malnutrition that often accompanies alcoholism rather than from the alcohol. Cirrhosis may have other causes: biliary tract obstruction, severe viral hepatitis, malnutrition, hemochromatosis, Wilson's disease, congestive heart failure, and syphilis. Symptoms include fatigue, weight loss, low resistance to infections, and gastrointestinal disturbances. As the disease progresses, other symptoms appear and may include jaundice, vomiting of blood, loss of libido, absence of menstruation. A backup of pressure because of poor circulation of blood through the liver vessels may lead to varices, or swollen veins, in the esophagus, which may rupture and drain blood into the stomach. Treatment includes a nutritious high-protein diet, strict ban on alcohol, often vitamin supplements. A corticosteroid drug such as prednisone may be used in some cases. Distention of the abdomen with fluids may require fluid and salt restriction and use of a diuretic drug to help increase fluid elimination. Surgery may sometimes be done for bleeding esophageal varices.

## CLAUDICATION, INTERMITTENT (see INTERMITTENT CLAUDICATION)

## COARCTATION OF THE AORTA

A congenital defect, coarctation is a pinching or constriction of the aorta, the great artery carrying blood from the heart to the body. The pinching usually occurs just beyond the point in the aorta at which arteries for the head and arms branch off, and since the narrowing obstructs blood flow, blood pressure increases (much as does water pressure in a hose when the nozzle is tightened). The pressure elevation affects vessels to arms and head, sometimes producing headaches and nosebleeds. Often, no symptoms develop and the diagnosis is made during a routine examination when elevated blood pressure is found in the arms but not in the legs. Surgery to remove the constricted aorta segment and join the healthy portions directly or with a synthetic graft is effective.

## COCCIDIOMYCOSIS (COCCIDIOIDOMYCOSIS)

Also known as *desert rheumatism* and *valley* or *San Joaquin fever*, coccidiomycosis is an infectious fungal disease. It is endemic in the U.S. Southwest, may be dustborne, affects men more than women. It occurs in two forms, primary and progressive. The *primary* is an acute, benign respiratory disease which in some cases may produce no symptoms; in other cases, it gives rise to one or more symptoms of fever, cough, chest pain, chills, sputum production, sore throat, coughing and spitting of blood, and, in some patients, arthritis and conjunctivitis. Commonly, the primary form is self-limiting and disappears on its own. But, in about 1 percent of white people and up to 20 percent of blacks, Mexicans, and Filipinos who get the infection, the progressive form develops. The *progressive* form involves spread of the disease and is chronic. Symptoms include low-grade fever, appetite loss, loss of weight and strength. Blueness, breathing difficulty, and bloody sputum also may occur in some cases, and as the disease spreads, joints, skin, bones, brain, and other areas may become involved. A potent antifungal agent, amphotericin B, is the only effective drug.

## COLD, COMMON

Also called *acute rhinitis,* a cold is a highly contagious infection of the upper respiratory tract that may be caused by any of several dozen viruses. It is spread by droplets from a victim as he coughs, sneezes or talks, and by contact with objects upon which the droplets may have fallen.

All colds are not identical because of different viruses and individual reactions. Commonly, the throat may feel irritated and other symptoms may include runny nose, sneezing, stuffy feeling in the head, slight headache, watering of the eyes, general aching and listlessness, and perhaps fever (especially in a child). A cold usually begins to subside after several days and, on average, lasts from seven to fourteen days.

There is no specific medication for an uncomplicated cold. Aspirin may provide some relief. Nose drops or a nasal spray may be used to help relieve congestion. The use of vitamin C in large doses—2 grams or more a day—remains controversial, both for prevention and relief, but may be helpful in some cases. Rest, large fluid intake, and moderate eating are useful measures.

By lowering body resistance, the common cold may lead to complications such as sinus infection, ear infection, laryngitis, pneumonia. A physician should be consulted whenever a cold shows signs of getting worse—for example, if there are prolonged chills, fever above 103°, aches in the chest, ears or face, shortness of breath, coughing up of blood-streaked or rust-colored mucus, or persistent hoarseness.

Antibiotics are not helpful for colds themselves but may be prescribed if complications occur.

## COLIC

When an infant screams excessively and flexes his legs on his abdomen, colic is considered present. No disease in itself, it may be symptomatic of any of a wide range of problems: swallowed air, underfeeding or overfeeding, intolerance of certain foods, hernia, intestinal disorder. Often, improved burping technique, or smaller and more frequent feedings, or a change in formula may help. In some cases, a sedative or antispasmodic may be used.

## COLITIS, CHRONIC ULCERATIVE

A chronic inflammatory disease that produces ulcerations and oozing of blood and pus in the lower colon, ulcerative colitis may extend upward, affecting much of the colon. It may appear at any age but most often affects the 20-to-40-year age group. It manifests itself usually as a series of bloody diarrhea attacks, with freedom from symptoms in between. If the disease extends upward, stools become looser and more frequent (10 to 20 a day), often consisting almost entirely of blood and pus. Other symptoms may include severe cramps, appetite loss, malaise, mild temperature rise in the evening, and, later, high fever, nausea, vomiting, severe appetite loss, anemia. Diagnosis can be made on the basis of symptoms, stool examination, instrument examination of the colon, and x-ray studies. As many as one in five patients recover completely after one attack. Others suffer chronically. Treatment may require medication to lessen cramps and stool frequency, a high-protein, high-calorie diet, blood transfusion if anemia is severe, antibiotics or other antibacterials. Corticosteroids such as prednisone and hydrocortisone, by mouth, injection, or enema, do not cure but do bring remission of symptoms in as many as 85 percent of patients, often rapidly. When medical measures do not suffice, surgical removal of the affected portion of the colon may be required.

## COLITIS, MUCOUS (see COLON, IRRITABLE)

## COLON, CANCER OF (see CANCER OF THE COLON)

## COLON, INACTIVE

Also called *atonic constipation* and *lazy colon*, this condition manifests itself as constipation with soft or puttylike rather than hard stools, with little or no abdominal discomfort. It may occur in the elderly and in people confined to bed, with feces accumulating as the colon fails to respond to the usual stimuli for bowel movement. It may also result from long-term abuse of laxatives or enemas. For an elderly patient or invalid, laxatives such as milk of magnesia, cascara sagrada, or sodium sulfate may be prescribed. For younger patients, treatment is directed at training the colon to work normally, through a regular visit to the bathroom soon after breakfast (as food intake tends to stimulate peristaltic contractions in the intestine), and includes a diet rich in fruits and vegetables. In some cases, in the beginning, as a training aid, a suppository or a drug such as bethanechol or neostigmine may be prescribed for use before bathroom time to stimulate evacuation.

## COLON, IRRITABLE

Also referred to as *spastic colon* and *mucous colitis,* the irritable colon is one of the most common digestive disorders. Symptoms are extremely variable and may include any or many of the following: abdominal pain that may be sharp and knifelike or deep and dull, on the left or right side, often relieved by passage of flatus or stool; constipation (with small hard or long ribbonlike stools), or diarrhea (with frequent semisolid stools) or constipation alternating with diarrhea; stools that may contain mucus but rarely blood unless hemorrhoids are present; lack of appetite in the morning; nausea; heartburn; excessive belching; headaches; faintness; weakness; insomnia. Diagnosis may require tests to exclude other possible problems such as ulcerative colitis and cancer; tests include blood and stool studies, colon examination, x-ray studies.

In treatment, a bland diet has long been recommended, with avoidance of raw fruits and vegetables. More recently, however, some physicians, believing that a major factor in irritable colon may in fact be lack of sufficient fiber or roughage in the diet, have been prescribing a high-fiber diet including wholemeal breads and cereals, and raw fruits and vegetables, with reports of excellent results. Some people tolerate whole milk poorly and some experience symptoms after using very hot or cold drinks, coffee, alcohol, and tobacco and benefit from avoidance of these. Regular physical activity is often helpful. When necessary, mild sedatives may be prescribed for tension and anxiety and agents for diarrhea.

## CONGESTIVE HEART FAILURE

In congestive heart failure, the heart's pumping efficiency is impaired, with reduction of blood flow to body tissues and congestion in the lungs or body circulation or both. Symptoms may begin suddenly and acutely or insidiously. Often, there is gradual loss of energy, increasing breathing difficulty on exertion, a tendency to ankle swelling. Later, breathing difficulty may become disabling, with breathing labored even at rest. Nausea, appetite loss, abdominal pain, blueness and, in older people, mental confusion may be other symptoms. In some cases, severe symptoms may appear suddenly after some severe stress. Causes of congestive heart failure include coronary heart disease, hypertensive heart disease, acute rheumatic heart disease, pericarditis (inflammation of the sac enclosing the heart), hypothroidism (low thyroid function), Paget's disease, some chronic lung diseases, severe anemia.

In treatment, as efforts are made to determine and if possible overcome the underlying problem, digitalis may be given to help increase heart pumping efficiency, salt restriction and diuretic drugs may be used to reduce fluid retention, bed or chair rest may be prescribed to reduce temporarily the heart's workload. If necessary, oxygen may be administered.

## CONJUNCTIVITIS, ALLERGIC

Producing itching, tearing, and redness of the eye, allergic conjunctivitis may be part of a larger allergic disturbance such as hay fever or may occur alone from contact with pollens, dusts, animal danders, and other airborne substances or from contact with such items as hair dye, nail polish, face powder, drugs carried by fingers to the eye. Avoidance of a known or suspected cause is advisable. Antihistamines may be helpful. In severe cases, an ophthalmic ointment containing a corticosteroid drug may be prescribed.

## CONJUNCTIVITIS, CATARRHAL

**Acute.** Highly contagious, caused by various bacteria, acute catarrhal conjunctivitis occurs most often in fall and spring. Symptoms include tearing of the eyes, watery discharge that later becomes mucus- or pus-laden and often seals the lid margins overnight, redness, itching, smarting, burning of the lids, sensitivity to light. In treatment, an antibiotic or sulfa ophthalmic preparation may be prescribed for use several times a day.

**Chronic.** Caused by the same agents as the acute form, chronic catarrhal conjunctivitis produces itching, smarting, redness, foreign body sensations, and tends to be worse at night, with exacerbations and remissions occurring over a period of months or years. Treatment requires elimination of any irritating factors such as wind, smoke and dust; a preparation combining an antibiotic and a corticosteroid may be given; special lid massage also may be prescribed.

## CONJUNCTIVITIS, INCLUSION

Also known as *swimming pool conjunctivitis* in adults and *inclusion blennorrhea* in newborns, this acute conjunctivitis is caused by an organism with some of the characteristics of both viruses and bacteria. In a newborn, it produces lid swelling, pinkness, edema of the conjunctiva and mucopurulent discharge, usually involving both eyes. In adults, symptoms are less severe, and commonly one rather than both eyes is affected. For newborns, application of an antibacterial ophthalmic preparation often leads to cure within a week. Adults may require antibiotic treatment by mouth as well.

## CONJUNCTIVITIS, VERNAL (SPRING)

Producing intense itching, tearing, light sensitivity, and a sticky mucoid discharge, this is a chronic conjunctivitis thought to be allergic in nature. Symptoms usually recur in spring, persist through summer, disappear in winter, although in some cases they may last year-round. In treatment, application of corticosteroid eye preparations, sometimes supplemented with small doses of corticosteroids by mouth, may be prescribed. In some cases, desensitization injections to increase tolerance for pollens may be helpful.

## CONSTIPATION

This symptom—difficult or infrequent passage of stools—has many possible causes. Among the organic causes are intestinal obstruction, diverticulitis, gastrointestinal cancer, megacolon, infections, thyroid or other gland disorders. Commonly, however, constipation is functional, related to poor bowel habits, poor diet, abuse of laxatives and enemas, inactive colon, irritable colon.

## CONTACT DERMATITIS (see DERMATITIS, CONTACT)

## CORNEAL ULCER

Ulceration of the cornea, the clear transparent front covering of the eye, is caused by bacteria that invade after injury of the cornea or by spread of infection from nearby infected areas. Symptoms include pain, light sensitivity, tearing, and eye muscle spasm. Treatment, which should be by an ophthalmologist, may consist of such measures as antibiotics applied to the eye and administered by mouth, cauterization of the base of the ulcer, hot compresses, local anesthetics, patching, and sometimes corticosteroid drugs.

## COR PULMONALE

An enlargement of the right ventricle of the heart which pumps blood to the lungs, cor pulmonale most commonly results from chronic bronchitis and emphysema. Other causes include sarcoidosis, berylliosis, and obesity. Symptoms may include one or many of the following: breathing difficulty which in some cases may be slight or absent at rest, cough, asthma, blueness, fainting attacks on exertion, chest pain similar to that of angina, distended jugular veins in the neck, leg swelling, clubbing of the fingers. Treatment is directed at the underlying disorder and may include digitalis and other medication to strengthen the pumping action of the heart if this has been impaired.

## CREEPING ERUPTION

Also known as *cutaneous larva migrans*, this disease, relatively common in the southeastern section of the country, is caused by the parasitic agent responsible for dog and cat hookworm. The parasite is deposited on the ground in animal feces, and the larva, capable of penetrating exposed skin on feet or legs, burrows under the skin and causes inflammation as it wanders in a winding trail, causing itching and commonly, as the result of scratching, a skin outbreak and bacterial infection. A drug, thiabendazole, may be given orally for two or three days and repeated after two weeks if necessary. Also often used: freezing briefly, with ethyl chloride spray or liquid nitrogen, a site just ahead of the burrow.

## CRETINISM

In this condition, which occurs in infants and children, the thyroid gland may be congenitally absent or greatly reduced in size. For lack of gland hormone secretion, the child may have thick, dry, wrinkled skin, enlarged tongue, thickened lips, broad face, flat nose, puffy feet and hands, and may be apathetic and mentally dull. If untreated, the child will become permanently dwarfed and probably mentally retarded and sterile. Treatment is lifetime administration of thyroid hormone. With such treatment, the outlook is excellent for normal growth and mental development.

## CROSS-EYE (STRABISMUS) (see STRABISMUS)

## CROUP (see LARYNGITIS, ACUTE OBSTRUCTIVE)

## CRYPTOCOCCOSIS

Most often affecting the middle-aged, and men more often than women, cryptococcosis occurs mainly in the southeastern area of the United States (but is worldwide). It is a fungal infection which may begin in the lungs but then spread to nervous system, kidney, and skin. Symptoms may include any or many of the following: cough, acnelike skin outbreak or ulcers, deep nodules under the skin, headache, vision blurring, confusion, depression, agitation, inappropriate speech or dress. Diagnosis is helped by recovery of the fungus from sputum, pus, or other material. Although once commonly fatal, especially when the nervous system was involved, cryptococcosis is now curable in about 85 percent of all cases with an antifungal drug, amphotericin B.

## CUSHING'S SYNDROME

In this condition, excessive amounts of hormones are produced by the adrenal glands atop the kidneys and lead to any or many of these symptoms: obesity, rounding of the face ("moon face"), fat accumulations in the back ("buffalo hump"), muscle wasting and weakness, thin and easily bruised skin, menstrual irregularities, excessive hairiness and sometimes baldness at the temples in women, thinning of bones, kidney stones, high blood pressure, mental and emotional disturbances. The overabundance of adrenal hormones may be caused by excessive stimulation of the glands by the pituitary gland at the base of the brain or by an adrenal gland tumor, which may be benign. Treatment depends upon the cause and with blood, urine and other tests, the cause often can be pinpointed. Treatment may include pituitary irradiation, surgical removal of an adrenal tumor, or removal of both adrenal glands followed by regular administration of adrenal hormone to compensate.

## CUTANEOUS LARVA MIGRANS (see CREEPING ERUPTION)

## CYST, SEBACEOUS

Also called a *wen*, this is a firm, movable, nontender mass with cheesy contents that may occur on the face, ears, scalp, back, scrotum. When small, a cyst may be treated simply by incision and removal of its contents. In other cases, injection of a corticosteroid such as triamcinolone or surgical removal of the entire intact cyst may be necessary.

## CYSTIC FIBROSIS

Also known as *fibrocystic disease of the pancreas, pancreatic cystic fibrosis,* and *mucoviscidosis,* cystic fibrosis is an inherited disease affecting the pancreas, sweat glands, and respiratory system. Abnormally thick mucus is produced and clogs the lungs and obstructs the flow of enzymes from the pancreas into the small intestine. Often, a first indication of the disease is the failure of an infant to regain birth weight despite good appetite. Chronic cough and rapid breathing, large, frequent and foul-smelling stools appear, often a protuberant abdomen, sometimes rectal prolapse. Other symptoms may include persistent respiratory infection, paroxysms of coughing and vomiting, barrel-like chest, blueness, digital clubbing, sinusitis, nasal polyps, lung abscess, empyema, spitting of blood, and cor pulmonale.

Although no cure is available, health often can be improved and life extended by continuous treatment which may include careful diet, replacement of pancreatic enzymes, use of mist tents for sleeping to help liquefy mucus, breathing exercises, postural drainage, bronchodilator drugs, antibiotics to control infection, and sometimes surgery to correct complications such as localized bronchiectasis and nasal polyps. With such treatment, about 70 percent of children with cystic fibrosis have been reaching adulthood.

## CYSTITIS (see URINARY TRACT INFECTIONS)

## CYSTOCELE

Muscles that support the bladder may sometimes be stretched during childbirth or may lose tone and become flabby with lack of adequate physical activity. With loss of firm muscular support, the bladder may become loose and bulging and may press down on the vagina. This is a cystocele. It may cause stress incontinence or loss of urine with sneezing, coughing, laughing, or straining. In corrective surgery, excess membrane is trimmed, muscles from the sides of the vagina are drawn together and tied beneath the urethra (or urinary channel), thus tightening the urethra and weak bladder-outlet muscle. The incision, made within the vagina, is not visible.

## DACRYOCYSTITIS

This is an inflammation of the tear sac of the eye which produces pain, redness and swelling about the sac, overflow of tears, fever, conjunctivitis, and inflamed edges of the eyelid margin. It results from dacryostenosis, or abnormal narrowing of the nasolacrimal duct (see below), or from injury to the nose, deviated septum, polyps, or other nasal problems. In treatment, hot compresses, penicillin by mouth or injection, and antibiotic ophthalmic preparations are employed and, in case an abscess has formed, incision and drainage may be necessary. If chronic dacryocystitis develops, it may be relieved by use of a probe under local anesthesia to dilate the nasolacrimal duct, and any nasal or sinus problems require treatment.

## DACRYOSTENOSIS

This is an abnormal narrowing of the nasolacrimal duct, the downward continuation of the tear sac, opening within the nose. It may result from congenital abnormality, chronic nasal infection and obstruction of the duct by inflammation, or fracture of the nose and bones of the face. Dacryostenosis produces persistent tearing of one eye, occasionally both. Often, in a child, fingertip massage twice a day to "milk" the tear sac, moving its contents through the duct, is effective. If this fails, a special probe may be introduced to open up the duct. Probes of increasing size are used in adults when the obstruction is not complete. For complete obstruction, surgery may be used to make an opening from the sac into the nasal passages.

## DANDRUFF (see DERMATITIS, SEBORRHEIC)

## DEFIBRINATION SYNDROME

This is a disorder resulting from abnormally rapid destruction of various blood factors needed for blood coagulation. It may produce profuse bleeding from all body openings along with purplish-red spots and bruises on the skin from bleeding into the skin. Suitable replacement blood factors may be administered to help control bleeding while treatment is directed at any underlying factor such as cancer, shock, sepsis (an illness resulting from disease-producing bacteria and their products), or oxygen deficiency in body tissues.

## DEHYDRATION

Abnormal dehydration, or loss of water from the body, may result from prolonged fever, diarrhea, and vomiting and occurs in severe injuries or surgical procedures involving loss of blood or body fluids. Water makes up more than half the body weight, and normally about 2½ liters (approximately 2½ quarts) are lost daily through urination, skin, and feces and must be made up for through liquids and foods in the diet. Depending upon the degree of dehydration, or excess of fluid loss over replacement, there may be one or more such symptoms as flushing, dry skin and mucous membranes, cracked lips, diminished urinary secretion, mental confusion, and low blood pressure. In severe dehydration, treatment may require replacement not only of fluid but also of specific electrolytes dissolved in body fluids and lost with them.

## DENGUE

Also known as *breakbone fever* and *dandy fever,* this is a painful viral disease often found in tropical climates, although epidemics have occurred in Gulf and southeastern sections of the United States. The causative virus is carried by a mosquito. Symptoms begin within a week after a bite by an infected mosquito, starting with severe headache and pain behind the eyes, followed within hours by back and joint pain, with fever up to 106°, and movement difficulty (the severe bone pain accounts for the name "breakbone fever"; the need to keep the neck rigid, for "dandy"). A pink rash, flushing of the face, and congested eyeballs develop. Usually, after a few days, fever falls and symptoms disappear for about 24 hours but then return along with a red rash on elbows, knees, and ankles that often leads to peeling of the skin. There is no specific drug for the disease; bed rest, fluids, and aspirin are used. The active disease usually disappears within six or seven days, and recovery is complete although convalescence is slow.

## DERMATITIS, ATOPIC

Also called *neurodermatitis*, this is a chronic itching inflammation of the skin occurring most often in people with a personal or family history of hay fever, hives, asthma, or other allergic disorder. The skin is generally dry, without blisters or other lesions, although scratching and rubbing may cause outbreaks and skin thickening. Although people with atopic dermatitis tend to be tense, it is not known whether emotions have an effect on the skin condition. In some cases, dust or wool causes flare-ups. Itching may be relieved by antihistamines. Corticosteroid ointment often helps. In some cases, striking improvement occurs with a change to a sunny, warm climate.

## DERMATITIS, AURAL ECZEMATOUS

The external canal of the ear is commonly affected by eczema, manifested by itching, redness, and discharge. A dilute aluminum acetate solution may be prescribed and often helps. Itching may be relieved by a mixture of a corticosteroid drug combined with solutions of alcohol, camphor, and menthol.

## DERMATITIS, CONTACT

An acute or chronic inflammation caused by substances that irritate or sensitize the skin, contact dermatitis may affect any area, most commonly the exposed portions of skin such as the forearms, face, neck and eyelids. The dermatitis produces redness, itching, sometimes crustiness, fissures, or other skin changes. Among the most common troublemakers are plants such as poison ivy, oak and sumac, primrose, ragweed, chrysanthemum; trees such as white pine, balsa, mahogany, teak; chemicals such as mercury, chromates, pyrethrum; drugs such as penicillin, sulfonamides, antihistamines, major tranquilizers; household items such as waxes, polishes, detergents; fabrics such as wool, silk, synthetic fibers, leather, fur; and cosmetics such as bleaches, hair dyes, deodorants. Patch tests may be used to pinpoint the causative agent. When the dermatitis is acute and markedly uncomfortable, a corticosteroid such as prednisone by mouth may be used or, in some cases, a corticosteroid lotion or ointment. For permanent benefit, the cause must be avoided.

## DERMATITIS, NUMMULAR

Of unknown cause, occurring most often in middle-aged people under stress, nummular dermatitis is an inflammatory skin condition in which itching, oozing, round patches may appear suddenly on arms, legs, sometimes on back and buttocks or generally over the body. Often an oral corticosteroid may control an acute outbreak. Trimeprazine or an antihistamine may be used for itching. Calamine lotion with menthol and camphor or a tar ointment may be prescribed, and moderate exposure to sunlight may help.

## DERMATITIS, SEBORRHEIC

When it affects only the skin of the scalp in mild form, producing scaling and moderate itching, this chronic inflammation is known as *dandruff* and is helped by more frequent shampooing with a conventional shampoo or one containing sulfur and salicylic acid or with a selenium sulfide preparation. In severe seborrheic dermatitis, yellowish greasy scaling may involve the hairline, other areas about the face, neck, central part of the trunk, and elsewhere. The cause is unknown although there is some belief a disorder of the sebaceous glands may be involved. For extensive seborrheic dermatitis, scrupulous cleansing is important. Dusting powder and a hydrocortisone lotion may be prescribed or, in extremely severe cases, a corticosteroid by mouth. Often, obese patients benefit from weight reduction.

## DERMATOMYOSITIS

Affecting women more often than men, this is a systemic disorder with inflammation and degenerative changes in skin and muscle. It may begin suddenly with fever, painful and swollen muscles, and prostration, or gradually with fatigability and progressive weakness in various muscles. Dermatomyositis may produce variable symptoms: reddening and edema of the skin on the face, about the eyes, and elsewhere; swelling, tenderness, weakness, stiffness, and sometimes pain of one or more muscle groups, most often those of the shoulders and pelvic girdle; swallowing difficulty; joint pain and stiffness; spleen and lymph node enlargement. Dermatomyositis is often subject to remissions and complete recovery may occur. Usually, though, the disease progresses up to a point and disability often remains at that level. Treatment may include a course of prednisone, aspirin, codeine, application of heat, splinting of painful muscles, sometimes methotrexate.

## DEVIATED SEPTUM

The nasal septum is a plate of bone and cartilage covered with mucous membrane that divides the nasal cavity. The septum may deviate, because of injury or malformation, so that one side of the cavity is smaller than the other. In addition to making for somewhat difficult breathing, the deviation sometimes may block normal flow of mucus from the sinuses during a cold and prevent proper drainage of infected sinuses. Surgery may be performed to relieve the obstruction and reduce irritation and infection in nose and sinuses.

## DIABETES INSIPIDUS

A disorder due to deficiency of a pituitary gland hormone, vasopressin, required by the kidneys for reabsorption of water from the urine, diabetes insipidus is marked by excessive urination and thirst, with as many as 5 to 40 quarts of fluid taken in and excreted daily. The disease may be congenital or may follow injury, infectious disease, or emotional shock. If a cause can be found, it should be treated. Otherwise, effective control of the disorder can be obtained with pituitary gland preparations or synthetic vasopressin. In some cases, a diuretic drug such as chlorothiazide may act to decrease free water clearance in diabetes insipidus and may be enough to control the condition.

## DIABETES MELLITUS

A disorder in which there is some degree of intolerance for carbohydrates (sugars, starches), diabetes results from inadequate production of insulin by the pancreas or from disturbance in the use of insulin. It occurs in some children and is relatively common after the age of 40, especially but not solely in the obese and in those with family histories of diabetes. Symptoms include excessive urination, thirst, itching, hunger, weakness, weight loss, dryness of the skin. In children and young adults, onset of diabetes often is abrupt, but in older people, the onset is commonly subtle and symptoms so relatively mild that medical help is not sought and diabetes may be discovered only on routine blood and urine examination.

Treatment may depend on severity of the disease, age of patient, and symptoms. Diet, exercise, and insulin administration are the primary measures for controlling the disease and returning carbohydrate metabolism toward normal. In milder forms of diabetes appearing in middle age or later, oral drugs may be used instead of insulin.

## DIAPHRAGMATIC HERNIA (see HERNIA, HIATAL)

## DIARRHEA, CHRONIC NONINFLAMMATORY

Also called *chronic enteritis,* this is a disorder in which intestinal motility is increased abnormally and transport of material through the bowel is very rapid. Symptoms include chronic or chronic relapsing diarrhea, with stools loose but free of blood or pus and sometimes containing undigested food residue, mild abdominal pain, nausea, heartburn, and fullness after eating with some relief from belching. Emotional strain may be a factor. Food allergy—to such foods as milk, wheat, rye, egg protein—also can be a cause. In some cases, elimination of a suspected food may bring improvement. In other cases, treatment with one or more drugs—such as methscopolamine, diphenoxylate with atropine, or phenobarbital—is often helpful.

## DIPHTHERIA

An acute, highly contagious bacterial disease of childhood, diphtheria usually affects the throat and sometimes the nose. It can be spread by coughing or sneezing and by handkerchiefs, towels, utensils, and other objects used by an infected person. After an incubation period usually of two to five days, the first symptoms commonly are sore throat, fever of 100° to 104°, headache, and nausea. Swallowing difficulty and prostration follow. Patches of a grayish or dirty-yellowish membrane appear in the throat and gradually coalesce into one membrane which, combined with edema of the throat and larynx, obstructs breathing and swallowing. Diphtheria can be prevented by immunization. In treatment, antitoxin is used to counteract the toxic reaction from the bacteria, and an antibiotic such as penicillin or erythromycin is prescribed.

## DIVERTICULITIS

Because of weakness of the muscles in the wall of the colon or large bowel, small blind pouches, or diverticula, may form in the lining and wall. Inflammation may occur as a result of bacteria or other irritating agents becoming trapped in the pouches. This is diverticulitis. Symptoms include muscle spasms and cramplike pains in the lower left side of the abdomen, often with distention, nausea, vomiting, unyielding constipation or diarrhea, or one alternating with the other. Depending upon the degree of inflammation, chills, fever and malaise may develop. Diagnosis can be made by barium enema which shows up the diverticula clearly on x-ray film.

Treatment for acute diverticulitis may include antibiotics and antispasmodics. In severe cases wih complications such as intestinal obstruction, perforation of the colon, or abscesses that do not respond to medical treatment, surgical removal of affected portions of the colon may be required. Recent studies suggest that diverticula may be formed as the result of high pressures produced in the colon when the colon walls must clamp down in an effort to move along stools that are small in volume for lack of bulk. Where once a low-bulk diet was used almost invariably for patients with diverticular disease, there is now an increasing tendency for physicians to prescribe just the opposite: a high-fiber, high-bulk diet which may prevent constipation and high pressures in the colon.

## DYSENTERY (see AMEBIASIS and BACILLARY DYSENTERY)

## DYSMENORRHEA

Dysmenorrhea, or painful menstruation, is characterized by pain that appears 24 to 48 hours before menses and persists for a variable period. It may be accompanied by headache, irritability, depression, malaise, fatigue, abdominal distention, nausea and vomiting, painful breasts. Dysmenorrhea is *primary* when it begins at puberty; the cause is not known. *Secondary* dysmenorrhea, which begins later in life, is usually associated with an organic cause such as pelvic inflammation, cervical stricture, abnormal position of the uterus, endometriosis, or tumor of the uterus or ovary. Primary dysmenorrhea may benefit from physical activity including sports, postural exercises, and medication, which may include a diuretic drug prior to the period to minimize abdominal distention, simple analgesics, or mild antispasmodics. Secondary dysmenorrhea requires correction of underlying problems.

## DYSTROPHY (see MUSCULAR DYSTROPHIES)

## EARDRUM INFLAMMATION (see MYRINGITIS)

## EAR INFECTIONS (see OTITIS)

## EDEMA, PULMONARY (see PULMONARY EDEMA)

## EJACULATION, PREMATURE

Occurring either before or after penis insertion in the vagina, premature ejaculation in some cases may be the result of inflammatory diseases such as those of the prostate or urethra and may be overcome with treatment for the disease. In some cases, sexual naiveté may be responsible and sexual counseling can help. Emotional problems may be involved and may be related to fear of failure; physician encouragement and counseling of both partners often are helpful. In some cases, application of a local anesthetic jelly such as 5 percent benzocaine to desensitize the penis during foreplay may be a useful aid.

## EMBOLISM, PULMONARY (see PULMONARY EMBOLISM)

## EMPHYSEMA, PULMONARY

A disease in which air spaces in the lungs become overdistended and undergo destructive changes, pulmonary emphysema is often preceded, accompanied, and complicated by chronic bronchitis. Although final proof is lacking that smoking causes emphysema, emphysema patients include a much higher proportion of heavy smokers than of others in the general population. Air pollution also may play a role. Symptoms of emphysema include wheezing, a chronic cough that is spasmodic, hard and tiring and may be brought on in severe cases by any exertion, even talking, expectoration of thick sputum, labored breathing with even mild exertion. Although the lung changes are irreversible, much can be done to increase comfort. Continued smoking is known to aggravate the disease and should be eliminated. Treatment may include bronchodilator drugs to enlarge the airways, expectorants and liquefying agents to help in removal of mucus and other obstructing materials, postural drainage to help clear air passages, special breathing exercises and, in some cases, antibiotics and corticosteroids.

## EMPHYSEMA, PULMONARY INTERSTITIAL

In this condition, rupture of air sacs in the lungs or in a bronchus or passage carrying air to or within the lungs allows air to escape and spread elsewhere in the chest and neck. Symptoms may include labored breathing, blueness, or pain behind the breastbone sometimes severe enough to simulate angina pectoris or a heart attack. In treatment, oxygen inhalation helps relieve blueness and breathing difficulty and sometimes, through effects on the blood, may allow the blood to absorb the escaped air. Drugs to relieve pain and cough are usually needed until the rupture seals off and air is absorbed.

## EMPYEMA

The presence of pus in the fluid between the membrane layers encasing a lung, empyema may arise as an occasional complication of pleurisy or other respiratory disease. Symptoms include chest pain on one side, coughing, fever, breathing difficulty, malaise. The condition is treated with antibiotics, rest, and often drainage with a tube to eliminate the pus collection.

## ENCEPHALITIS, VIRAL

Also known as *sleeping sickness*, encephalitis is an acute inflammation of the brain caused by viruses. Symptoms may include headache, fever, drowsiness, vomiting, and stiff neck. Muscle twitching, tremors, mental confusion, convulsions, and coma may develop. Occasionally paralysis of the extremities occurs. Although no effective specific drugs for the disease are available, bed rest, cold compresses, intravenous feeding if necessary, and other supportive measures often help, and although the patient appears desperately ill, recovery may follow and be complete.

## ENDOCARDITIS, BACTERIAL

An infection of the endocardium, the membrane lining the chambers of the heart, bacterial endocarditis can be either subacute or acute. The symptoms in either case—fever, chills, malaise, joint pains, lassitude, appetite loss, sometimes tender small nodules about the tips of the digits—are generally similar, but in the acute form the course is more rapid. If untreated, endocarditis can be fatal. In the great majority of cases, adequate treatment with the right antibiotic— determined by tests to establish the kind of bacteria involved and their sensitivity to various antibiotics—is successful.

## ENTERITIS, CHRONIC (see DIARRHEA, CHRONIC NONINFLAMMATORY)

## ENTERITIS, REGIONAL (see REGIONAL ENTERITIS)

## ENTEROCOLITIS, PSEUDOMEMBRANOUS

A serious disease in which the lining of small and large intestines is replaced by a mixture of white blood cells, mucus and fibrin, pseudomembranous enterocolitis may occur with shock following a heart attack, in very ill patients after injury or surgery, and sometimes in ill patients with various infections treated with broad-spectrum antibiotics that may, in the gut, kill off enough useful bacteria to allow other disease-producing bacteria to multiply. Symptoms usually appear abruptly and include high fever, watery and sometimes bloody diarrhea, prostration, abdominal distention, dehydration, and shock. In treatment, blood or plasma is used to combat shock, intravenous fluids for dehydration, and a corticosteroid for prostration; a suitable antibiotic may be required after discontinuation of any previously used antibiotics.

## ENURESIS (see BED-WETTING)

**EPIDIDYMOORCHITIS** (see under SCROTAL MASS in Symptoms Section)

## EPILEPSY

A disorder of the nervous system, epilepsy affects almost two million Americans. Brain damage or mental deterioration occurs only rarely. Epilepsy is mainfested by brief or prolonged loss of consciousness and by involuntary movements. In *petit mal*, loss of consciousness lasts only a few seconds, and although there is often twitching about the eyes or mouth, the patient remains standing or seated and appears to have had no more than a moment of absent-mindedness. Petit mal occurs more frequently in children. In *grand mal*, the victim falls to the floor unconscious, often with foaming at the mouth, biting, violent limb shaking. Often a grand mal patient has a warning such as ringing in the ears, spots before the eyes, or finger tingling before an attack, giving him time to lie down and avoid falls. In *psychomotor epilepsy* there is very brief clouding of consciousness with some repeated purposeless movement such as hand clapping, followed by brief periods of forgetfulness. Epilepsy may result from injury to the brain at birth, a blow on the head, a wound, or a tumor. But most commonly no cause is known. Most victims have their first seizures before age 18. Many anticonvulsant drugs, including Dilantin, Zarontin, phenobarbital, Mysoline, are available for treatment of epilepsy and are effective for the great majority of patients, permitting virtually normal living.

## ERYSIPELAS

An acute streptococcal infection of the skin, erysipelas often begins with chills and fever, sometimes nausea and vomiting, followed in a day or so by appearance of round or oval patches on the skin that enlarge, spread, become swollen, tender, and red, with the skin hot to the touch. An antibiotic such as penicillin or erythromycin cures the infection. Cold packs relieve local discomfort, and aspirin, with codeine if needed, can be used for pain relief.

## ERYTHEMA MULTIFORME

Its cause unknown, although allergy or sensitivity may be involved, erythema multiforme is an inflammatory skin eruption, primarily on the hands, feet, and mucous membranes. It usually appears suddenly, usually lasts two or three weeks but sometimes longer, tends to be more frequent in spring and fall, and may recur. The eruption may take the form of red spots, circumscribed solid elevations, wheals, blisters, sometimes large blisters or bullae, and is often accompanied by fever, joint pain and malaise. Compresses and ointments prescribed by a physician may be useful. In severe cases, corticosteroids may be needed.

*Oral erythema multiforme,* which produces multiple blisters and eroded areas throughout the mouth, with fever to 104° or 105°, bloody and crusted lips, largely affects infants, adolescents, and young adults. It may be treated by oral corticosteroids or in some cases by application of a triamcinolone ointment in dental paste. Healing usually occurs without any scarring.

## ERYTHRASMA

A bacterial skin infection that may sometimes be mistaken for psoriasis or other skin disease, erythrasma may produce scaling, fissuring, and maceration in the toe webs, genital and upper thigh area, underarms, and sometimes the trunk and the extremities. Diagnosis can be made with the aid of a special (Wood's) light. Erythrasma often responds quickly to the antibiotic erythromycin.

## ERYTHROMELALGIA

A relatively rare condition, erythromelalgia involves attacks of blood vessel dilation that lead to burning pain, heat and redness in the feet, less often in the hands. The cause is unknown and the symptoms may remain relatively mild, or the attacks may sometimes become so severe as to cause invalidism. The episodes may be triggered by exercise, standing, or exposure to heat. Often they may be avoided or abbreviated by rest, elevation of legs, and cold applications. Aspirin is often effective in relieving pain. Drugs such as ephedrine or methysergide that have a constricting effect on blood vessels may also provide relief. In a few cases, when all else fails, injection of alcohol into nerves in the legs or a nerve-cutting procedure may be needed.

## ERYTHROPLASIA OF QUEYRAT

An area of reddish pigmentation on the glans penis or at the corona of the penis, erythroplasia of Queyrat may be a precancerous lesion and should be investigated carefully.

## ESOPHAGEAL ULCER

Its cause not clear, an ulcer of the esophagus is similar to a peptic ulcer but, unlike the latter, rarely ruptures. Symptoms may include severe pain under the breastbone, sometimes radiating to the back, occurring soon after eating, heartburn, appetite loss, sometimes excessive salivation. Treatment may include bland diet, antacids, frequent use of milk, avoidance of hasty eating and reclining after meals.

## ESOPHAGITIS

An inflammation of the esophagus lining, esophagitis may be caused by infection, acid reflux from the stomach, smoking, irritation from some foods or drugs. Symptoms may include burning pain behind the breastbone, swallowing difficulty, and heartburn. In treatment, a bland diet may be prescribed along with antacids and avoidance of hasty eating and reclining soon after meals.

## ESOPHAGUS, ZENKER'S DIVERTICULUM OF

An abnormal pouch or diverticulum in the esophagus wall, this condition causes swallowing difficulty, especially after the first few mouthfuls of food. Other symptoms may include a gurgling noise during eating or drinking, cough, and regurgitation. Often, when the diverticulum is small, eating while leaning to one side helps food get by without becoming trapped. In severe cases, surgery can be performed.

## EUSTACHITIS

An inflammation of the eustachian tube, which leads from throat to ear, eustachitis produces pain in the ear, fullness, impaired hearing, sometimes ringing in the ears, dizziness, often with cough or symptoms of influenza. Factors in producing eustachitis include colds or other upper respiratory infections, overgrowth of the adenoids in children, septal deviation, and blowing the nose vigorously without opening the mouth so that infected material may be forced into the tube. Relief may be obtained with a vasoconstrictor such as ephedrine sulfate or phenylephrine, decongestants, and antihistamines.

## EXOPHTHALMOS

This is a protrusion of the eyeball which may result from varied causes, including hyperthyroidism, cavernous sinus thrombosis, inflammation, edema, tumors, and injuries. Treatment is determined by the cause. When hyperthyroidism is involved, its control may cause the exophthalmos to subside. Tumors must be removed. Corticosteroids often help control edema.

## EYELID EDEMA

Edema or fluid congestion of one or both eyelids can be due to TRICHINOSIS but is commonly the result of allergies to eyedrops, nail polish, other cosmetics or drugs. Elimination of the cause is necessary. Compresses of cold water over the closed lids are helpful. Corticosteroid treatment may be used in some cases.

## FARMER'S LUNG AND BAGASSOSIS

Inhalation of moldy hay, moldy vegetables, bagasse (the moldy pulp of sugarcane), and other materials such as flax and mushroom compost can lead to sensitivity that produces abnormal changes in the lungs. Symptoms—which include labored breathing, fever, rapid pulse, sometimes faintness for lack of adequate oxygenation of body tissue—occur in acute episodes that may last several weeks after exposure. With repeated exposure, irreversible lung changes may occur. During acute attacks, treatment is the same as for acute bronchitis. In very severe acute attacks, corticosteroid treatment may be needed.

## FEVER BLISTER (COLD SORE)

Fever blister, also called cold sore, is an itching or stinging sore on the skin or mucous membrane due to a virus infection. It is most common on the lip or mouth. The medical name for the eruption is *herpes simplex.*

The sore may be triggered by a respiratory infection, or by strong sunlight, gastrointestinal upset, or emotional distress. It usually lasts several days, then dries up and forms a crust.

A drying lotion such as calamine may be helpful. Zinc oxide applied to the crust may speed recovery.

## FIBROADENOMA, BENIGN

Also called *adenofibroma*, this is one of the most common breast tumors, occuring most often in young women. The lump is firm, well circumscribed, rubbery in consistency, and readily popped about. Treatment is surgical removal of the lump.

## FIBROIDS AND FIBROID TUMORS OF THE UTERUS (see UTERUS, MYOMA OF)

## FIBROMYOSITIS

An inflammation of muscle tissue and the connective tissue of muscles and joints, fibromyositis is usually caused by injury, strain, exposure to damp or cold, occasionally by infection. It produces muscle pain, tenderness, stiffness. The condition usually subsides within a few days. Rest, heat, massage, and aspirin often provide relief.

## FISH SKIN DISEASE (see ICHTHYOSIS)

## FISSURE-IN-ANO

Intensely painful, a fissure-in-ano is an ulcerated crack in the anal canal. It may start as a superficial crack caused by passage of hard stools. When the crack fails to heal because of distention and contraction of the canal with stool passage, it may deepen, become inflamed, and cause painful spasm or involuntary contracture of the anal sphincter. Distress can be especially intense when the anus is stretched during defecation. Cure is often possible in several weeks with medical treatment that may include use of a low-residue diet, stool softener, anesthetic ointment, and sitz baths after bowel movements to help relax spasm. When a fissure becomes chronic, it may be repaired by a relatively minor surgical procedure.

## FISTULA-IN-ANO

Producing a purulent discharge near the anus, often with skin irritation and recurring abscess formation, a fistula-in-ano is an abnormal tunnel from inside the rectum to the skin outside. Usually, it results from an infection that may start in the rectal or anal wall. The infection leads to abscess formation. The abscess breaks the skin near the anal opening and discharges pus. It may seem to heal but then may open and discharge over a period of weeks or months, forming a tunnel or fistula. Surgery is required.

## FLATFOOT

An absence of the normal arch of the sole of the foot, flatfoot may produce no symptoms in some cases. When it does, they may include pain in the arch extending to calf muscles and sometimes to the knee, hip, and lower back, with discomfort increased by extended walking or standing. Arch supports help by supporting the foot during walking. Warm foot baths also help reduce discomfort. In an acute flare-up of symptoms, aspirin and bed rest are usually helpful.

## FLU (see INFLUENZA)

## FOLLICULITIS

An inflammation of hair follicles which occurs most often in the beard area, producing itching and pain when the hairs are touched or moved as in shaving, folliculitis can become chronic if not treated promptly. Antibiotics to be taken by mouth or applied locally or sulfur ointment may be prescribed. Use of an electric instead of safety razor and avoidance of close shaving is helpful. In some cases, growing a beard eliminates folliculitis.

## FOOD INFECTION OR STAPHYLOCOCCUS TOXIN
GASTROENTERITIS (see GASTROENTERITIS, FOOD INFECTION or STAPHYLOCOCCUS TOXIN)

## FOOD POISONING, NONBACTERIAL

Various foods containing naturally occurring poisons are capable of causing gastroenteritis (or inflammation of the lining of the stomach and intestines) and sometimes systemic or body-wide adverse effects. Mushroom (toadstool) poisoning may produce, within a few minutes to two hours, tearing of eyes, salivation, sweating, pupil contraction, vomiting, abdominal cramps, diarrhea, thirst, dizziness, confusion, collapse, coma, sometimes convulsions. In another type of mushroom poisoning, symptoms, beginning within 6 to 12 hours, or more, may include abdominal pain, nausea, vomiting, and diarrhea, with blood-streaked stools and vomitus. In poisoning from immature or sprouting potatoes which contain a toxic agent, solanine, symptoms develop within a few hours and may include nausea, vomiting, abdominal cramps, diarrhea, pupil dilation, dizziness, throat constriction, and prostration. In fish poisoning—from Pacific-type trigger fish, sea bass, eel, black ulna, red snapper, and barracuda; Caribbean-type sierra, cavalla, great barracuda, grouper, amberjack; and *Tetraodon*-type globe and balloon fish, and puffers—symptoms may appear immediately or up to 24 hours after a meal and may include tingling around the mouth, limb numbness, nausea, vomiting, diarrhea, abdominal pain, joint aches, chills, fever, sweating, itching, muscle weakness. Mussel poisoning may, within half an hour, produce abdominal cramps, nausea, vomiting, muscle weakness and paralysis. In ergot poisoning, caused by rye or other grain contaminated with the ergot fungus, symptoms may include chest pain, racing pulse or slow pulse, headache, nausea, vomiting, diarrhea, weakness, drowsiness, itching, dizziness, cramps in the extremities. Fava bean poisoning in people who are susceptible may produce vomiting, dizziness, diarrhea, prostration, anemia.

In treatment, bed rest is required. Stomach washing may be needed if there has been no violent vomiting or diarrhea. An emetic, such as syrup of ipecac, may be used to induce vomiting if necessary. Fluids may be given by vein in some cases. Various drugs—such as atropine, papaverine, sodium amobarbital, or others—may be needed to combat specific symptoms.

## FROSTBITE

Sometimes generalized but commonly affecting toes, fingers, nose and ears, frostbite, or injury by cold, produces disturbances of smaller surface blood vessels, with tingling, numbing sensations that may be followed by burning, itching, and swelling. In generalized cold injury, blankets may be used to prevent any further body heat loss and to permit natural, slow rewarming of the body. In local frostbite, an often-recommended treatment is application of warm water to encourage rapid rewarming, with the water kept between 100° and 104° degrees Fahrenheit, never warmer or colder, and a thermometer used to check its temperature. Other parts of the body are kept warm and whiskey or a drug such as papaverine which dilates blood vessels may be used.

# FURUNCLE

An inflamed lump on and under the skin with a central core, a furuncle (or *boil*) is caused by bacteria which enter through hair follicles or sweat glands. Like a boil, a *carbuncle* is caused by pus-forming bacteria but is larger, more deeply rooted, and has several openings. A carbuncle is most frequent in men, commonly on the nape of the neck. A single boil may be treated with moist heat to bring it to a head so it can be incised and the core removed. Sometimes, single boils, and commonly multiple boils and carbuncles, require antibiotic treatment.

## FURUNCULOSIS OF THE EAR

Either alone or as part of an outbreak of boils elsewhere, a boil may develop in an ear, producing fullness of the ear, pain, impaired hearing, and neck gland swelling. Treatment may be the same as for boils elsewhere (see above), or when the boil is in the ear canal, an aluminum acetate solution may be applied through a gauze wick.

## GALACTOSEMIA

This is an inherited disorder in which an enzyme is lacking. The enzyme is needed for the proper handling of galactose, a sugar derived from lactose in milk. In its absence, galactose accumulates in the blood and tissues. An infant with galactosemia appears normal at birth but within a few days, after relatively mild feeding problems, begins to vomit. Diarrhea, abdominal distention, liver enlargement, mental retardation, and cataracts may develop. The disorder can be detected by test, and when diagnosed early before damage to the nervous system, all symptoms can be overcome by eliminating milk and milk products. Milk substitutes are used and the diet is planned to provide necessary nutrients from products containing no lactose or galactose.

## GALLSTONES (see also CHOLECYSTITIS, ACUTE)

A gallstone is a stonelike mass, called a *calculus*, that forms in the gallbladder, and the presence of gallstones is known as *cholelithiasis*. Cause is unknown although there is evidence of a connection between gallstones and obesity. Women tend to be more often affected than men. Gallstones may be present without causing trouble or they may produce such symptoms as upper abdominal discomfort, bloating, belching, and nausea, especially after eating fatty foods. But such symptoms also may occur with dyspepsia or indigestion and so may not necessarily be attributable to stones, even when stones are revealed by x-ray.

There is no present available medical treatment for gallstones, although currently under investigation is a method of dissolving the stones over a period of time. Since inflammation (*acute cholecystitis*) occurs in up to one third or more of patients with gallstones at some point, removal of the gallbladder (cholecystectomy) may be done even in the absence of symptoms. Symptoms like those mentioned may occur in *chronic cholecystitis,* which can result from repeated attacks of acute cholecystitis, leaving the gallbladder shrunken, scarred, and sometimes but not always with stones present. If stones are found, gallbladder removal may be carried out; if gallstones are not present, a low-fat diet or use of antispasmodics may be helpful.

## GANGLION

A painless lump on the back of the wrist, a ganglion is a cyst (or liquid-containing sac), which often disappears spontaneously. Sometimes, disappearance may be speeded by a blow, such as from a book, that may break the cyst and allow the fluid to escape.

## GASTRIC DILATION, ACUTE

Its precise cause unknown, dilation of the stomach and accumulation of large amounts of fluid and gas may sometimes follow surgery, severe abdominal or chest injury, or severe or chronic illness. Symptoms may include sensation of abdominal fullness, pain over the stomach area, vomiting or regurgitation of large quantities of bile-stained fluid, severe thirst, and breathing difficulty. In treatment, the stomach is emptied by mild suction through a tube, usually producing cure within 48 hours. Intravenous solution may be needed to overcome dehydration and restore lost minerals.

## GASTRITIS, ACUTE AND CHRONIC

An inflammation of the mucous membrane lining of the stomach, acute gastritis is a common disorder.

An acute *erosive* form may result from drugs (especially aspirin), heavy alcohol intake, hot spicy foods, foods to which an individual may be allergic (milk, eggs, fish, among others), food poisoning by bacteria or their toxins, viral and other acute illness. Symptoms include appetite loss, malaise, abdominal pressure, sensation of fullness, nausea, vomiting, dizziness, headache, sometimes vomiting of blood. Because the stomach lining is usually renewed every 36 hours, acute erosive gastritis is often short-lived unless the cause is not removed. A normal diet can be used and, if necessary, a drug such as prochlorperazine may be prescribed for nausea and vomiting.

Acute *corrosive* gastritis results from swallowing strong acids or alkalis, heavy metal salts, iodine, or potassium permanganate. Symptoms may include corrosion of the lips, tongue, mouth, and throat, inflammation of the esophagus with pain and swallowing difficulty, severe stomach pain, vomiting of blood, blueness, collapse. Prompt treatment, usually in a hospital, is needed and may include antidotes, drugs to induce vomiting, use of a stomach tube to remove the causative agent, and other measures.

*Chronic* gastritis, with chronic stomach lining inflammation, is of unknown cause but may occur with pernicious anemia, diabetes, chronic aspirin intake, stomach cancer, thyroid, adrenal or pituitary gland disorders. Commonly, chronic gastritis produces no symptoms but in some cases there may be mild nausea, pain or discomfort on eating, a burning sensation over the stomach area. Although there is no specific treatment for chronic gastritis, correction of any underlying disease is important. Antacids and avoidance of any foods that seem to increase symptoms are often helpful.

## GASTROENTERITIS, ACUTE

An inflammation of the stomach and intestinal lining, acute gastroenteritis causes malaise, nausea, vomiting, appetite loss, gas sounds in the intestines, diarrhea, sometimes fever and prostration, with symptoms usually appearing suddenly. Causes are many: excessive alcohol intake, "intestinal grippe" virus, food allergy, food poisoning, drastic cathartics, drugs such as aspirin and related compounds, colchicine, and quinacrine, and infectious diseases such as typhoid fever and amebic dysentery. Pinpointing of cause may be aided by stool and blood tests and instrument examination of the colon.

In treatment, bed rest is helpful. Nothing is usually given by mouth until nausea and vomiting disappear (or, if necessary, are controlled by scopolamine, sodium phenobarbital, or other drugs); then light fluids such as tea, strained broth, cereal, gruel or bouillon with salt may be taken, and when these are well tolerated, other foods may gradually be added.

## GASTROENTERITIS, FOOD INFECTION

Caused by food contaminated with *Salmonella* bacteria, food infection gastroenteritis is manifested, generally after about 12 hours (the range is 6 to 48 hours), by sudden headache, chills, fever, muscle aches, nausea, vomiting, abdominal cramps, severe diarrhea, sometimes with blood-streaked vomitus and stools. It usually lasts one to two days. Treatment is the same as for acute gastroenteritis (see above). In severe cases, an antibiotic may be used.

## GASTROENTERITIS, STAPHYLOCOCCUS TOXIN

The most common type of food poisoning, this form of gastroenteritis is produced by foods such as custards, cream-filled pastries, milk, fish, and processed meat contaminated with a toxin formed by staphylococcal bacteria, usually by food handlers with staphylococcal skin infections. Within two to four hours after eating contaminated food, nausea, vomiting, abdominal cramps, diarrhea, sometimes headache and fever appear. Symptoms usually last only six hours or less. Treatment is the same as for acute gastroenteritis (above).

## GASTROINTESTINAL ALLERGY

Individual sensitivity to a specific food or foods may lead to some degree of crampy abdominal pain, nausea, vomiting, and diarrhea when the culprit food is eaten. Hives sometimes may appear. Occasionally food allergy may cause anal itching and eczema around the anal area. Some people with food allergy become aware of the food involved. For others, an elimination diet may be needed and operates on the principle of eliminating most or all of the most common food allergens and gradually restoring them until the culprit becomes obvious by return of symptoms. Some physicians advocate oral desensitization in which the offending food is avoided for a time, then used in small, gradually increasing amounts to try to build up tolerance. Medication is usually not helpful for GI allergy.

## GAUCHER'S DISEASE

Affecting Jewish families more often than others, this is a relatively rare familial disorder involving abnormal handling of fats. It may lead to spleen, liver, and sometimes lymph gland (node) enlargement, bone pain, joint swellings, brown pigmentation of the skin, anemia, blood disturbances. No specific treatment is known, but blood transfusions or spleen removal or both may be carried out when necessary. Patients who survive beyond childhood may live for many years.

## GIARDIASIS

A disease caused by an intestinal parasite, *Giardia*, giardiasis is transmitted through human feces and produces mucous diarrhea, abdominal pain, and weight loss. Diagnosis is aided by stool examination. Treatment is with quinacrine or metronidazole.

## GINGIVITIS

An inflammation of the gums which produces redness, swelling and bleeding, gingivitis is most often due to local causes such as tartar, food impaction, malocclusion, faulty dental work, and mouth breathing. Other causes include vitamin deficiencies, blood disorders, diabetes, allergic reactions, pregnancy, leukemia, and some drugs such as diphenylhydantoin used over long periods. If unchecked, gingivitis may lead to PERIODONTITIS with gum recession and loss of bone and teeth. In treatment, any local or systemic contributing disorders must be controlled, and tartar and faulty dental work eliminated. In some cases, removal of excess gum tissue (gingivectomy) may be needed.

## GINGIVOSTOMATITIS, NECROTIZING ULCERATIVE

Also known as *trench mouth* and *Vincent's disease,* resulting from infection, this disease produces painful, bleeding gums, gum ulceration, painful swallowing and talking, salivation, unpleasant breath. It is most likely to occur in people with poor oral hygiene, heavy smokers, and those with nutritional deficiency. In treatment, smoking is stopped for several days, and rinses of warm peroxide along with soft diet, vitamins, and drugs for pain may be used. In some cases, anti-biotics may be prescribed. Debridement, or removal of some of the infected tissues, is often needed.

## GLAUCOMA

An eye disease characterized by increased pressure within the eye resulting in damage to the retina and optic nerve, glaucoma accounts for almost half of all cases of adult blindness; it rarely occurs before age 40 but affects more than 2 percent of the U.S. population after that. One form, acute, may cause sudden dimming of vision, with severe eye pain. Chronic glaucoma, which is more common, affects vision very gradually. Symptoms include loss of side vision so that objects may be seen much as if they were viewed through a rifle barrel, blurred or fogged vision, and appearance of colored rings or halos around bright objects. Treatment varies with type and severity of glaucoma. Early detection often permits satisfactory treatment with miotics and other drugs that help reduce intraocular pressure. In some advanced cases, relatively simple surgery may be done to improve drainage of pressure-raising fluid.

## GLOMERULONEPHRITIS, ACUTE

An inflammatory disease of the kidneys, acute glomerulonephritis is usually related to previous strep infection of the throat, sinuses or tonsils, sometimes of the skin or ear. Symptoms include blood in the urine, change in urine color, or reduced volume of urine, with edema or fluid retention appearing as puffiness of face and eyelids and later extending to legs and other parts of the body, and blood pressure elevation. Treatment may include bed rest; penicillin; restriction of protein, salt and water intake; use of diuretics. Most patients recover completely, although recovery time may range from a few weeks to two years.

## GLOSSITIS

An inflammation of the tongue, glossitis may result from local in-fection, mechanical injury, excessive use of alcohol, tobacco, hot foods, spices, allergy (to toothpaste, mouthwash, candy dyes, some-times dentures), vitamin deficiency, anemia, skin diseases that may also affect the tongue. Symptoms may include reddening of tip and edges, sometimes with painful ulcers, whitish patches, smooth area, hairy tongue, burning, tenderness or pain with swelling. In addition to being directed at removing the cause, treatment may include a mouthwash containing an antiinfective agent such as benzalkonium chloride or cetylpyridinium chloride, an anesthetic solution used before meals, direct application of a corticosteroid such as triamcinolone in a dental paste.

## GLUCOSE-GALACTOSE MALABSORPTION

Manifesting itself soon after birth with unyielding diarrhea, this is an inherited defect in intestinal and kidney handling of the sugar glucose which, if undiagnosed, can lead to death. Treatment involves elimination of all dietary sugar except fructose (fruit sugar). Other sugars may be added later, after age 3 to 5, and normal growth and development follow.

## GOITER

An enlargement of the thyroid gland with swelling in the front part of the neck, goiter results from iodine deficiency from any cause, including inadequate intake in the diet or the effect of some drugs such as aminosalicylic acid, sulfa drugs, or iodine in very large doses. In treatment, iodized salt may be used, or if some drug is involved, its use may be discontinued. In some cases, thyroid hormone may be prescribed to block the stimulation that causes the gland to enlarge.

## GONORRHEA

Caused by a bacterial organism, the *gonococcus,* gonorrhea inflames the mucous membranes of the genital and urinary systems. In a man, symptoms include painful burning sensation during urination and discharge of a whitish fluid. In some women there may be no early symptoms; others experience lower abdominal pain with or without a burning sensation during urination and whitish vaginal discharge. If neglected, gonorrhea may lead to serious complications, including arthritis, urethral stricture, meningitis. Penicillin in most cases, another antibiotic in others, is effective.

## GOODPASTURE'S SYNDROME

An uncommon disease of unknown cause, Goodpasture's syndrome is a serious illness affecting membranes of lungs and kidneys. It occurs most often in young men, produces coughing and spitting of blood, breathing difficulty, blood in the urine, anemia. Corticosteroid treatment may be helpful for patients whose disease is predominantly centered in the lungs. In some cases, removal of the kidneys followed by kidney transplantation has prolonged life.

## GOUT

Affecting mostly men, gout is a recurring arthritis, usually affecting a single joint in the beginning but sometimes later affecting two or more at the same time. An attack produces throbbing, crushing pain, most often in the big toe, sometimes in the ankle, instep, knee, wrist, or elbow. Gout is a disorder of body handling of purines, substances found in many high-protein foods, leading to accumulation of uric acid in excess amounts in the blood and deposition of uric acid crystals in the joints. A first attack may follow surgery, an infection, a minor irritation such as tight new shoes, or may have no apparent cause. Without treatment, attacks usually last a few days or weeks, with all symptoms then disappearing completely until a recurrence. Without treatment, chronic gout may develop with degeneration of joints as in rheumatoid arthritis. In treatment, colchicine in most cases relieves symptoms in 72 hours or less. For prevention of attacks, regular use of a drug such as probenecid (which prevents uric acid retention) or allopurinol (which prevents formation of the acid) may be prescribed. In some cases, moderate diet restrictions may be needed.

## GUM DISEASE (see GINGIVITIS)

## GYNECOMASTIA

Gynecomastia, or enlargement of the male breast, occurs most often either during adolescence or after the age of 40. In adolescents, the enlargement may be due to the increase in hormone secretions at that point and may later disappear. When it occurs later in life, it may involve one or both breasts. When it involves one, it may lead to some worry about the possibility of cancer of the breast. Such cancer is infrequent. When it occurs, surgery for removal of the malignancy is the same as for breast cancer in women. Enlargement should receive medical attention. Rarely, it may be associated with liver disease or a tumor of the testicle. Some drugs may produce gynecomastia as a side effect, which disappears when the drugs are stopped. Often gynecomastia occurs for unknown reasons in men who are normal in every other respect. If the enlargement should be marked, persistent, and a cause of embarrassment, surgery can be performed. In the relatively minor operation, excess breast tissue is removed through an incision about three inches long or a little longer.

## HAY FEVER (see RHINITIS, ALLERGIC)

## HEART ARREST (see CARDIAC ARREST)

## HEART FAILURE, CONGESTIVE (see CONGESTIVE HEART FAILURE)

## HEAT CRAMP

Physical exertion under conditions of high temperature, leading to profuse sweating and loss of body salt, can cause spasms of excruciatingly painful cramps, most often of arm and leg muscles, with relative comfort between spasms. Heat cramp may be prevented by drinking salt-containing water. In treatment, administration of salt and water is essential and, in severe cases, treatment may have to begin with administration by vein followed by oral intake until symptoms are relieved.

## HEAT HYPERPYREXIA (SUNSTROKE, HEATSTROKE)

Prolonged exposure to heat or sunshine, often combined with exercise, may cause body temperature to rise to 106° or higher, with flushing, hot and dry skin, sometimes with muscular twitching or cramps, sometimes convulsions. Heat hyperpyrexia (excessively high fever) can threaten life and constitutes an emergency, requiring immediate medical attention. Treatment may include ice-water tub bath or covering with water-soaked blanket and vigorous skin massage to bring rectal temperature down to 101° but not lower, with cold applications discontinued then but massage continued. Other measures including use of intravenous fluids with bicarbonate and medication may be employed.

## HEAT PROSTRATION

Resulting from failure to adjust to prolonged exposure to high heat, heat prostration may begin with warning symptoms of weakness, dizziness, headache, nausea, dimming or blurring of vision, and muscular cramps, followed by profuse sweating, cold damp ashen skin, a semicomatose or unconscious state. In treatment, the patient is moved to a cool environment, placed in reclining position with clothing loosened, and cool water is given by mouth. Intravenous fluid administration, oxygen, heart stimulants and other medication may be needed. With prompt medical attention, outlook for recovery is good.

## HEAT RASH (see MILIARIA)

## HEATSTROKE (see HEAT HYPERPYREXIA)

## HEEL PAIN

Painful heel may result from bursitis due to ill-fitting shoes or ligament bruising or inflammation from strain. Often, the underlying problem is FLATFOOT, which should be treated. Proper shoes, sometimes with adjustment of heel height, may be prescribed. For pain under the heel, a ring of felt or sponge rubber may be used to minimize pressure on the painful area. If necessary, the painful area may be injected with hydrocortisone.

## HEMOCHROMATOSIS

A relatively rare disease in which the body becomes overloaded with iron, hemochromatosis may be inherited or caused by some anemias, liver disorder, or excessive intake of iron. Symptoms include pigmentation of the skin and those of diabetes and liver disease, along with loss of libido and sometimes heart failure. Treatment requires removal of excess iron, often by weekly bleeding until blood iron drops toward normal, and measures for diabetes; testosterone may be used to restore libido.

## HEMOPHILIA

An inherited disorder, transmitted by females and limited to males, hemophilia involves impaired ability of the blood to coagulate or clot. Symptoms include excessive bleeding from minor cuts and wounds, often with spontaneous bleeding under the skin and in the gums, gastrointestinal tract, joints and muscles, sometimes leading to joint stiffening. Treatment requires replacement of the missing blood factor for coagulation. Serious bleeding episodes may require transfusion to replace lost blood.

## HEMORRHOIDS

Hemorrhoids, also called *piles,* are enlarged, varicose veins in the mucous membrane either just inside the rectum (internal hemorrhoids) or outside (external hemorrhoids). They may result from increased pressure transmitted from the abdominal circulation and caused by pregnancy, obesity, coughing, sneezing, straining at stool, and abdominal tumors. Symptoms may include sense of rectal fullness, bleeding, painful defecation. Small hemorrhoids causing only slight and infrequent bleeding may require no treatment; avoidance of constipation and straining at stool often is helpful. Painful hemorrhoids may be relieved by heat applications, cold compresses, warm sitz baths, or analgesic ointment. In some cases, if necessary, simple bleeding internal hemorrhoids without complications may be treated by injection. Surgical removal (hemorrhoidectomy) usually is not required unless bleeding is enough to cause anemia, the hemorrhoids protrude in a large mass, or anal itching is intolerable.

## HEPATITIS

An inflammation of the liver, hepatitis produces such symptoms as appetite loss, nausea, fever, tenderness in the region of the liver, and liver enlargement. As the disease progresses, jaundice may develop and there is rapid loss of weight and strength. Hepatitis may stem from another disorder such as amebic dysentery, cirrhosis, or infectious mononucleosis. It may be caused by toxic materials such as carbon tetrachloride, phosphorus, anesthetic agents, antibiotics and other medications. It also may be a viral infection. The virus may be transmitted through contaminated foods or liquids or by transfusion of infected blood. There is no specific drug for hepatitis. Once, strict bed rest and a low-fat, high-carbohydrate diet were considered essential but no longer are, and diet and activity are adapted to the individual patient's condition. In very severe, life-threatening cases, prednisone and growth hormone have been used although their value is uncertain. Exchange blood transfusion is credited with enabling some severely afflicted patients to recover. When hepatitis is due to a toxic material, the substance must be removed.

## HEPATITIS, ALCOHOLIC

Occurring only in alcoholics, alcoholic hepatitis is a severe disturbance in liver function. Symptoms, which may appear suddenly, include fever, jaundice, abdominal fluid accumulation and distention, and fluid accumulation elsewhere. The disease can be fatal. Some patients recover completely, some develop cirrhosis of the liver. Treatment includes bed rest, avoidance of alcohol, dietary care.

## HEPATITIS, AMEBIC (see AMEBIASIS)

## HERNIA

A hernia is a weakening of tissue surrounding an organ so that a portion of the organ bulges at the weak point.

Inguinal hernia. In this, the most common type, much more frequent in men than in women, the groin (the abdominal wall near where thigh joins trunk) weakens and the intestine pushes out. There may be no symptoms, but discomfort is usual. Occasionally, a hernia is strangulated as a loop of intestine is caught and constricted in the bulge, with risk of gangrene. Any hernia needs medical attention; a painful one, immediately. Some half-million hernia repair operations are performed annually in the United States, with more than 90 percent bringing permanent cure.

Femoral hernia. More frequent in women than in men, this hernia occurs high up in the thigh, about an inch or so below the groin. It, too, may become strangulated. Repair surgery is effective.

**Umbilical hernia.** This herniation or protrusion through the navel occurs most often in infants and may also appear in women after pregnancy. As weak muscles pull away, the abdominal membrane protrudes under the skin and the navel may appear to be inflated. Many small umbilical hernias require no surgery, tend to disappear gradually over the first years of life, and adhesive tape to hold the muscles together or other support may be used during that time. Repair may be advised, however, when a child is about a year old if the hernia remains or has become large enough to admit an adult little finger.

**Incisional hernia.** This is a protrusion through the scar of a surgical incision, almost always in the abdomen, which may occur soon after surgery or years later. For repair, the incision is opened and muscle layers overlapped for added strength, sometimes with a plastic fabric mesh inserted for support.

**Hiatal hernia.** A protusion of the stomach above the diaphragm through an enlarged opening in the diaphragm, hiatal hernia is common and often produces no symptoms. When it does, they may include distress under the breastbone, heartburn, swallowing difficulty, vomiting of blood, darkening of stools with blood. Relatively simple measures are often effective and include sleeping with the head of the bed raised on eight-inch blocks, weight reduction if obesity is present, avoidance of lifting, bending over, and straining at stool, all of which increase pressure within the abdomen and, in so doing, exacerbate hiatal hernia. Antacids may be used. When necessary, surgical repair can be employed.

## HERPES SIMPLEX VIRUS, TYPE 2

Herpes simplex virus has long been known to produce fever blisters. A recent discovery is that there is another form of the virus, Type 2, which is transmitted by sexual contact and produces painful blisters on the penis, within the vagina or cervix, and in the pubic area, thighs and buttocks. Although the blisters may disappear within a week or so without treatment, recurrences are frequent. The disease, if present during pregnancy, may cause damage to the child.

## HERPES ZOSTER (SHINGLES)

Caused by the virus of chickenpox, herpes zoster is an acute nerve inflammation which often begins with chills, fever, malaise and gastrointestinal complaints, followed within a few days by an eruption of blisters along the course of the affected nerve which, about five days later, begin to dry and scab. Most patients recover without any aftereffects except for some scarring, but in some, especially older people, neuralgic pain may persist for years. There is no specific treatment. A corticosteroid such as prednisone given early may relieve symptoms and shorten the duration of the disease. Large doses of vitamin $B_{12}$ have been reported to be helpful in some cases. Local applications of calamine or other lotions are helpful.

**Aural.** Herpes zoster infection may affect the ear, producing fullness, pain, ringing in the ear, hearing impairment, fever to 102°, sometimes with vomiting and dizziness. Treatment is the same as for shingles (above).

**Ophthalmic.** When the viral disease affects the eye, it will produce marked swelling of the eyelids, eye pain, congestion of the conjunctiva. In some cases, glaucoma may develop later. In treatment, corticosteroid drugs are used both systemically and topically.

## HIDRADENITIS SUPPURATIVA

An inflammation of sweat glands, most often in the underarm area, this disease produces boil-like outbreaks and can spread and disable. Treatment includes antibiotics, rest, moist heat. In advanced cases, surgical removal of the affected area may be needed.

## HISTOPLASMOSIS

Caused by a fungus inhaled in contaminated dust, histoplasmosis occurs throughout the United States, in urban as well as rural areas, with greatest incidence in areas north of the Ohio River and west of the Mississippi. An acute form, resembling common upper respiratory infections, produces fever, cough, and malaise. In a small number of cases, the disease may spread from the lungs, producing liver, spleen, and lymph gland (node) enlargement, sometimes mouth or gastrointestinal ulcers, less often ADDISON'S DISEASE. A third form, chronic in the lungs, produces cough and increasing breathing difficulty. Diagnosis is helped by recovery of the fungus in blood, urine, or other tests. Only rarely does the primary acute disease need treatment. In other cases, drug treatment, including amphotericin B, is helpful, sometimes producing dramatic response.

## HIVES (AND GIANT HIVES OR ANGIOEDEMA)

In hives, also known as *urticaria*, slightly elevated patches appear on the skin, redder or paler than surrounding areas, accompanied by itching. The outbreak may be caused by insect stings or bites, by allergy to drugs or certain foods (among the most common: eggs, shellfish, nuts, fruits), or may follow some strep and viral infections. Often, the patches come and go, and after remaining at one site for some hours may disappear only to reappear elsewhere. A more serious form of hives—known as *giant hives, angioneurotic edema,* or *angioedema*—appears as large swellings on the lips, tongue, eyelids, genitalia, or other parts of the body and, when they affect the upper airway, may produce breathing distress and wheezing. The appearance of giant hives is an emergency, calling for immediate medical help and, when the airway is affected, injection of epinephrine and sometimes a throat incision to permit breathing. Ordinary acute hives usually subsides within a week or much less and may be helped by antihistamine tablets. Any suspected factor such as a drug is stopped until the hives disappear.

## HODGKIN'S DISEASE

Also called *malignant granuloma* and *lymphogranuloma*, this disease may occur at any age but most often affects young adults between 20 and 40, men about twice as often as women. Its cause remains unknown, with some cases suggesting a familial tendency. Symptoms include painless enlargement of the lymph glands (nodes), usually first on one side of the neck, then the other, later under the arms and in the groin, often with severe itching. As the disease progresses, it is often marked by sweating, fever, weakness, loss of appetite and weight. Diagnosis is aided by lymph node biopsy. Treatment is by radiation with high-voltage x-rays. Drug therapy also may be used. If treatment is begun early, there usually is remission of symptoms and prolongation of life. Some recent reports suggest that prompt, aggressive treatment may even be considered curative in many, possibly most cases.

## HOOKWORM INFESTATION

Particularly common in the southern United States, hookworm may enter through the mouth but more commonly penetrates through the skin, usually the feet in children who walk barefoot. The source of infection is fecal contamination of the soil. After gaining entry through the skin, the worm migrates to the small intestine, attaches to the intestinal wall, and feeds on blood. The worm can produce darkening of the stool with blood pigments, anemia, retarded growth. Diagnosis is aided by the finding of immature eggs in the stool. Effective medication includes tetrachloroethylene, hexylresorcinol, bephenium hydroxynaphthoate, and thiabendazole.


## HOUSEMAID'S KNEE (see BURSITIS)


## HUNTINGTON'S CHOREA

A rare hereditary disease that leads to degenerative brain changes, Huntington's chorea produces marked personality changes including moodiness, irascibility, obstinacy, and spitefulness, along with irregular jerky movements of the face, neck and arms, speech disturbances, shuffling gait, memory and judgment impairment. Symptoms may occur at other times but most commonly do so after age 30 and before 50. No specific treatment is known. Tranquilizers such as reserpine and chlorpromazine may have some usefulness but do not halt mental deterioration.


## HYDATIDIFORM MOLE

A degeneration of pregnancy, a hydatidiform mole is a mass of cysts, most of them benign, which produces a rapid increase in the size of the uterus shortly after conception, with vaginal bleeding. The condition is revealed by x-ray studies. Removal of the mole is essential and, depending upon such factors as size of the uterus and age of patient, may be achieved with suction curettage, oxytocin followed by dilatation and curettage, incision (hysterotomy) or removal (hysterectomy) of the uterus.


## HYDROCELE (see under SCROTAL MASS in Symptoms Section)


## HYDRONEPHROSIS

In hydronephrosis, the kidney becomes distended with urine as the result of obstruction in the urinary tract, causing recurrent attacks of pain in the kidney region that may be dull, nagging or sharp, sometimes with fever and with blood and pus in the urine. The obstruction may result from stones, tumors, prostate enlargement, urinary tract infections, cancer of bladder, urethra, or glans penis. In treatment, the urinary tract is drained by catheter or other means; any infection is treated with antibiotics and urinary antiseptics. In some cases, surgery may be required.

## HYPERALDOSTERONISM

In this disorder, in which the adrenal glands atop the kidneys secrete excessive amounts of a hormone, aldosterone, symptoms may include episodic weakness, burning or tingling sensations, transient paralysis, muscle spasms and cramps, excessive urination and thirst, and blood pressure elevation. In one type of hyperaldosteronism, the fault lies with overgrowth of the adrenal glands or a benign or malignant tumor; in another, the disorder results from hypertension, heart failure, cirrhosis, or kidney disease. In some cases, surgery may be required to stop the excessive secretion; in others, a drug, spironolactone, may be helpful.

## HYPERHIDROSIS

Often occurring in healthy individuals, hyperhidrosis—excessive sweating in palms, soles, underarm, groin, or underbreast areas—is of unknown cause although tension and anxiety may be involved. Treatment may include use of aluminum chloride solution and potassium permanganate compresses, with a drying powder applied once a day for a time thereafter. In *bromhidrosis,* the excessive perspiration has an unpleasant odor caused by the action of bacteria and yeasts on the sweat. Treatment is the same as for hyperhidrois. Shaving the underarm area is often helpful. In some cases, a germicidal soap may be used along with a topical antibiotic such as neomycin as an underarm deodorant.

## HYPERKALEMIA

Meaning abnormally high levels of potassium in the blood, hyperkalemia may cause paralysis of skeletal muscles. It may result from kidney failure, acidosis, burns, inflammation, heart attack, diuretic drugs, adrenal gland insufficiency. When moderate, it may respond to decreased potassium intake in the diet. More severe hyperkalemia may require infusion of glucose solution containing insulin, sometimes with sodium bicarbonate added, or use of an exchange resin to remove potassium via the bowel. In some cases, cleansing of potassium from the blood by a kidney machine may be required.

## HYPERLIPOPROTEINEMIA, TYPE 1

This is a relatively uncommon disorder caused by a deficiency of an enzyme needed for proper handling of fats (triglycerides). It is manifested by abdominal pains, by pinkish-yellow skin deposits of fats, and sometimes by liver enlargement, with the symptoms intensified by increased amounts of fatty foods in the diet. Treatment consists of greatly restricting all common dietary sources of fat. Special fats, made up of medium-chain fatty acids, which are absorbed in a different way than conventional fats, can be prescribed for use as supplements.

## HYPERPARATHYROIDISM

Overactivity of the parathyroid glands may cause such symptoms as appetite loss, nausea, constipation, abdominal pain, excessive urination, calcium stones in the urinary tract. The excessive gland activity may be caused by overgrowth or benign tumor, rarely a cancer, of the glands. Other possible causes include cancer of lung, kidney or other organs; other endocrine gland disturbances; chronic kidney disease; intestinal malabsorption. Surgical treatment removes excess parathyroid tissue to reduce the gland secretions.

## HYPERTENSION

A common disorder, affecting upward of 23 million Americans, high blood pressure often is silent for many years. Symptoms, when they finally occur, may include one or more of the following: headaches, nervousness, dizziness, palpitation, insomnia, weakness. When uncontrolled for long periods, hypertension may cause heart enlargement, anginal chest pain, heart attack, stroke, eye changes, kidney disturbances. In about 10 percent of cases, the pressure elevation can be traced to a physical cause such as a narrowed kidney artery, benign adrenal gland tumor, narrowing of the aorta, which may be cured by surgery. The remaining cases, 90 percent of the total, are *essential* or of unknown cause, but can be treated effectively with one or a combination of drugs that lower blood pressure and markedly reduce risks of hypertension complications. If treatment produces side effects, a change of dosage or of drugs often helps.

## HYPERTHYROIDISM

Hyperthyroidism—overactivity of the thyroid gland—may produce weakness, heat sensitivity, sweating, overactivity, restlessness, weight loss with increased appetite, tremor, palpitation, stare, abnormal eye protrusion, sometimes with headache, nausea, abdominal pain, diarrhea. The cause is unknown, although there is some familial tendency to the condition. Diagnosis is made by blood and other tests of thyroid function. Treatment to suppress the excess hormone secretion by the gland may include antithyroid drugs such as propylthiouracil and methimazole, radioiodine therapy, or surgical removal of part of the gland.

## HYPERVITAMINOSIS A

The hypervitaminosis, or excessive intake of vitamin A, may cause sparse and coarse hair, eyebrow loss, dry rough skin, cracked lips, severe headaches, generalized weakness, all of which subside within several weeks of discontinuation of the vitamin.

## HYPERVITAMINOSIS D

Excessive intake of vitamin D produces such symptoms as appetite loss, nausea, vomiting, weakness, nervousness, itching, excessive urination and thirst. When long continued, it may lead to irreversible kidney damage. Treatment includes discontinuing use of the vitamin, a low-calcium diet, and keeping the urine acidic.

## HYPOGAMMAGLOBULINEMIA

Almost all antibodies produced in defense of the body are gamma globulin molecules. In hypogammaglobulinemia, gamma globulin levels in the blood are abnormally low and there may be repeated episodes of pneumonia, skin infections, middle ear infections, or meningitis. The disorder may be congenital or acquired following use of certain drugs for cancer or transplantation. In treatment, monthly injections of immune serum globulin, rich in antibodies, may be needed throughout life. Avoidance of exposure to others with known infections is important. Antibiotics are used to combat any infections that do occur.

## HYPOGLYCEMIA

A condition in which the blood sugar level is abnormally low, hypoglycemia may produce, several hours after meals, flushing or pallor, chilliness, numbness, hunger, trembling, headache, dizziness, weakness, palpitation, faintness, sometimes convulsions. It may result from organic disorders such as pancreatic tumors, liver disorders, inadequate pituitary gland function, deficient adrenal gland secretions due to infections or other causes. It may also have functional causes such as poor nutrition, severe muscular exertion. For an acute attack, 10 to 20 grams of dextrose or its equivalent in sugar, candy, orange juice, or honey may be taken by mouth, and bread or other food containing protein and starch helps to prevent relapse. If the hypoglycemia has an organic cause, that must be treated. In functional hypoglycemia, a high-protein, high-fat, low-carbohydrate diet with a snack on waking and another on retiring often helps. If diet alone fails, small doses of corticosteroids may help.

## HYPOKALEMIA

Hypokalemia—abnormally low levels of potassium in the blood—may produce muscular weakness, sometimes with paralysis, breathing difficulty, failure of bowel contraction leading to distention and abdominal pain. Hypokalemia may result from use of diuretic drugs, abuse of cathartics, diarrhea, vomiting, excessive adrenal gland activity. Treatment may require carefully prescribed doses of potassium chloride.

## HYPOPITUITARISM

The pituitary gland at the base of the brain releases numerous hormones involved in varied activities: water conservation, release of milk, growth, thyroid and other endocrine gland activity, ovulation, sperm formation. In hypopituitarism, one or more hormones may be deficient, leading to one or many symptoms including poor appetite, weight loss, easy fatigue, cold intolerance, diminished libido, scantiness or absence of pubic and underarm hair, scanty menstruation, failure to lactate after childbirth. The disorder may result from various types of brain growths, ballooning of an artery feeding the brain, hemorrhage or shock after childbirth, or other causes.

In treatment, hormones ordinarily produced by other glands under the control of pituitary hormone secretions—and not produced for lack of the pituitary hormones—may be prescribed. They may include thyroid and adrenal gland hormones, estrogens, testosterone, and others. When hypopituitarism is due to a tumor, treatment must be directed at the growth and may involve its irradiation or surgical removal.

*Growth failure in a child* may be due to lack of growth hormone from the pituitary, in which case human growth hormone may be administered, although the hormone, because of current difficulty in obtaining it, is expensive and not available in adequate quantities. But growth failure also may be due to other factors, alone or in combination, including nutritional deficiencies (of vitamins, minerals or protein); diseases of liver, kidneys, pancreas, heart, or lungs; malabsorption disorders; deficiencies of thyroid, adrenal, and gonadal hormones. Correction of the deficiencies and treatment of any underlying disease often results in a growth spurt that may make up for previously retarded growth.

## HYPOSPADIAS

In this birth defect in a male baby, the urethral urinary channel, instead of running the full length of the penis, is short and opens to the exterior on the underside, an inch or more from the penis tip. In some cases, the opening is far enough forward so surgical correction is not needed. In other cases, directing the urinary stream is a problem. Also, there may be a fibrous band which curves the penis so sexual intercourse later in life will be difficult. Surgical correction usually is carried out between 1 and 2 years of age.

## HYPOTHYROIDISM (see also CRETINISM)

Hypothyroidism—underfunctioning of the thyroid gland—may result from many causes, including lack of iodine in the diet, deficient pituitary gland secretion of thyrotropin (which activates the thyroid), wasting of the thyroid, or its destruction by radioactive iodine. Symptoms may include dry, cold skin, puffiness of hands and face, decreased appetite, weight gain, slow speech, mental apathy, drowsiness, constipation, hearing loss, poor memory, menstrual disturbances. Symptoms can be abolished with regular use of thyroid hormone.

## ICHTHYOSIS

Sometimes called *fish skin disease,* this is a congenital disorder which may run in families. It is usually mild or moderate, affecting skin over elbows, knees, upper arms and thighs, producing dryness, roughness, scaliness. In more severe cases, skin may thicken, fissures develop, the face become glazed and sometimes red. Some patients who improve in summer may benefit from exposure to sunlight or ultraviolet rays. Often helpful: lubricating the skin with a bland grease such as hydrogenated cooking fat. Vitamin A may be used. A lotion containing urea is sometimes beneficial.

## IMPETIGO

A highly contagious skin infection, usually occurring in infants and young children, occasionally in adults, impetigo is manifested by pustules (or pus-filled lesions) that may rupture or crust within a few hours to several days, sometimes spreading all over the body. If not treated, impetigo may lead to systemic infection. It usually can be cleared with appropriate antibiotics applied to the skin.

## IMPOTENCE (see in Symptoms Section)

## INACTIVE COLON (see COLON, INACTIVE)

## INDIGESTION

Also called *dyspepsia,* indigestion is a complex of symptoms that may include nausea, heartburn, upper abdominal pain, flatulence, belching, feelings of fullness and distention of the stomach, all developing during or after a meal. Although it can result from disease in the gastrointestinal tract or elsewhere, commonly it involves no organic problem. Frequent causes include rapid eating, overeating, eating during emotional upsets, swallowing large amounts of air, excessive smoking, constipation, poorly prepared foods and foods high in fat content, or gas-forming vegetables such as beans, cabbage, turnips, and onions. Fats tend to increase the time before the stomach empties its contents into the small intestine. Although moderate distention of the stomach stimulates stomach activity, overeating that leads to marked distention slows the activity and may cause nausea. Smoking, fear, depression, fatigue, and pain slow stomach activity.

Treatment may require a normal balanced diet, eaten unhurriedly, in a relaxed atmosphere, in moderate amounts, with no smoking beforehand, and avoidance of any foods which, in individual experience, cause trouble.

## INFECTIOUS MONONUCLEOSIS (see MONONUCLEOSIS, INFECTIOUS)

## INFLUENZA

A viral infection, influenza, or "flu," often begins suddenly with chills or chilly sensations and fever. In mild cases, temperature rises to 101° or 102° and fever lasts two or three days; in severe cases, fever may reach 103°–104° and continue for four or five days. Other symptoms include generalized aches and pains most pronounced in the back and legs, headache, weakness, appetite loss, anxiety, moderate sore throat, nonproductive cough, mild distress below the breastbone, sometimes nasal discharge. Acute symptoms usually begin to subside as temperature falls, although weakness, sweating, and fatigue may continue for several days, sometimes longer. Persistence of fever, cough, and other respiratory symptoms may indicate a complication, bacterial pneumonia, which leads to increased cough and sputum production and requires antibiotic treatment.

## INTERMITTENT CLAUDICATION

Associated with atherosclerosis or artery clogging, intermittent claudication produces leg pain and weakness on walking. The pain, absent at rest, begins soon after walking starts, intensifies until walking further becomes impossible, disappears after rest. In severe cases, surgery to bypass obstructed arteries may be performed.

## INTERTRIGO (CHAFING)

Caused by wetness, heat, and friction when skin surfaces rub together, intertrigo, with reddening and skin maceration, may occur in underarm, groin, and anal areas, under the breasts, or in spaces between fingers and toes. Cold compresses often help. In some cases, topical applications of corticosteroids may be used.

## INTESTINAL OBSTRUCTION, MECHANICAL

Mechanical obstruction, blocking the passage of intestinal contents partially or completely, can occur in either the small or large intestine. In complete small intestine obstruction, symptoms include severe intermittent cramplike pain in the navel area, soon followed by vomiting, which at first occurs with but then later independently of the pain, becoming fecal in nature, with no passage of gas or feces. Similar but less severe symptoms occur with partial obstruction, and cramps may be followed by diarrhea. In complete obstruction of the large intestine, or colon, pain is similar but less severe, with infrequent vomiting and slowly developing abdominal distention. In partial colonic obstruction, there are intermittent cramps low in the abdomen and constipation, or constipation alternating with diarrhea.

Intestinal obstructions can result from adhesions after abdominal surgery, hernia, pressure from tumors, impacted feces or foreign bodies, inflammatory narrowings, intussusception (telescoping of one part of the gut into another), volvulus (twisting of a loop of intestine). Other possible causes include a clot in a gut artery or vein and paralytic ileus (failure of peristalsis, or bowel contractions) accompanying peritonitis, gallstones, kidney stones, or following surgery.

Objective of treatment is to overcome the obstruction as quickly as possible. To begin with, fluids may be administered by vein, constant suction applied via a stomach tube, and pain relieved. In complete obstruction, surgery may be required and is often successful. In partial obstruction, a long intestinal tube may be used to try to remove the obstruction; if unsuccessful, surgery is performed.

## IRRITABLE COLON (see COLON, IRRITABLE)

## IRITIS

An inflammation of the iris, the colored portion of the eye with the pupil in its center, iritis can produce severe eye pain, often radiating to the forehead and becoming worse at night, with the eye red and the pupil contracted and sometimes irregular in shape, extreme sensitivity to light, blurring of vision, and tenderness of the eyeball. The inflammation may be acute, with sudden pronounced symptoms, or chronic, with less severe but longer-lasting symptoms. It may be associated with rheumatoid arthritis, diabetes, syphilis, tonsillitis, other infection, or injury. In treatment, the pupil is dilated with atropine drops, and local corticosteroids may be applied frequently to reduce inflammation. Systemic corticosteroids also may be used while the cause is sought and if possible eliminated.

## JUVENILE RHEUMATOID ARTHRITIS (see ARTHRITIS)

## KERATITIS, DENDRITIC

An ulceration of the cornea caused by the herpes simplex "cold sore" virus, dendritic keratitis produces foreign body sensation, tearing, photophobia, congestion of the conjunctiva. A drug, idoxuridine, is usually effective.

## KERATITIS, DISCIFORM

This is a disc-shaped inflammation of the cornea that may follow injury or dendritic keratitis. In treatment, atropine is used to dilate the pupil, and corticosteroids may be used systemically or in the eye, along with idoxuridine.

## KERATITIS, SUPERFICIAL PUNCTATE

Producing photophobia, pain, tearing, and diminished vision, this is a disorder of the cornea (the transparent membrane in the middle of the white of the eye) which may affect one or both eyes. It may accompany eye or eyelid infections or be a reaction to local medication, and may last for as long as several months before virtually complete healing takes place. In treatment, antibiotics or sulfa drugs may be given both systemically and in the eye. Corticosteroids in the eye also may be used.

## KERATOSIS, PLANTAR (see PLANTAR KERATOSIS)

**KIDNEY, CANCER OF** (see CANCER OF THE KIDNEY)

**KIDNEY DISEASE** (see GLOMERULONEPHRITIS, POLYCYSTIC KIDNEY DISEASE, PYELONEPHRITIS, and RENAL FAILURE, ACUTE)

## LARYNGITIS

An inflammation of the larynx, or voice box, laryngitis is accompanied by hoarseness or loss of the voice, often with throat tickling and rawness and constant effort to clear the throat. It can be caused by colds and other respiratory infections and by misuse of the voice. When it is severe, fever, throat pain, swallowing and breathing difficulty may occur. When it stems from infection, laryngitis usually disappears with cure of the infection. Often helpful: rest of the voice, steam inhalation, warm fluids, anesthetic lozenges. Similar but less marked symptoms may occur in chronic laryngitis and may result from repeated attacks of acute laryngitis or from excessive alcohol intake, smoking, abuse of the voice, exposure to irritating fumes or dusts, or chronic inflammation of nose, tonsils, or sinuses.

## LARYNGITIS, ACUTE OBSTRUCTIVE (CROUP)

Occurring chiefly in infants and young children, croup produces a "barking" cough, croaking sound (stridor) during breathing, and spasms of choking. It may result from larynx obstruction due to infection, allergy, or a foreign body. A foreign body, if present, may be removed by bronchoscopy. Steam, humidification, and a mild sedative often are helpful, and a corticosteroid may be valuable in some cases. In very severe cases, tracheostomy—surgically creating an opening in the windpipe through the neck—may be needed to facilitate breathing.

## LARYNGOTRACHEOBRONCHITIS, ACUTE

This is an acute infection that inflames mucous membranes of the larynx, windpipe, and lung passages, leading to tissue congestion and secretion of large amounts of sticky mucus which may threaten to block breathing passages. Symptoms include severe breathing difficulty, violent efforts to breathe, high fever, almost constant but nonproductive cough, hoarseness, flushing followed by pallor and blueness. The infection may occur at any age but most often affects infants and children, most commonly in late winter and early spring. Treatment includes antibacterial agents, oxygen, humidification via vaporizer, nebulizer, or humidifier. Tracheostomy—surgical creation of an opening in the windpipe through the neck—may be needed in some very severe cases to bypass obstruction and permit removal of mucus.

## LARYNX, CANCER OF (see CANCER OF THE LARYNX)

## LARYNX, CONTACT ULCER OF

Occurring almost solely in men, this is a superficial ulceration which may be caused by explosive, tense speech. Symptoms include a sticking sensation and pain sometimes extending to an ear. Treatment consists of resting the voice followed by instruction to correct faulty speech techniques.

## LARYNX, PAPILLOMA OF

A papilloma is a benign tumor that may occur in children as well as in adults, causing loss of voice, sometimes breathing difficulty. Treatment requires removal of the tumor.

## LEPROSY

Also called *Hansen's disease,* leprosy is caused by a bacillus, *Mycobacterium leprae.* The source of infection is believed to be discharge from sores of persons with active disease, yet leprosy is one of the least contagious conditions, with fewer than 5 percent of those exposed ever contracting it. Most of an estimated 10 million cases are in tropical and subtropical regions of Africa, Asia, and Latin America. Of about 2,600 known United States cases, 70 percent were acquired outside the country. An early symptom is appearance of pink or brown patches on the skin. Loss of sensation, appearance of nodules (or small solid swellings), fever, loss of body hair, and painful neuritis may occur and, in some cases, open sores appear on face, forehead, and ear lobes. Treatment is with a sulfone drug, such as dapsone; antibiotics also may be used.

## LEPTOSPIROSIS

Variously known as *Weil's disease, mud fever, autumn fever,* and *swineherd's disease,* leptospirosis is a group of diseases caused by spiral organisms, *Leptospira,* that infect the kidneys of cattle, swine, dogs, cats, rats, and other animals. Infection may be transmitted through direct contact with an afflicted animal's urine or through contaminated water or soil. Although considered an occupational problem, leptospirosis affects most victims through accidental exposure to infected dogs or other animals and through swimming in contaminated water. In the United States, most infection occurs from June through September. After an incubation period of 2 to 20 days, fever, acute headache, chills, sometimes nausea and vomiting appear. Subsequently, jaundice, skin rash, bleeding of skin and mucous membranes, eye inflammation, blood in the urine, and diminished urination may develop. Most cases tend to be mild, lasting one to two weeks. Penicillin or another antibiotic may be used.

## LEUKEMIA, ACUTE

A malignant disease affecting tissues of the bone marrow, spleen and lymph nodes, acute leukemia causes uncontrolled proliferation of white blood cells, reduced numbers of red cells and blood platelets, leading to anemia and increased susceptibility to infections and hemorrhage. Symptoms may include abrupt high fever; mouth, throat, or lung infection; joint pains; small purplish-red skin sores and bruises; bleeding from the mouth, nose, bowel, kidneys. In some cases, however, the disease begins more insidiously with progressive pallor and weakness. There are two major types of acute leukemia: *ALL (acute lymphoblastic),* which predominantly affects children under 10, although a significant number of patients are in the teens and a few are adults up to about age 40; and *AML (acute myeloblastic),* which occurs at all ages but most often affects those from 25 to about 60. Either is rapidly fatal unless treated. Especially in children with ALL, new drugs and drug combinations have been achieving remission in as many as 90 percent of cases, and long-term survivals, which may well be cures, are increasing. In AML, results have been less dramatic, with remissions occurring in fewer cases, but intensive experimentation with new drug combinations lends hope for remission rates that may match those for ALL.

## LEUKEMIA, CHRONIC

One form, *chronic lymphocytic leukemia*, leads to accumulation of white cells that arise in lymph nodes and may move into the bone marrow, replacing normal blood-forming elements there. Occurring most often in the 50-to-70-year age group, more often in men than in women, CLL leads to increasing weakness, fatigue, appetite loss, lymph node swellings, and mild pallor. Onset is insidious, and in one fourth of patients the disease is discovered from a blood count during a routine checkup. Often, no treatment is needed until the disease begins to actively progress; in some patients, it may be present for many years without symptoms. In treatment, x-ray therapy, radiophosphorus, anticancer drugs, and corticosteroids such as prednisone may be used to destroy most of the abnormal leukemic tissue and may cause all indications of disease to disappear for long periods.

Another form, *chronic myelocytic leukemia*, leads to white blood cell accumulation in bone marrow, spleen, liver and blood, and later in the intestinal tract, lungs, kidneys, lymph nodes, and gonads. Symptoms may include weakness, fatigue, appetite loss, weight loss, vague upper abdominal distress or heaviness, breastbone tenderness. In therapy, anticancer drugs and sometimes radiation or radiophosphorus may be used and may keep a patient in almost normal health, but often the patient becomes less responsive in time and may succumb to anemia, hemorrhage, fever, exhaustion, and infection. Currently about 20 percent of patients survive for more than five years, a few for more than ten. There is increasing hope of further gains.

## LEUKOPLAKIA

In leukoplakia, thickened white patches appear on gums, lips, tongue, or other mucous membranes, tend to grow into larger patches or ulcerate, and may in time grow malignant. Affecting men more often than women, they result from prolonged irritation that may be caused by repeated injury, poor dentures, sharp tooth surfaces, tobacco, highly seasoned foods. Treatment is aimed at removing any possible cause and may require avoidance of tobacco, alcohol, some foods, and attention to teeth or dentures. Surgical removal of affected areas is relatively simple and often is the best means of preventing further development.

## LEUKORRHEA

The vaginal and cervical glands normally secrete a mucuslike fluid to moisten vaginal membranes. The discharge often increases at ovulation, before menstruation, and with sexual excitement. Excessive discharge, with or without odor, may indicate an abnormality. A yellowish or creamy white discharge often contains pus, indicating infection. An excessive thinner or seemingly clear mucous discharge may indicate a chronic disorder. A frequent leukorrhea cause is trichomonas infection, with usually yellowish discharge, unpleasant odor, itching. Other infectious organisms, including bacteria and fungi, may be responsible. Infection of the cervix may occur during childbirth, or infection may result from contraceptive devices left in the vagina too long or from venereal disease. Leukorrhea also may result from other causes, including pelvic congestion associated with heart disease and polyps or myoma of the uterus. Sometimes, it is an early indication of cervical malignancy. Treatment is directed at the cause and, in case of infection, will include suitable antiinfective agents.

## LICE INFESTATION (see PEDICULOSIS)

## LICHEN PLANUS

Of unknown cause, lichen planus is an inflammatory eruption of itching patches of pimplelike, violaceous lesions on wrists, front and back leg surfaces, trunk, genital area, and sometimes the mouth. The eruption may persist for weeks or months and recur for years. Treatment may include use of cyproheptadine or trimeprazine to relieve itching and, in severe cases, corticosteroid drugs.

## LIP CANCER (see CANCER OF THE LIP)

## LIVER CANCER (see CANCER OF THE LIVER)

## LOEFFLER'S SYNDROME

A lung inflammation sometimes caused by parasitic worms but often of unknown cause, Loeffler's syndrome may produce cough, with or without a stitch in the side, sometimes with slight fever, and exacerbation of symptoms in an asthmatic. The disorder is usually benign and self-limited. If a parasite is the cause, it may be detected in sputum and a deworming drug used. Otherwise, if symptoms are severe, a corticosteroid may be prescribed.

## LUNG ABSCESS

A lung abscess—with purulent sputum, sweats, chills, fever, appetite loss, and sometimes chest pain—may develop because of bronchial obstruction due to pneumonia, malignancy, a foreign body or foreign material that may get into the lung during regurgitation. Antibiotic treatment, which may be continued for as long as six to eight weeks, is usually effective. Surgery may be performed in other cases and may involve removal of a lobe of a lung or, sometimes, if multiple abscesses are present, removal of a whole lung.

## LUNG CANCER (see CANCER OF THE LUNG)

## LUPUS ERYTHEMATOSUS

Of unknown cause, occurring most often in young women in their 20s, lupus erythematosus takes two forms. One, *chronic discoid*, is limited to the skin, producing a red eruption of nose and cheek shaped somewhat like a butterfly, with itching and scaling. The other, more serious form, *systemic*, is an inflammatory connective tissue disorder which, in addition to skin manifestations, can affect the joints and produce arthritislike joint pains, the lungs and produce recurrent attacks of lung inflammation, or the kidneys and produce inflammation there. A patient with systemic lupus erythematosus may have fever, abdominal, muscle and joint pains, spleen enlargement, congestive heart failure. Treatment for the chronic discoid form may include avoidance of exposure to sunlight, use of topical applications of triamcinolone or another corticosteroid, or oral doses of an antimalarial drug. For the systemic form, treatment may include aspirin, corticosteroids, sometimes antimalarial and other drugs.

## LYMPHANGIECTASIA, INTESTINAL

Causing dilation of lymph vessels within the lining of the small intestine, this disorder affects mostly children and young adults. In some cases, it may be congenital, in others the result of pancreatitis or other disease. Intestinal lymphangiectasia produces massive edema or waterlogging of body tissues, abdominal pain, nausea, vomiting, mild intermittent diarrhea. Some patients recently have benefited from a diet low in fat or one including medium-chain triglycerides (fats). If the disorder is limited to a small area of the intestine, surgical removal of the area may be indicated.


## LYMPHEDEMA (see also under SCROTAL MASS in Symptoms Section)

Producing painless chronic swelling of the whole or part of an arm or leg, lymphedema is caused by abnormalities in lymph vessels or nodes which impair circulation of lymphatic fluid. It may be congenital or may follow an infectious tropical disease, filariasis, or irradiation or radical surgery for breast cancer. In treatment, diuretic drugs are used to promote fluid elimination, and a low-salt diet, elastic compression and frequent elevation of the affected arm or leg are used to minimize fluid accumulation.


## LYMPHOGRANULOMA VENEREUM

A venereal disease, lymphogranuloma venereum produces, usually within 7 to 12 days after infection, a small hard sore in the genital area. The disease soon spreads to lymph nodes, particularly those in the groin, which swell to walnut size. In women, the vulva may become enlarged, the rectum narrowed. In early stages of the disease, joint inflammation, skin rash, and fever may be present. The disease usually can be treated successfully with an antibiotic such as tetracycline.


## LYMPHOSARCOMA

A malignancy that may arise in lymph nodes or in lymphatic tissue in the gastrointestinal tract, lymphosarcoma produces gland (node) enlargement in the neck, under the arms, or in the groin, usually on one side. Late in the disease, fever, sweating, lack of strength, and debility develop. Diagnosis depends upon microscopic study of biopsied tissue. Treatment is similar to that for HODGKIN'S DISEASE.

## MACROGLOBULINEMIA

Occurring most often in elderly people, this is a disease in which macroglobulins, proteins of unusually high molecular weight, appear in the blood. It begins usually with vague symptoms of ill health and weight loss, followed by repeated infections, bleeding of mucous membranes, anemia. In treatment, a drug such as melphalan or cyclophosphamide is used and, when necessary because of abnormal blood thickening, some blood plasma may be withdrawn.

## MADUROMYCOSIS

This fungal disease of the foot, occasionally of the hand, may begin with a small solid elevated lesion or an abscess that ruptures and produces a fistula, or tubelike passage. Half a dozen or more elevations or abscesses may appear successively and disappear. The foot becomes swollen and deformed with many fistulas producing an oily fluid containing colored granules. Unless diagnosed and treated, the disease persists for years and may involve muscles, tendons, and bone. In treatment, penicillin or sulfa drugs may be used.

## MALARIA

Found mostly in tropical and subtropical regions, malaria is caused by a mosquito-transmitted parasite, *Plasmodium*. Symptoms include chills followed in a few hours by fever up to 105° which subsides and is followed by profuse perspiration. Other symptoms are headache, nausea, body pains, and, after an attack, exhaustion. Quinine was once the standard treatment for malaria, but more recently superior synthetic drugs such as chloroquine, pentaquine, and quinacrine have become available and can be used to relieve attacks and cure the infection. No vaccine for malaria is available, but antimalarial drugs can be given in advance to anyone traveling to malaria-prone areas.

## MASTITIS, CHRONIC CYSTIC

The most common breast disease, this is a benign condition in which cysts develop, usually in both breasts, often multiple and of many sizes, giving the breasts a "cobblestone" feel, in some cases without symptoms, in others with tenderness and premenstrual breast discomfort. Treatment is simple removal of the diseased area.

## MASTOIDITIS, ACUTE

A complication that may occur in untreated or inadequately treated middle ear infection, acute mastoiditis produces pain over the mastoid bone behind the ear, usually with discharge from the ear. Antibiotic treatment is usually effective. In a few cases, mastoid surgery may be needed.

## MEASLES

A highly contagious childhood viral disease, also called *rubeola*, measles is spread by droplet infection and can be acquired by touching any article that an infected person has recently used. The incubation period ranges from about 9 to 14 days and the disease can be transmitted to others about 3 or 4 days prior to rash appearance and until the rash begins to fade, a total of approximately 7 or 8 days. One attack usually provides lifetime immunity. Often the disease begins with a tired feeling, slight fever, pains in head and back, reddening of the eyes, sensitivity to light. The fever rises a little each day, and about the third or fourth day reaches 103° or 104°. Small white dots often can be seen on the gums and inside of the cheeks. A rash starts at the hairline and behind the ears, spreads downward, and covers the body in about 36 hours. At first the rash consists of separate pink spots, about one-fourth inch in diameter; later the spots may run together. Fever usually goes down after the rash has spread, and the rash fades after 3 or 4 days. Treatment consists of bed rest as long as rash and fever continue, fluids, and aspirin for fever. Nose drops and cough medicine may be prescribed. For itching, calamine lotion, cornstarch solution, or cool water may be used and, if necessary, an antihistamine drug.

## MEASLES, GERMAN

Also known as *rubella* and *three-day measles*, German measles is a mild viral disease that begins with fever, slight cold, and sore throat. A rash, similar to that of measles except that the spots do not run together, appears on the face and scalp and the same day spreads to body and arms, usually fading after two or three days. Other than bed rest, no special treatment usually is needed. German measles, almost invariably of little consequence in a child, can be dangerous in a pregnant woman because the chances are great that during the first three months of pregnancy the virus can cause serious defects in the fetus. A vaccine is available.

## MEGACOLON

Usually occurring in children, megacolon may be congenital, in which case it is also called *Hirschsprung's disease*, and is the result of absence of normal nerve supply to the wall of the colon so that the colon fails to propel feces for evacuation, leading to severe constipation, abdominal distention, vomiting, appetite loss. Surgery may be performed to remove the area of colon lacking the nerve supply and connect up the remaining portions. Megacolon may be acquired rather than congenital in some cases, usually in retarded or mentally ill children who refuse to try to move their bowels, and psychiatric treatment may be needed, along with laxatives and enemas.

## MENIERE'S DISEASE

This is a disturbance of the labyrinth of the inner ear, most often affecting one ear. It may develop after head injury or ear infection but often has no apparent cause. Symptoms may include repeated episodes of hearing impairment, ringing in the ears, dizziness, nausea and vomiting, sometimes oscillation of the eyeball (nystagmus). During acute attacks, medication such as dimenhydrinate is often effective. A vasodilating drug such as niacin may be useful. In severe, incapacitating cases, ultrasound (high-frequency sound waves) may be used to destroy the labyrinth while preserving hearing. Other surgical techniques are sometimes used.

## MENINGITIS

An inflammation of the meninges, the membranes that cover brain and spinal cord, meningitis may produce stiff neck, persistent headache, vomiting, fever, and, in infants, convulsions. It results from infection by bacteria, viruses, or fungi. An epidemic type, meningococcemia, is caused by meningococcal bacteria and is very contagious because the bacteria also are present in the throat as well as cerebrospinal fluid. Tuberculous meningitis is produced by the same organisms that cause lung TB. Aseptic meningitis, which occurs mainly among young children during the warm months, is caused by viruses and often is accompanied by a skin rash. Most viral meningitis in the United States results from mumps and polio viruses, less frequently from other viruses such as herpes simplex, which is also responsible for cold sores. Diagnosis of meningitis is confirmed by identification of organisms in a sample of cerebrospinal fluid. Treatment is with a suitable antibiotic often administered by vein. Corticosteroids also may be used. In fungal meningitis, a special antibiotic, amphotericin B, is often used.

## MENSTRUATION, ABSENCE OF (see AMENORRHEA)

## MENSTRUATION, PAINFUL (see DYSMENORRHEA)

## METABOLIC ACIDOSIS

This is a condition in which acid accumulates in blood and body tissues, bicarbonate levels fall, and other chemical changes take place. Symptoms may include weakness, headache, malaise, sometimes abdominal pain, nausea, vomiting. Metabolic acidosis may result from large losses of bicarbonate in diarrhea; from excessive acid production as in diabetic ketoacidosis (when diabetes is uncontrolled); from interference with normal handling of acids that may result from poisoning with aspirin, aspirinlike compounds, methyl alcohol, and ethylene glycol; from impaired kidney excretion of acid in kidney failure; or from severe dehydration. Severe acidosis can be corrected with sodium bicarbonate administered by vein. Correction of an underlying problem, such as providing insulin in diabetic acidosis, is vital.

## METABOLIC ALKALOSIS

This is a condition in which the blood becomes alkaline and contains increased levels of bicarbonate. Symptoms may include irritability, shallow or irregular breathing, prickling or burning sensations in the fingers, toes, or lips, muscle cramps. Metabolic alkalosis may be caused by excessive vomiting, treatment with diuretics, Cushing's syndrome, hyperaldosteronism. The alkalosis can be remedied by correction of fluid, sodium, potassium and chloride deficiencies.

## MIGRAINE

Although the cause is not completely understood, migraine is believed to be associated with constriction and then dilation of brain arteries. It is also thought to have a psychologic aspect, since it often follows emotional disturbances. It also tends to run in families. Symptoms of migraine can vary. Typically, an episode may begin with changes in vision, such as flickering before the eyes, flashes of light, or blacking out of part of sight. The headache is severe, often on one side of the head, sometimes accompanied by nausea and vomiting. Aspirin is usually of little help. Ergotamine tartrate is often used. Some success in helping migraine patients with biofeedback has been reported. Recently, too, the drug propranolol, often used for heart patients, has been showing promise in reducing the frequency and severity of attacks and, in some cases, eliminating them.

## MILIARIA (HEAT RASH, PRICKLY RASH)

The result of obstruction of sweat ducts, miliaria is characterized by pinhead-size itching eruptions, sometimes with small vesicles or blisters, on the chest, back, waistline, underarms, or other areas. It may be triggered by skin irritation from adhesive tape, sunburn, wet compresses, diapers, exercise. The eruption disappears within days, sometimes hours, if the cause is eliminated. A starch bath is often soothing. A drying lotion may provide relief. When necessary, a corticosteroid lotion or cream may be prescribed.

## MILK LEG (see VENOUS THROMBOSIS)

## MITRAL INSUFFICIENCY

The mitral valve within the heart controls movement of blood from the left atrium, where it arrives freshened from the lungs, into the left ventricle below which pumps it out to the body. In mitral insufficiency, which may be an aftermath of rheumatic fever, the valve fails to close properly so blood can leak backward from ventricle to atrium. With severe backward flow, weakness and fatigue develop, and replacement of the valve with an artificial one may be needed.

## MITRAL STENOSIS

The mitral valve functions as indicated immediately above. In mitral stenosis, which may be an aftermath of rheumatic fever, the valve is unable to open properly. As a result, the flow of blood from atrium to ventricle is reduced; and since the atrium, in contracting, cannot push most of its blood through to the ventricle, pressure builds up in the atrium and is transmitted back through the pulmonary veins to the lungs, affecting lung function, causing, at first, labored breathing on severe exertion and later limiting exercise ability. There may be spitting of blood as small vessels in the lungs and airways rupture. Surgery to snip apart the fused leaflets of the valve to permit improved blood flow may be required.

## MONONUCLEOSIS, INFECTIOUS

Mainly a disease of children and young adults, infectious mononucleosis is believed to be viral in nature with its transmission not fully understood. It occurs most frequently in the spring. It commonly begins with malaise, fatigue, headache and chilliness. Gland (lymph node) swellings in the neck and elsewhere are common, giving the disease its other name of *glandular fever*. Mononucleosis may affect many areas of the body, producing one or many other symptoms: sore throat, fever, abdominal pain, nausea, jaundice, faintly red skin eruptions, eyelid swelling, severe headache, stiff neck, photophobia, eyeball tenderness, chest pain, breathing difficulty, and cough. There is no specific drug treatment. Bed rest, liberal fluids, aspirin to reduce temperature, gargles and anesthetic lozenges for sore throat may be used; and if secondary infection develops, an antibiotic may be needed. The disease is usually benign, departing within one to three weeks, although in some cases it may hang on much longer. There is no aftermath.

## MOTION SICKNESS

Caused by excessive stimulation of inner ear apparatus, motion sickness may produce cold sweating, yawning, pallor, sometimes headache and dizziness, nausea and vomiting. It is best treated before nausea and vomiting appear. Before any activity (such as air, car, train, or other travel) likely to cause motion sickness, phenobarbital or another drug such as dimenhydrinate, meclizine, cyclizine, or hyoscine is often effective. Once vomiting begins, medication must be given by injection or per rectum.

## MOUTH CANCER (see CANCER OF THE MOUTH)

## MULTIPLE SCLEROSIS

Of unknown cause, MS generally occurs in young adults and leads to formation of hardened patches in the brain and spinal cord which interfere with normal nerve activity. Symptoms may be any or many of the following: double vision or loss of part of the visual field, weakness, fatigue, tremor or shaking of limbs, slowing and monotony of speech, impaired balance, unsteady walking, unbending knees, stiff gait, loss of bladder and bowel control, paralysis in any part of the body. Although not a killer, the disease can be extremely disabling. It is subject to spontaneous improvement and exacerbation. No specific treatment is known. Physiotherapy and muscle training may be helpful.

## MUMPS

A viral disease spread by droplet infection, mumps causes swelling of a parotid gland, one of the salivary glands located on either side of the face, just below and in front of the ears. Early in the disease, temperature may reach 100° to 104°. Other common symptoms include appetite loss, headache, and back pain. The gland swelling increases for two or three days, then diminishes, disappearing by the sixth or seventh day. Usually, swelling appears first on one side, then the other, with as many as 10 or 12 days intervening. Occasionally, both sides swell simultaneously or the second side does not swell at all. In boys past puberty, the testes may become inflamed in some cases and this can, but does not necessarily, present further complications. Other complications that sometimes develop include pancreas inflammation, prostatitis, and kidney inflammation. Treatment for mumps itself and any complications is directed at symptoms and may include bed rest, soft diet, aspirin, phenobarbital, ice packs.

## MUSCULAR DYSTROPHIES

These are several related muscular disorders that are progressively crippling, involving loss of protein in affected muscles and its replacement by fat and connective tissue, leading to muscle wasting and weakness. Muscles of pelvis, shoulder, legs, or eyes may be affected. There is no specific drug therapy. Treatment may include exercises to strengthen muscles, braces, corrective surgery.

## MYASTHENIA GRAVIS

A chronic disease characterized by muscular weakness thought to be due to a chemical defect at the sites where nerves and muscles interact, myasthenia gravis may occur at any age in either sex but is most common in young adult women. Symptoms may include drooping of eyelids, double vision, swallowing and speaking difficulty. Drugs such as neostigmine and pyridostigmine have been used with some success. Additional benefit sometimes is achieved with ephedrine. In some cases, removal of the thymus gland, situated behind the upper part of the breastbone, has been found valuable.

## MYELOMA, MULTIPLE

Originating in the bone marrow, most commonly affecting people over 40, with men predominating two to one, multiple myeloma is a progressive, malignant disease. It most often affects bones of pelvis, spine and rib, causing persistent pain, weight loss, and recurrent bacterial infections. Although the disease is usually fatal, various measures may make the patient more comfortable and extend life. They include pain-relieving agents, splints, x-ray therapy, and anti-cancer chemotherapy with drugs such as melphalan and cyclophosphamide.

## MYOMA OF THE UTERUS (see UTERUS, MYOMA OF THE)

## MYRINGITIS

An inflammation of the tympanic membrane (or eardrum), myringitis may be caused by infection or injury (from bobby pins, toothpicks). It produces severe ear pain, hearing impairment, fever. Treatment may include aspirin or codeine for pain, systemic antibiotics, and ear drops containing antibiotics and corticosteroids.

## NAIL INFECTIONS (see PARONYCHIAL INFECTIONS)

## NARCOLEPSY

Of unknown origin, narcolepsy is more frequent in men than in women and usually begins during adolescence or young adulthood. It can produce sleep attacks, a few to many a day, that may last only minutes and are almost impossible to resist even in the midst of eating or driving a car; weakness or momentary limb paralysis, especially during emotional reactions such as anger, fear or joy; sleep paralysis, a momentary inability to move just upon falling asleep or waking up; hallucinations at the beginning of sleep. Treatment, often effective in abolishing the symptoms, involves the use of stimulant drugs such as amphetamine, dextroamphetamine, or methylphenidate in doses calculated not to interfere with normal sleep.

## NEPHROTIC SYNDROME

Also called *nephrosis*, this is a disorder in which kidney tissue malfunctions without inflammation, failing to properly regulate the body's water content. It is marked by accumulation of fluid in the body, loss of protein in the urine, and decreased albumin in the blood. The disease sometimes follows acute kidney infection but may also occur without previous kidney disorder. The edema and swelling may be massive, affecting arms, face, and torso. A low-salt diet and diuretic drugs can be used to reduce edema, and in some patients a corticosteroid such as prednisone leads to remission of the disorder. Other drugs such as azathioprine and cyclophosphamide have been successful in some patients not responding to corticosteroids.

## NEURALGIA

Neuralgia means paroxysms of severe, throbbing or stabbing pain along the course of a nerve for which no cause usually can be found. A neuralgia may subside after a time or may persist. Hot or cold applications and aspirin or other pain-relieving agents may help. In very severe, otherwise unyielding neuralgia, a drug such as diphenylhydantoin provides relief in some cases, while another agent, carbamazepine, reduces attack frequency in more than two thirds of patients. When necessary, injection of alcohol into an affected nerve or cutting of the nerve may be done.

One form of neuralgia sometimes may seem like heart trouble. This is neuralgia of the intercostal nerve which is distributed to the muscles and skin of the chest, back, and upper abdomen. *Intercostal neuralgia* can produce pain in the chest wall. In *glossopharyngeal neuralgia*, pain usually begins in the throat and base of the tongue, radiates to the ears and sometimes down the side of the neck. In the best known neuralgia, *trigeminal*, also called *tic douloureux*, pain occurs in the face and forehead.

**NEURITIS** (see POLYNEURITIS)

**NEUROBLASTOMA**

The most common solid malignancy of childhood, neuroblastoma may originate in nerve cells in the adrenal glands or elsewhere in the nervous system, usually within the abdomen, sometimes in the chest. Symptoms, which come from pressure exerted by the growth, may include a usually firm but not tender abdominal mass, obstruction of urine flow, breathing difficulty, fever, weight loss. When possible, surgery is performed in treatment. Radiation and drug therapy are also employed. There is some chance for cure.

**NEURODERMATITIS** (see DERMATITIS, ATOPIC)

**NEUTROPENIA** (see PRIMARY SPLENIC NEUTROPENIA)

**NIACIN DEFICIENCY** (see VITAMIN DEFICIENCIES)

**NYSTAGMUS**

This is involuntary rhythmic, horizontal, vertical or rotatory oscillation of the eyeball. It may result from poor vision caused by congenital abnormalities or, when it appears in later life, may stem from inner ear disease, multiple sclerosis, prolonged use of eyes with bad light and in strained position, fatigue of eye muscles from myopia or astigmatism. Nystagmus may be relieved in some cases by correction of refraction error and other causes of eyestrain or by treatment of underlying disease; in other cases, eye muscle surgery may be needed.

## OPHTHALMIA, SYMPATHETIC

In sympathetic ophthalmia, after one eye is injured, the other becomes involved, with symptoms such as blurring of vision, tearing, pain, tenderness, sensitivity to light. The disorder often can be prevented by prompt, effective treatment for the injured eye.

## OPTIC ATROPHY

A degeneration of the optic nerve which may cause moderate to total loss of vision, optic atrophy may result from syphilis, glaucoma, injury, optic neuritis, or any drug that may injure the nerve. Treatment is directed at any underlying cause. In some cases large doses of the vitamin nicotinic acid (niacin) or of corticosteroids may be of value.

## OPTIC NEURITIS

An inflammation of the optic nerve, optic neuritis almost always affects only one eye and may produce vision disturbances ranging from only slight contraction of the vision field to blindness. Possible causes include meningitis, encephalitis, syphilis, acute fever-producing diseases, multiple sclerosis, and poisoning with various substances such as methyl alcohol and carbon tetrachloride. Immediate use of corticosteroids, either systemically or injected behind the eyeball, often helps.

## ORBITAL CELLULITIS

An inflammation of the tissues of the orbit, the bony cavity containing the eyeball and its muscles, nerves and blood vessels, and other structures, orbital cellulitis may cause severe pain, impaired eye motion, lid swelling, and edema of the conjunctiva. It may be caused by injury to the orbit or by extension of infection from nasal sinuses or teeth, or from elsewhere. Treatment includes suitable antibiotics and sulfa drugs, bed rest, hot applications to localize infection, medication for pain.

## OSTEITIS DEFORMANS (see PAGET'S DISEASE)

## OSTEOARTHRITIS (see under ARTHRITIS)

## OSTEOMALACIA

Like rickets in a child, osteomalacia in adults results from vitamin D deficiency. In a child, the deficiency may lead to bone softening, nodules on ribs, bending of bones, bowleg, knock-knee, misshapen skull. In adults, it may cause bending, flattening or other deformation of bones in the spine, pelvis, and legs. In both cases, cure can be achieved gradually with prescribed doses of vitamin D along with adequate dietary intake of calcium and phosphorus. There is a type of vitamin D–resistant rickets, often familial, which responds only to massive doses of the vitamin and calcium supplements.

## OSTEOMYELITIS

A bone inflammation caused by invading bacteria that may reach the bone through a compound fracture or other injury, from a nearby infection, or through the blood, osteomyelitis may produce sudden pain in a bone anywhere, with fever, tenderness over the bone, painful movement, swelling. The disease usually can be controlled by prompt treatment with suitable antibiotics, greatly reducing the risk of chronic osteomyelitis. In the now-rare chronic cases, destroyed bone must be removed.

## OSTEOPOROSIS

Osteoporosis—loss of bone density with bones becoming porous and brittle—is most common in women after menopause but may be present to some extent in both men and women at younger ages. Symptoms may include pain in the vertebrae, often from the mid-back down, sometimes with rounding of shoulders, height loss, vertebral fractures. Causes include lack of physical activity, lack of estrogens or other hormones, possibly chronic low intake of calcium in the diet. Osteoporosis may occur in Cushing's disease and in liver disease. Many measures may be used in treatment, with some benefit, but with still some question as to which may be most effective. The measures include calcium and vitamin D supplements, fluoride supplements, estrogen administration, and, more recently, newly available calcitonin, a thyroid gland hormone.

## OTITIS, ACUTE EXTERNAL

An inflammation of the skin of the ear canal, acute external otitis often follows swimming and may produce severe pain in the outer ear, sometimes with fever and enlargement of neck lymph nodes. Treatment with antibiotics and a corticosteroid ear-drop preparation often produces prompt relief.

## OTITIS MEDIA, ACUTE

An inflammation of one or both middle ears, otitis media may stem from disease organisms which spread from nose and throat through the eustachian tubes or from eardrum injury. Symptoms include earache, fullness, fever, chills, sometimes ringing in the ear and impaired hearing. Treatment may include antibiotics or sulfa drugs, heat, and antihistamines and decongestants to keep eustachian tubes and nasal passages open and help drainage from the middle ear. In some cases, incision of the eardrum may be needed.

## OTITIS MEDIA, CHRONIC CONGESTIVE

Producing gradual hearing loss, ringing in the ear, dizziness but rarely pain, this condition may follow repeated attacks of acute otitis media or nose and throat infections involving the eustachian tube. Treatment may involve inflation of the eustachian tube, insertion of a plastic tube in the middle ear for a period of time, sometimes surgery to break up any adhesions that may be present in the middle ear.

## OTITIS MEDIA, CHRONIC PURULENT

Usually preceded by acute otitis media or acute mastoiditis, this condition produces a chronic purulent discharge from the ear, sometimes with pain, low-grade fever, impaired hearing, and ringing in the ear. Treatment may include systemic antibiotics, ear drops containing antibiotics and corticosteroids, other local applications.

## OTITIS MEDIA, CHRONIC SECRETORY

This disorder results from an inflammation of the middle ear, an allergic reaction, or changes in ear pressure after high-altitude flying or deep-sea diving. Symptoms are ear pain, fullness and deafness, with pain disappearing in a few days but fullness and deafness persisting and often accompanied by a sensation of water in the affected ear. Treatment may include withdrawal of fluid through an eardrum incision, eustachian tube inflation, antihistamines, and decongestants.

## OTOMYCOSIS

This is a fungal infection of the external ear that may produce severe itching, pain, or stinging sensation in the ear canal. Treatment is with a suitable antifungal agent.

## OTOSCLEROSIS

In otosclerosis, spongy bone forms in the internal ear, fixing the stapes bone so it cannot conduct sound. Producing progressive loss of hearing, otosclerosis is the prime cause of conductive deafness in young adults, usually appearing between the ages of 18 and 40, affecting women more often than men. Most patients benefit from surgery carried out through the ear canal and middle ear, in which the stapes (stirrup bone) may be replaced with a prosthetic device, reestablishing sound conduction.

**OVARIAN CANCER** (see CANCER OF THE OVARY)

**OVARY, POLYCYSTIC** (see POLYCYSTIC OVARY SYNDROME)

## PAGET'S DISEASE

Also called *osteitis deformans,* this is a slowly progressive bone disorder of unknown cause, usually occurring after age 40 and affecting men and women equally. Symptoms may include bone pain (commonly of pelvis, skull, spine, legs), with bone softening, thickening, enlargement and deformity, sometimes with hearing impairment from temporal bone involvement. In treatment, estrogens, male sex hormones, and fluoride may be used. Recently, promising results have been obtained with the thyroid hormone calcitonin.

## PANCREATITIS, ACUTE

An inflammation of the pancreas, acute pancreatitis sometimes occurs with gallstones, is more common in alcoholics, may follow injury, abdominal surgery, a penetrating peptic ulcer, infectious disease, pregnancy, use of corticosteroid or diuretic drugs. Symptoms may include severe abdominal pain (steady, boring, sharpest in the area about the stomach, extending to the back and chest, often relieved by sitting up), with fever, nausea, vomiting. In treatment, intravenous fluids are given to overcome dehydration; in some cases blood transfusions are needed. Suction of the stomach helps reduce both distention and stimulation of the pancreas. Atropine or another drug may be used to inhibit pancreatic secretion, along with a pain-relieving agent, and antibiotics if infection develops. Any underlying disease requires treatment, and in some cases, as with gallstones, surgery may be needed.

## PANCREATITIS, CHRONIC

Chronic inflammation of the pancreas may lead to such symptoms as abdominal pain (constant or intermittent, mild or severe, beginning in the stomach area and sometimes radiating to back, left shoulder), sometimes with fever and jaundice. The disease may begin as a series of acute attacks after a first episode of acute pancreatitis or may appear as an insidious chronic disorder. No specific curative treatment is known. Alcohol is banned. A diet high in carbohydrates, low in fat, with vitamin B supplements may be used. Pancreatin, a substance containing pancreatic enzymes, may be helpful. Any underlying condition, such as diabetes or gallbladder disease, must be treated. If pain cannot be otherwise relieved, removal of part of the pancreas may be indicated.

## PANOPHTHALMITIS

This is an infection that produces intense eye pain, rapid vision loss, lid swelling, spread of pus throughout the interior of the eye.

For treatment, large doses of antibiotics or sulfa drugs may be used both systemically and within the eye; corticosteroids, often given simultaneously, are also helpful.

## PAPILLOMA, BENIGN INTRADUCTAL

Producing a clear or bloody discharge from the nipple, a benign intraductal papilloma is a tumor within the ducts of the breast. It is relatively rare and may occur at any age from puberty to old age. Surgical removal of the affected duct or ducts is the treatment. Much more rarely, an intraductal papilloma may be malignant, particularly if the discharge is bloody. Surgery is required and may be coupled with radiotherapy and chemotherapy.

## PARKINSON'S DISEASE (SHAKING PALSY)

A chronic nervous system disorder occurring in later life, Parkinson's disease may, in some cases, result from viral infection or carbon monoxide poisoning, but usually the cause is unknown. Symptoms may include tremor of the hands and nodding of the head, loss of mobility in the face, with tremors increasing and sometimes involving the whole body, stiffening of muscles so movement is increasingly difficult, shuffling gait, stooped position with back bent forward. A drug, levo-dopa, is often effective in relieving parkinsonian symptoms. Other drugs, such as diphenhydramine and biperiden, may be used. Brain surgery has sometimes been performed to relieve tremor and rigidity.

## PARONYCHIAL INFECTIONS

Produced by bacteria or fungi that may gain entrance through a hangnail or break in the skin due to improper manicuring, these infections involve the folds of tissue surrounding the fingernail. Acute infections are treated with hot compresses and an antibiotic or antifungal ointment. A pocket of purulent material may require incision to promote drainage and healing. Chronic infections are more difficult to clear and may require use of a corticosteroid ointment. If infection is widespread and difficult to treat topically, nail removal may be needed.

## PAROXYSMAL TACHYCARDIA

This is a condition in which the heart rate suddenly shoots up to 100 or more beats a minute. Symptoms may include fluttering sensation in the chest, weakness, faintness, nausea. Paroxysmal tachycardia may occur in rheumatic or other heart disease but also may appear in a normal heart and may be induced by anxiety, fatigue, tobacco, tea or coffee, and sometimes by gastrointestinal, nervous system, or genitourinary system disturbances. An episode may last for minutes or hours, or even days, ending as suddenly as it began. In some cases, the fast beat may be interrupted by exhaling or trying to inhale with the glottis (the opening between vocal cords) closed; lying down with feet in air; bending over; or vomiting induced mechanically or with a warm solution of sodium bicarbonate. When necessary, a normal rate may be restored by drugs such as neostigmine, quinidine, procainamide, digitalis, or others.

## PATENT DUCTUS ARTERIOSUS

Before birth, the ductus arteriosus, a channel conducting blood between pulmonary artery and aorta, is needed. No longer necessary after birth, it normally closes off. In some children, however, the duct remains open, or patent. As a result some of the fresh blood flowing from heart to aorta is shunted back to the lungs needlessly, causing the heart to work harder and lose pumping efficiency. Symptoms may include blueness of the lower half of a baby's body and clubbing of the toes. A typical murmur helps in diagnosis. Surgical closure of the ductus corrects the anomaly completely. The operation is relatively simple since the ductus is located outside the heart. Recently, early results with medical treatment to close the ductus appear promising and suggest that in some cases surgery may be unnecessary.

## PEDICULOSIS (LICE INFESTATION)

Lice—grayish, wingless insects as small as one sixteenth of an inch in length—are parasites that live on human blood obtained by biting the skin. Infestation, particularly common on the shoulders, buttocks, and abdomen, but occurring elsewhere as well, produces intense itching. Small red marks may be noticed. For treatment, a safe insecticide is employed. One commonly used is gamma benzene hexachloride. Additional measures may sometimes be needed, including an antibiotic ointment or corticosteroid lotion.

## PEMPHIGUS

A potentially grave disease of unknown cause, pemphigus leads to development of clusters of large "water blisters" which may appear first near or inside the nose and mouth and gradually spread over the skin of the rest of the body, bursting, leaving patches of raw, tender skin, with itching, burning, offensive odor. Untreated, pemphigus can be fatal. Relief of symptoms to some extent may be obtained with oatmeal or starch baths and potassium permanganate compresses. But, beyond this, corticosteroids by mouth, in individualized high and then later lower maintenance doses, can often eliminate symptoms and prolong life.

## PEPTIC ULCER

A peptic ulcer, an area of erosion, may occur in the stomach or first portion of the duodenum, which is the beginning of the small intestine. Symptoms typically are pain in the upper abdomen, over the stomach region, occurring from one to three hours after a meal and usually relieved by eating or an antacid, with nausea and vomiting sometimes following a severe pain episode. Although the cause is not entirely clear, excessive secretion of acid gastric juice is a factor in ulcer production. The diagnosis is aided by x-ray examination.

Cure is possible but not easy. Smoking and alcohol may be banned. In early treatment stages, meals may be frequent and small (bland diets, once universally used, are no longer considered essential by many physicians). Antacids are used to counteract acidity, sedatives to reduce tension, belladonna, atropine or other agents to reduce stomach activity and secretion. If they live up to promise and prove safe in the long term, new investigational compounds, including burimamide, cimetidine and metiamide, belonging to a new class of drugs known as $H_2$-receptor antagonists, could revolutionize treatment of peptic ulcer because of their marked ability to reduce gastric acid secretion and give the stomach or duodenal lining a chance to heal.

*Complications* sometimes may occur with peptic ulcer. One is *perforation* of the ulcer, producing agonizing abdominal pain, shallow breathing, beads of sweat on the forehead, boardlike and tender abdomen over the ulcer site, fever. Perforation is a surgical emergency.

Another complication is *massive hemorrhage,* with early symptoms consisting of faintness, weakness, dizziness, profuse sweating, later followed by vomiting of blood and passage of tarry stools. If hemorrhage fails to stop within 24 hours, surgery may be required. Another complication, *obstruction of the stomach outlet* by scarring, spasm, inflammation, edema or other causes, is often manifested by foul belching and vomiting of food from previous meals. Supportive treatment, with medication to relieve pain and vomiting, correction of dehydration, liquid feedings, and continuous suction through the nose, may be beneficial. If the obstruction fails to disappear, surgery may be necessary.

## PERIAPICAL ABSCESS

Causing gnawing pain and swelling of the face near the affected tooth, periapical abscess usually results from infection of the pulp due to decay. Extraction or root canal treatment is required.

## PERICARDITIS

An inflammation of the pericardium (the sac enclosing the heart), acute pericarditis produces dull or sharp chest pain, under the breastbone or in the region over heart and stomach, often with fever, chills, weakness, anxiety, sometimes quick, shallow breathing and nonproductive cough. The inflammation may follow a bacterial infection such as osteomyelitis, pneumonia, or lung abscess. It may also be caused by a tumor, rheumatic heart disease, uremia or heart attack, or by a chest wound involving piercing of the sac. Occasionally, pericarditis appears to result from what seems to be a viral infection, and is called acute nonspecific pericarditis. Treatment may require use of antibiotics or corticosteroids, or both, and sometimes drainage of the sac.

## PERIODONTITIS (PYORRHEA)

In periodontitis, the gums are inflamed, may show some recession, bleed when the teeth are brushed, and may become infected. If unchecked, periodontitis can lead to destruction of supporting bony tissues and loosening of the teeth. Periodontitis is treated with cleansing and scraping of the affected area, drainage, antibiotic drugs if necessary. Proper home care, with instruction from a dentist, may help limit further advance of the disease. In some cases, surgical removal of diseased gum tissue and other dental procedures may be needed.

## PERITONITIS

An acute inflammation of the membrane lining the abdominal cavity and covering abdominal organs, peritonitis can produce severe abdominal pain (constant, diffuse, prostrating, intensified by movement, so breathing is shallow), with fever, chills, nausea, vomiting, sometimes diarrhea. The inflammation can result from infection or irritation from bacteria or chemicals reaching the membrane through an inflamed, burst appendix, perforated ulcer, ruptured gallbladder, perforated bladder, or ruptured spleen. Antibiotics are used and surgery is usually essential to repair the perforated area.

## PERSPIRATION, EXCESSIVE (see HYPERHIDROSIS)

## PERTUSSIS (see WHOOPING COUGH)

## PEYRONIE'S DISEASE

Of unknown cause, this disease involves a fibrous contracture that usually results in deviation of the erect penis to one side, sometimes with painful erection and inability to engage in coitus. Radiation sometimes may arrest the disease. In some cases, local injections of corticosteroids have been successful.

## PHARYNGITIS

An inflammation of the pharynx—the cavity about five inches long behind the nose, mouth, and larynx—*acute* pharyngitis may occur with the common cold or be caused by bacterial or other viral infection. Symptoms may include burning, dryness or lump in the throat, chills, fever, swallowing difficulty, hoarseness, swelling of neck glands. In treatment, antibiotics, an ice collar, lozenges containing a local anesthetic, and pain-relieving medication may be used. *Chronic* pharyngitis may result from excessive or improper use of the voice, excessive alcohol consumption, or smoking. Symptoms may include chronic cough, dryness, tickling and, in some cases, secretion of thick, sticky mucus which is difficult to expectorate and may cause gagging, nausea, and vomiting. Lozenges may be used for palliation but the basic cause must be eliminated.

## PHENYLKETONURIA

An inborn error of metabolism which prevents proper handling of phenylalanine, an amino acid constituent of protein, phenylketonuria may be manifested early in infancy by unusual irritability, vomiting, and seizures. If untreated, it can lead to mental retardation. The disorder is now commonly detected early in life by a simple test and can be controlled by reduction of phenylalanine in the diet, using a preparation such as Lofenalac, supplemented by fruits, vegetables, and cereals low in protein.

## PHEOCHROMOCYTOMA

This is a relatively rare, usually benign adrenal gland tumor that produces such symptoms as palpitations, pallor, sweating, headache, high blood pressure, abdominal pain, and apprehension. Potentially fatal if neglected but curable if diagnosed before irreparable damage, pheochromocytoma can be detected by relatively simple tests such as use of a drug, phentolamine, which can reduce elevated blood pressure to near normal within three to four minutes in pheochromocytoma. Surgical removal of the tumor is necessary for complete elimination of symptoms.

## PHLEBITIS (see VENOUS THROMBOSIS)

## PHOTOSENSITIVITY

An abnormal sensitivity to sunlight which can lead, after only a few minutes of exposure, to varied skin reactions such as areas of redness, hives, and large watery blisters, photosensitivity may be due to a disease such as lupus erythematosus, sensitivity to drugs such as some antibiotics, sulfa compounds, and diuretics, or sensitivity to even externally applied compounds such as some soaps, perfumes, and toilet water. Any discoverable cause should be treated or avoided. In some cases, an antimalarial drug, hydroxychloroquine, may reduce or eliminate photosensitivity.

## PIEBALD SKIN (see VITILIGO)

## PINWORMS

Pinworm infection, the most common worm infection in children and often present in whole families, occurs in the intestine. The tiny worms, measuring under half an inch in length, often come out at night, causing itching around the anal area and perineal area (the region between anal opening and vagina or scrotum). The infection can be treated with piperazine, pyrvinium pamoate, or thiabendazole.

## PITYRIASIS ROSEA

A mild inflammatory disease occurring most often in children, pityriasis rosea produces pinkish oval patches (often accompanied by itching) on the trunk, although in some cases the arms may be primarily affected. It commonly disappears on its own within a month. Itching may be relieved by a drying lotion or a sulfur–salicylic acid ointment. Sunlight often helps. If necessary, a corticosteroid may be used.

## PLAGUE

An acute infectious disease transmitted from rats to humans via fleas, *bubonic plague* strikes suddenly from a few hours to a week or more after exposure, with chills, fever of 103° to 106°, acutely inflamed, painful swelling of lymph nodes, usually in the groin. Children may have convulsions. Vomiting, thirst, generalized pain, headache, and delirium may develop. The disease has been called the *black death*, from the black spots that appear after the third day. If untreated, 30 percent of patients die. Another form of plague, *pneumonic*, produces cough, blood-specked sputum, and rapidly progressing pneumonia; until recently it was almost invariably fatal. Now, for both types of plague, prompt treatment with antibiotics such as the tetracyclines, chloramphenicol, and streptomycin is usually effective, with mortality reduced to less than 5 percent.

## PLANTAR KERATOSIS

An abnormal, sometimes disabling thickening of the soles of the feet at the site of an injury, with some individuals seeming to have an inherited predisposition to develop the problem, plantar keratosis may be helped by use of soft-lined shoes and callus pads to relieve pressure and application of salicylic plaster followed by soaking.

## PLEURISY

An inflammation of the pleura, the membrane investing the lungs, pleurisy can produce sharp, sticking chest pain, worse on inhaling, fever, cough, chills, rapid shallow breathing. The inflammation may result from infection, injury or tumor, and may be a complication of pneumonia, influenza, lung abscess, or other lung disease. The membrane encasing each lung consists of two close-fitting layers with lubricating fluid between. If the fluid content remains unchanged by the disease, the pleurisy is called *dry*. If fluid increases abnormally, it is *wet pleurisy* or *pleurisy with effusion*. In dry pleurisy, the two membrane layers may become swollen and congested, rubbing against each other as the lungs inflate and deflate, causing pain. Wet pleurisy is less likely to produce pain, but the fluid may compress the lungs and interfere with breathing. If the excess fluid becomes infected and pus forms, the condition is called *empyema* or *purulent pleurisy*. Effective measures against pleurisy include antibiotics, heat applications, bed rest, and, if pain should become extremely severe on breathing, strapping of the chest to limit its movement. In some cases, drainage may be used as in EMPYEMA.

## PNEUMONIA

Pneumonia is an acute inflammation or infection of the lung. Symptoms may include a shaking chill followed by fever up to 105°, headache, chest pain, breathing difficulty, production of pinkish sputum that becomes rusty. In *lobar pneumonia,* a segment or an entire lobe is affected. When both lungs are involved, the disease is called *bilateral* or *double pneumonia*. Antibiotics and sulfa drugs have greatly reduced the seriousness of lobar pneumonia. *Bronchial pneumonia* or *bronchopneumonia,* more common than lobar, is less dramatic, with the infection localized in or around the bronchi, symptoms milder, temperature lower, and no crisis as in lobar pneumonia. If the infection is caused by bacteria, penicillin or another antibiotic can be used effectively. If viral in origin, antibiotics are not effective, and the disease runs its course, with the patient receiving supportive treatment for symptoms. *Primary atypical pneumonia,* most common in young adults, is due to viruses or mycoplasma organisms. Symptoms are much like those of a cold, including headache, fever, dry cough, generalized aches, and fatigue. Antibiotics are used. Other types of pneumonia include *chemical,* from inhalation of toxic gases; *aspiration,* from accidental inhalation of food or liquid; *traumatic,* from a blow or injury to the chest that may interfere with normal breathing; and *lipid pneumonia,* from inhalation of oily materials.

## PNEUMOTHORAX

Pneumothorax, or collapsed lung, occurs when air or gas gets between the membrane lining the chest wall and the membrane surrounding the lung, preventing the lung from expanding with each breath. Symptoms may include difficulty in breathing, dry hacking cough, and sharp chest pain that may be referred to a shoulder or down over the abdomen, sometimes simulating a heart attack. Pneumothorax may occur spontaneously in the course of a lung disease or may follow injury to and perforation of the chest wall. Spontaneous pneumothorax may require no treatment other than bed rest and oxygen to relieve breathing difficulty. In some cases, air may have to be removed from the pleural cavity.

## POLIOMYELITIS

A contagious viral disease affecting the nervous system, poliomyelitis may produce early symptoms of fever, headache, vomiting, sore throat, pain and stiffness in the back and neck, and drowsiness. In the *nonparalytic* type of polio, the fever usually lasts about seven days and the stiffness fades in three to five days. In *paralytic* polio, some weakness or paralysis of arms or legs begins one to seven days after the first symptoms. The first indication of *bulbar* polio, which affects the muscles of swallowing and breathing, is difficulty in swallowing, speaking and breathing, which usually occurs in the first three days of illness. No cure is available for polio; once the disease strikes, it must run its course, although symptomatic treatment including application of warm packs often reduces pain and promotes relaxation, and good posture in bed can help avoid deformities. Preventive vaccination, of course, is available, but many people still have not been immunized.

## POLYARTERITIS

Of unknown cause, polyarteritis is an inflammation of small and medium-size arteries with disturbances in the tissues supplied by those arteries. Symptoms can include weight loss and one or many others such as severe abdominal pain, diffuse muscle pains, joint pains, bloody diarrhea, heart failure, wheezing, pneumonia, skin reddening, hives. Corticosteroids are often used in treatment.

## POLYCYSTIC KIDNEY DISEASE

An inherited disorder in which multiple cysts develop on the kidney and cause gradual deterioration of kidney function, polycystic kidney disease is present from birth but symptoms do not occur until the cysts have enlarged enough to distort the kidneys and diminish function, usually in early or middle adult years. Symptoms include episodic kidney pain, blood in the urine, abdominal discomfort. No specific treatment is available. The disease may predispose to urinary infections and high blood pressure, which can be treated successfully to prolong life. Surgery may sometimes be used to drain cysts that have become obstructive in size. When kidney failure occurs, transplantation may be used.

## POLYCYSTIC OVARY SYNDROME

In this condition, which is also called the *Stein-Leventhal syndrome* and is of unknown cause, the ovaries are enlarged by multiple cysts. Symptoms include infertility, absence of menstruation or infrequent or scanty flow, and in about 50 percent of cases progressive facial hairiness and acne. In most cases, removal of wedges of both ovaries overcomes the symptoms.

## POLYCYTHEMIA VERA

In this disorder of unknown cause, blood-forming tissues in the bone marrow overgrow, leading to abnormally high amounts of red cells in the blood, with thickening of the blood and increased clotting tendency. Symptoms which develop gradually include headache, dizziness, breathing difficulty, disturbances of vision, itching, numbness and tingling sensations, and lassitude. Treatment is aimed at reducing the red cell numbers and blood viscosity. Venesection, or bloodletting, is often used and may be done at first once or twice a week, later every three or four months. In some cases, in addition to or instead of venesection, injections of radiophosphorus may be used to irradiate the rapidly dividing red cells. Sometimes, drugs such as busulfan or melphalan may be of value.

## POLYNEURITIS

An inflammation of nerves, polyneuritis may be caused by injury, pressure on nerves, infection, poisoning with various substances such as arsenic, lead, mercury, tin, alcohol, carbon monoxide, carbon tetrachloride. Symptoms of pain or numbness and tingling may begin in fingers and toes and extend elsewhere. Treatment, in addition to being directed at eliminating the cause, includes analgesics and heat, passive exercises, and, as acute symptoms begin to subside, active exercises.

## POLYPOSIS OF THE VOCAL CORDS

A progressive condition in which polyps develop on one or both vocal cords, polyposis produces voice change, including drop in pitch and volume. It may occur in women but frequently affects men who are heavy smokers and use their voices to excess. Treatment includes smoking reduction, voice instruction, and stripping of the vocal cord thickening.

## POLYPS

Polyps are growths extending out from a mucous membrane. They may occur in the nose, ears, mouth, lungs, heart, and gastrointestinal tract. Usually, they are overgrowths of normal tissue but sometimes they are new tissue and are true tumors, usually benign, but occasionally capable of becoming malignant.

Polyps in the nose may be produced by local irritation or allergy. If they grow large enough, they may produce stuffiness and headaches. Treatment for allergy or other sources of irritation is often helpful. If the polyps continue to cause trouble, their surgical removal may be needed.

Occasionally polyps occur on the gums between teeth, and in the ear, and when they cause discomfort can be removed.

Intestinal polyps occur mostly in middle and later life, although occasionally an infant may be born with them. In most cases, they produce no symptoms unless they become large enough to obstruct the intestine or ulcerate and bleed. Symptoms then may include cramping lower abdominal pain, diarrhea, blood and mucus in stools. Most often, polyps in the large intestine are discovered on routine physical examination, and whether or not they cause symptoms, many physicians believe they should be removed, since there is a chance they may eventually become malignant.

Men sometimes develop polyps in the urethra, the canal extending from the bladder to outside the body. They may cause a discharge and make urination difficult or frequent but do not affect vigor or sexual potency. They can be removed by surgery or treatment with an electric current (fulguration).

In women, polyps may occur in the uterus, causing excessive menstrual flow or sterility. They can be removed surgically.

*Rhinosporidiosis* is an infectious fungal disease which causes large polyps on the nose, eyes, larynx, vagina, occasionally on skin of ears or penis. It is most common in India and Ceylon but cases have occurred in the United States. Rhinosporidiosis may lead to secondary infections that may be serious. Cure is achieved by early removal of the polyps.

## PORPHYRIA, ACUTE INTERMITTENT

This is a genetic disorder which causes a disturbance in the body's handling of porphyrins, compounds that, with iron, form hemes which combine with various proteins to form hemoproteins such as hemoglobin, the pigment in red blood cells. Affecting women more often than men, acute intermittent porphyria usually appears between the ages of 20 and 40, producing episodes of colicky abdominal pain, distention, vomiting, and diarrhea or constipation, with extended periods of freedom from symptoms in between. In some cases, there may be convulsive seizures, muscle pain, and one or more of the following: anxiety, confusion, irritability, restlessness, delirium, hallucinations. A high-carbohydrate, high-protein diet often relieves symptoms. During a severe attack, a drug such as chlorpromazine may be helpful. In some women whose attacks are related to the menstrual cycle, oral contraceptives may be valuable.

## PORPHYRIA CUTANEA TARDA

An inherited disorder that usually develops in middle age, more commonly in men than in women, and is often associated with alcoholism, porphyria cutanea tarda causes excessive hairiness and skin pigmentation, sometimes with episodes of colicky abdominal pain and neurologic disturbances. Repeated phlebotomy (or bloodletting) as often as every two weeks for as long as eight months is effective treatment.

## PREMATURE CONTRACTIONS

Producing what may seem to be a skipped heartbeat to some people while others feel as if they had received a "shock" in the chest or as if something were "turning over" in the chest, premature contractions occur in heart disease but also in normal hearts and can be caused by fatigue, anxiety, smoking, the caffeine in coffee or tea. Treatment is directed at removing the cause whenever possible. If the contractions are persistent and troublesome, a sedative may be helpful or if necessary, quinidine or another drug useful in some heart rhythm irregularities may be tried.

## PREMATURE EJACULATION (see EJACULATION, PREMATURE)

## PREMENSTRUAL TENSION

Occurring most often in women between the ages of 24 and 40, premenstrual tension is believed to be due to fluid accumulation resulting from increased hormone activity during the latter portion of the menstrual cycle. It may cause such symptoms as breast pain, nervousness, irritability, depression, headache, generalized edema during the week to ten days prior to menstruation, with disappearance a few hours after menstruation begins. In mild cases, only an analgesic such as aspirin may be needed. In more severe cases, at about the time symptoms are to be expected, limited salt intake and a diuretic drug such as hydrochlorothiazide may be used and often provide relief.

## PRIAPISM

Producing painful, persistent penile erection without sexual excitement, priapism is of unknown cause although it may be associated with sickle cell disease or trait, leukemia or other blood disorders, infections and inflammations such as prostatitis, urethritis, and cystitis. Treatment is often difficult. In some cases anticoagulant drugs may help. Surgical measures may be tried. Treatment for any associated disorder is important.

## PRIMARY SPLENIC NEUTROPENIA

Producing fatigability, joint pains, or chronic ill health, with repeated mild or severe infections, primary splenic neutropenia is a rare condition in which the numbers of certain cells in the blood are reduced and the spleen is enlarged. A similar condition can be related to leukemias, lymphomas, or agranulocytosis, and this possibility has to be considered before the diagnosis of primary splenic neutropenia is made. No specific treatment for the latter is available. Removal of the spleen may sometimes be necessary.

## PROCTITIS

An inflammation of the mucous membrane lining of the rectum, proctitis produces such symptoms as rectal discomfort, repeated urge to defecate, painful diarrhea with blood, pus, and mucus in stools. It may be caused by ulcerative colitis, regional enteritis, accidental or radiation injury, broad-spectrum antibiotics, infections such as amebiasis, tuberculosis, gonorrhea, actinomycosis, schistosomiasis, and lymphogranuloma venereum. In addition to treatment for the specific cause, a corticosteroid such as hydrocortisone may be used in suppository form or in retention enemas. Also helpful in some cases: use of stool softeners, drugs to reduce spasm, codeine or paregoric to avoid diarrhea.

## PROLAPSE OF THE RECTUM

This is a protrusion of the rectal mucous membrane through the anus. In children, it usually results from straining or sitting too long at stool and improves with use of mild laxatives and normal toilet habit development. In adults, prolapse may be due to internal hemorrhoids, and excess tissue is removed during removal of the hemorrhoids. In some cases in adults, the prolapse may involve the rectal wall as well as mucous membrane and may be due to weakening of supports as the result of childbirth, aging, or pelvic surgery. A wire loop may be inserted to strengthen the anorectal ring or in some cases other surgery may be needed.

## PROLAPSE OF THE UTERUS

Protrusion of the uterus through the vaginal orifice may result from stretching and weakening of muscles and ligaments holding the uterus in place as the result of an inherited condition, numerous pregnancies, or age. Excessive coughing sometimes may be a factor, as may straining at stool. Symptoms may include lower abdominal cramps, vaginal discharge and pain, frequent and urgent urination, painful intercourse. A pessary to provide support may be used. Permanent correction requires surgery.

## PROSTATE CANCER (see CANCER OF THE PROSTATE)

## PROSTATE ENLARGEMENT (BENIGN PROSTATIC HYPERTROPHY)

Of unknown cause, enlargement of the prostate gland is a common complaint in men over 50. Because of the prostate's position around the urethra, which carries urine from the bladder, the gland's enlargement interferes with normal flow and may cause increasing frequency, urgency, and difficulty of urination, excessive urination at night, hesitancy and intermittency of the stream and decreased size and force. Sometimes, blood may appear in the urine because of rupture of superficial veins of the prostatic urethra during straining to void. When urinary infection also occurs, it is indicated by burning on urination and fever and chills. Prostatectomy, or excision of the prostate, produces excellent results.

## PROSTATITIS

Infections of the prostate are relatively common in men. Acute infection may produce painful, frequent urination and severe fever, with the prostate becoming swollen and tender. Treatment with a suitable antibiotic, bed rest, and fluids usually brings the infection to an end within five to ten days. Chronic prostatitis may develop with or without previous acute infection, producing milder symptoms of frequency, discomfort, and during-the-night urination. Treatment may require long-term use of antibiotics, hot sitz baths, and prostatic massage.

## PROTEIN DEFICIENCY

Chronic protein deficiency can produce edema or swelling of the legs which may become generalized, digestive disturbances, weight and appetite loss, weakness and lethargy. The deficiency may sometimes stem from inadequate intake of protein, but it may also result from impaired intestinal absorption in some diseases such as sprue and chronic inflammatory diarrhea; liver diseases which interfere with utilization of protein; excessive protein breakdown as in hyperthyroidism; or loss of protein from draining wounds. A prescribed high-protein diet may be used and in some cases protein may be administered by vein.

## PSEUDOMEMBRANOUS ENTEROCOLITIS (see ENTEROCOLITIS, PSEUDOMEMBRANOUS)

## PSITTACOSIS (PARROT FEVER)

A form of pneumonia caused by organisms transmitted by birds, psittacosis produces fever, chills, malaise, appetite loss, and a cough, dry at first, that becomes productive with mucopurulent sputum. It can be treated effectively with a tetracycline antibiotic.

## PSORIASIS

A chronic recurrent skin disease of unknown cause, psoriasis tends to run in families, may occur at any age, but is most severe between ages 10 and 50. It produces bright red patches on the skin covered with silvery scales, most often affecting knees, elbows, scalp, chest, abdomen, backs of arms and legs, palms of hands, soles of feet, and may sometimes appear as dot-shaped marks on the fingernails. Although acute attacks often clear, permanent clearance is rare. Many treatments are employed, some of value in some cases, others in other cases. They include topical corticosteroids, anthralin ointment, nightly tar ointment application and daily exposure to sunlight or ultraviolet radiation, methotrexate.

## PSORIATIC ARTHRITIS (see ARTHRITIS, PSORIATIC)

## PULMONARY ALVEOLAR PROTEINOSIS

A disease of unknown cause in which granular proteinaceous material fills air spaces in the lungs, impairing respiration, pulmonary alveolar proteinosis affects men more often than women, most frequently appearing between the ages of 20 and 50. Symptoms include progressive breathing difficulty, with productive cough, thick yellow sputum that in some cases may contain bits of firm yellow-gray material, weight loss, malaise. In some cases, there is spontaneous gradual relief. Treatment may include use of iodides, which sometimes produce clearing, irrigation of the lungs with potassium iodide solution through a catheter or tube, and antibacterial drugs if needed.

## PULMONARY EDEMA

In pulmonary edema, fluid fills the lungs, most often as a complication of coronary heart disease, hypertension or aortic valve disease, sometimes as a complication of head injury. Symptoms may include cough, wheezing, labored breathing, sometimes with ability to breathe only in the upright position; there may also be a sense of oppression in the chest. Treatment includes rest, sitting position to help free the lungs of fluid, and elimination of excess fluid from the body with digitalis or diuretic drugs.

## PULMONARY EMBOLISM

A pulmonary embolism is a blood clot which after developing elsewhere, commonly in a deep leg vein, breaks off and is carried by the blood to a lung artery. Symptoms may include labored breathing, cough, chest pain, sometimes coughing and spitting of blood. Predisposing factors to a pulmonary embolism include extended bed rest, heart disease, chronic obstructive lung disease, hip fracture, cancer, blood disorders, surgery. Diagnosis—to distinguish pulmonary embolism from pneumonia, heart attack, congestive or respiratory failure—may be made with the aid of chest x-ray and other tests such as radioisotope lung scanning. Treatment may include sedation, a potent analgesic if needed, oxygen, anticoagulants. In some extreme cases, surgery to remove the embolism may be required.

## PULMONARY EMPHYSEMA (see EMPHYSEMA, PULMONARY)

## PULMONARY GRANULOMATOSES

A group of lung diseases involving nodules and other lesions in the lungs, cause unknown, pulmonary granulomatoses may produce breathing difficulty, sometimes with blueness after exercise, rapid pulse, fever, dry nonproductive cough, weight and appetite loss, malaise, easy fatigability. In many patients, symptoms are slight; the disease process does not advance and may regress. In severe cases, a corticosteroid such as prednisone may bring improvement within a few weeks.

## PULMONARY STENOSIS

This is a congenital narrowing of the pulmonary valve which regulates blood flow from the heart to the lungs. With the narrowing, flow to the lungs is reduced and body tissues get a reduced supply of fresh oxygenated blood. Symptoms may include shortness of breath, fatigability, fainting episodes. Some children, however, have no symptoms, and when stenosis is minor, no treatment may be needed. When major, surgery to relieve the narrowing provides permanent cure.

## PULPITIS

Producing sharp, throbbing, shooting, intermittent pain sometimes difficult to localize, pulpitis is an inflammation of the dental pulp, the soft tissue within a tooth. It most often results from infection and inflammation following tooth decay. In early pulpitis, removal of food debris from the cavity and application of clove oil or clove oil mixed with zinc oxide powder may provide relief. In advanced cases, removal of the diseased pulp or extraction of the tooth may be required.

## PURPURA, ALLERGIC

An allergic reaction in which there is effusion of blood into surfaces under the skin and mucous membranes, allergic purpura produces red spots which gradually darken and become purple, with itching, often with fever and malaise, sometimes with joint and abdominal pain. Except for eliminating any suspected allergy-producing agents, treatment is symptomatic to relieve fever and pain. The condition usually lasts one to six weeks and may or may not recur.


## PURPURA, IDIOPATHIC THROMBOCYTOPENIC

Producing bleeding into the skin and formation of small, round, purplish-red spots, sometimes also with nosebleeds and bleeding in the gastrointestinal or genitourinary tract, this is a disease of unknown cause in which the spleen removes too rapidly from the blood the platelets that help prevent bleeding. Spontaneous disappearance of the disorder is common. If bleeding is severe, a corticosteroid such as prednisone may reduce bleeding and increase the platelet count. If the disorder persists and is severe, spleen removal often produces complete, permanent remission. In some cases, a similar type of purpura, with the same symptoms, may result from exposure to a drug or from infection; treatment then is directed at the cause and its elimination.


## PYELONEPHRITIS (PYELITIS)

Producing painful urination, with frequency and urgency, sometimes with chills, fever, headache, pain in one or both sides of the lower back, pyelonephritis is a kidney infection. It is most common in young children, much more so in girls than in boys because the female urethra is shorter, making it easier for organisms from outside to ascend the urinary tract. Often, girls not properly toilet-trained may rub toilet tissue from anus toward vagina instead of vice versa and, in so doing, permit bacteria common in fecal matter to move into the urinary bladder and from there to the kidney. Any urinary obstruction may predispose to kidney infection by interfering with the kidney's ability to eliminate harmful bacteria. Treatment includes antibiotics or sulfa drugs, sometimes urinary antiseptics; prompt treatment usually leads to early and complete recovery. *Chronic* pyelonephritis, in which the kidneys are chronically inflamed, may be the result in some cases of repeated urinary infections. Symptoms are variable; they include intermittent fever and urinary disturbances. Treatment includes vigorous use of suitable antibacterial agents for the specific organisms involved. If obstruction is present, surgery may be needed.


## PYORRHEA (see PERIODONTITIS)

**Q FEVER** (see ROCKY MOUNTAIN SPOTTED FEVER AND OTHER
RICKETTSIAL DISEASES)


## RABIES

An acute viral infection from an animal bite, with an incubation
period averaging a month or a little more, rabies is commonly first
manifested by a short period of fever, mental depression, restlessness, and malaise. Restlessness progresses to uncontrollable excitement. Salivation becomes excessive and painful spasms of muscles of
the larynx and throat develop. Immediate treatment for an animal
bite includes thorough washing with soap and water. A physician
should be consulted without delay. Preventive treatment is based on
immunization by a series of vaccine injections along with immune
serum.


## RAT-BITE FEVER

Rat-bite fever is actually two distinct diseases, similar in symptoms, that may follow the bite of a rodent or other animal—most
often a rat, less commonly an infected squirrel, dog, cat, or pig. One,
*Haverhill fever*, which occurs in the United States, produces a fluid
filled sore at the bite site within ten days. At intervals of one to two
days, high fever alternates with normal temperature. Lymph nodes
swell and large joints redden, swell, and become painful. There may
be back pain and a measleslike spotty rash. In the other disease,
*sodoku*, rarely found in the United States, symptoms are similar except that the bite heals quickly and then, within 5 to 28 days, the site
swells and becomes purplish. Both forms of the fever respond
promptly to treatment with antibiotics such as penicillin, tetracycline, and streptomycin.


## RAYNAUD'S DISEASE

Of unknown cause, most common in young women, this disease
manifests itself as attacks of pallor and blueness of the fingers of both
hands, sometimes of the toes as well, with the attacks triggered by
cold or emotional disturbances and often relieved by warmth. Along
with pallor and blueness, there may be numbness, and as an attack
passes off, redness and throbbing pain may occur. Mild cases can be
controlled by avoidance of cold, use of mild sedatives, and, since the

disorder involves blood vessel constriction, elimination of smoking, which tends to constrict vessels. A drug, reserpine, often decreases the number and severity of attacks.

## RECTAL PROLAPSE (see PROLAPSE OF THE RECTUM)

## REGIONAL ENTERITIS

Also called *Crohn's disease*, regional enteritis, of unknown cause, involves inflammation usually of the lower ileum, the last portion of the small intestine, but sometimes other areas of the gastrointestinal tract. Symptoms are chronic diarrhea, with several loose, nonbloody stools daily, abdominal pain, fever, weight loss. In some cases, colic is added, producing what may seem like appendicitis. In other cases, partial obstruction of the intestine leads to repeated episodes of severe intestinal colic, vomiting, and abdominal distention. Diagnosis is aided by x-ray studies. Although in some cases complete recovery occurs after a single attack, in most cases the disease progresses. In treatment, a high-calorie, low-residue diet may be used, along with mild sedatives and anticholinergic drugs. Corticosteroids are often valuable in acute stages, lowering fever, decreasing diarrhea, and improving appetite. Surgery may sometimes be needed to overcome obstruction or to remove the diseased area, eliminating symptoms for a period of years. Recurrences occur in more than half of cases after surgery.

## RELAPSING FEVER

Also known as *tick, recurrent, spirillum,* and *famine fever,* this is an acute infectious disease caused by bacteria transmitted by ticks and lice. In the United States, it occurs largely in western states. After a week of incubation, the disease begins suddenly with chills, high fever, severe headache, vomiting, muscle and joint pain, frequently delirium. A reddish rash may develop over the trunk and extremities, followed by rose-colored spots. Jaundice sometimes occurs. Within several days to a week or more, all symptoms may disappear, only for a second attack of the same symptoms, with increased jaundice, to occur, and recurrences and remissions may follow at one- to two-week intervals, with the attacks becoming less severe until recovery occurs. Antibiotics are effective, and drugs may be used to relieve headache and nausea and vomiting.

## RENAL FAILURE, ACUTE

Acute renal (kidney) failure may be caused by kidney disease, crushing injuries, severe burns or shock, septicemia (bacteria or their toxins in the blood), mismatched blood transfusion, obstetric difficulties, or poisoning. It is manifested by marked decline in urination or failure to void, sometimes with low back pain or tenderness. In treatment, fluid intake is matched to urine output, and intake of sodium, potassium, and protein is eliminated. If necessary, dialysis (or machine cleansing of the blood) may be used to prevent uremia until the kidneys have a chance to recover.

## RESPIRATORY ACIDOSIS

When carbon dioxide is not exhaled normally, its accumulation in the blood causes chemical changes including a change in the blood's acid-base balance toward acidity. Drowsiness results and may progress, if acidosis continues, to stupor and coma. Respiratory acidosis may occur in severe emphysema, pneumonia, congestive heart failure, edema of the larynx, weakening of breathing muscles from injury or disease, or drug depression of the brain's breathing center. Treatment requires measures to combat the underlying cause and may include use of antibiotics, bronchodilators, expectorants and, in some cases, mechanical respiration.

## RESPIRATORY ALKALOSIS

Producing tingling and burning sensations, light-headedness, agitation, and fainting, respiratory alkalosis results from excessive exhalation of carbon dioxide. It may be caused simply by hyperventilation (or overbreathing) or by fever, nervous system disturbances, poisoning with aspirin or aspirinlike compounds. When hyperventilation is the cause, breathing into and out of a paper bag for a time returns exhaled carbon dioxide and often quickly relieves symptoms. In other cases, appropriate treatment for the cause is required.

## RETINAL DETACHMENT

Producing light flashes, often with the sensation that a curtain is being drawn across the eye, detachment of the retina at the back of the eye may occur after accidents and some eye diseases. It tends to be most common in people with severe myopia. The detachment is usually partial at first but may become complete if not treated promptly. Early surgery is usually effective.

## RETINITIS

An inflammation of the retina of the eye, retinitis may be caused by injury, drugs, smoking, or excessive use of alcohol. Loss of visual acuity, distortion of size and shape of objects, and eye discomfort are symptoms. Corticosteroid drugs often help. The vitamin thiamine may be prescribed along with elimination of tobacco and alcohol.

## RETINITIS PIGMENTOSA

An inherited disease in which there is progressive degeneration of the retina, retinitis pigmentosa may appear in childhood or later in life and is manifested by narrowing of side vision that produces a "looking through a tunnel" effect. No cure is available. Central vision often remains clear for a long period, sometimes a lifetime.

## RETINOBLASTOMA

A cancer of the retina which appears early in life and is often diagnosed before the age of two, retinoblastoma manifests itself in whitishness of the pupil of the eye and squinting. Vision changes and loss, which the child may be unable to report, commonly occur, and there may be enlargement of the eyeball. In early cases, radiation therapy may be effective. Chemotherapy also may be used. In advanced disease, the eye must be removed.

## RETINOPATHIES

Noninflammatory diseases of the retina, retinopathies may be caused by severe high blood pressure, arteriosclerosis, diabetes, excessive smoking. Symptoms include blurring of vision, blood spots in the eyes, sometimes a bloodshot appearance. If high blood pressure is involved, it can be reduced effectively. Elimination of smoking may be advisable. Corticosteroids are useful. Treatment with a laser beam to coagulate hemorrhaging retinal blood vessels may be used.

## RHEUMATIC FEVER

Called rheumatic fever because its two most common symptoms, fever and joint pains, are similar to those of rheumatism, this disorder is a complication of a tonsil, throat, ear, or other infection caused by streptococcal bacteria. It occurs most commonly among children 5 to 15 years of age but may affect young adults as well. The first symptoms, which usually appear one to four weeks after a strep infection, most often consist of slight fever, tiredness, vague pain in the limbs, and nosebleeds. Fever may remain mild or may climb to 104° by the second day, usually lasting about two weeks. At any point, from a few hours to some weeks after first symptoms, joints may swell and become tender to the touch. Pain often disappears in one group of joints only to start up in another. There may also be other symptoms: spasmodic twitching movements (Sydenham's chorea, also called St. Vitus' dance) may occur, a rash may appear on the body, and nodules may develop below the skin at elbows, knees, and wrists.

A serious complication, more likely with repeated attacks of rheumatic fever, is endocarditis, an inflammation of the heart which may affect a heart valve. The valve, upon healing, may have its edges scarred so it cannot close properly or the valve may be thickened so as to restrict blood flow.

Treatment is directed at reducing the pain and fever of rheumatic fever, and may include bed rest, analgesics, and a corticosteroid. Antibiotics may be used if there is ongoing strep infection. Valve damage may require surgery later for correction. Prevention is especially important for rheumatic fever. After one occurrence, there is a tendency for recurrence, which often can be prevented by prophylactic antibiotic therapy to prevent strep infections.

## RHEUMATOID ARTHRITIS (see ARTHRITIS, RHEUMATOID)

## RHINITIS, ALLERGIC

Known as *hay fever* when it is seasonal and *perennial allergic rhinitis* when it occurs year-round, this disorder may produce itching of the nose, roof of the mouth, throat, and eyes, with tearing of the eyes, sneezing, nasal discharge, and, in some cases, headaches, irritability, appetite loss, depression, insomnia, wheezing, and coughing. In the perennial form, symptoms often vary in intensity, commonly becoming worse in fall and winter. Avoidance of the causes of allergy if known (pollens, dust, feathers, animal dander) is, of course, advisable when possible. To some extent, filtered air conditioning may help hay fever victims. Antihistamines, sometimes combined with decongestants, may provide relief. When necessary, sprays of a corticosteroid such as dexamethasone may be prescribed. Desensitization treatment, using gradually increasing doses of offending materials given by injection to build up tolerance, helps some patients.

## RHINITIS, ATROPHIC

This disorder of unknown cause leads to progressive atrophy of the internal nose, producing obstruction of breathing, crust formation, offensive nasal odor, dryness and irritation, disturbances of smell. Treatment may include irrigation of the nose with warm salt and bicarbonate solution, and sprays of a neostigmine solution.

## RHINITIS, CHRONIC

Chronic rhinitis is a chronic inflammation that produces thickening of the nasal mucous membrane and enlargement of the turbinate structures in the nose. It may be caused by repeated upper respiratory infections, abuse of nose drops, chronic sinusitis, deviated septum, polyps, poor nasal hygiene. Symptoms may include obstructed breathing, continuous discharge, postnasal drip, throat tickle, dry lips, coated tongue, intermittent headache. Any causes that can be eliminated should be. Injections of corticosteroids into the turbinates often help. Silver nitrate, phenol, or electrocautery may be used to contract tissues.

## RHINOSCLEROMA

A chronic infectious disease, rhinoscleroma leads to hard patches or nodules in the nose, sometimes dark purple or ivory. In some cases, obstruction and sinusitis may be complications. Streptomycin and x-ray therapy often provide good results.

## RHINOSPORIDIOSIS (see POLYPS)

## RICKETS (see OSTEOMALACIA)

**RICKETTSIALPOX** (see ROCKY MOUNTAIN SPOTTED FEVER AND OTHER RICKETTSIAL DISEASES)

## RINGWORM

Caused by related fungi of different types, ringworm may affect the scalp, body, genital area, nails, and areas between the toes, producing reddish patches, often scaly or blistered, sometimes becoming ring-shaped as the infection spreads out. Other manifestations are itching and soreness. The fungi are highly contagious, spread by humans, animals, combs, towels, and other objects handled by the infected. Scratching often spreads the infection. Ringworm may be treated with an antifungal antibiotic such as griseofulvin. A sulfur-salicylic ointment may be used. For some ringworm infections, a corticosteroid lotion and aluminum acetate or potassium permanganate compresses may be prescribed. When ringworm affects the nails, the nails thicken, lose luster, and the nail plate may become separated and the nail destroyed. The nail infection may require extended treatment with griseofulvin until the nail has grown back. Months of treatment may be required for fingernails, more than a year for toenails.

## ROCKY MOUNTAIN SPOTTED FEVER AND OTHER RICKETTSIAL DISEASES

Insect-borne microscopic parasites called *rickettsiae* are responsible for Rocky Mountain spotted fever and a number of other diseases.

The strain responsible for Rocky Mountain spotted fever is transmitted from rodent to man by the wood tick. Principal areas for the disease are eastern and northwestern United States.

Other rickettsial disease are *epidemic typhus*, which occurs worldwide and is transmitted by the human body louse; *scrub typhus*, found mainly in the Asiatic-Pacific area and transmitted by chiggers from field mice and rats; *trench fever*, which occurs in central Europe, Africa, and North America, and is transmitted by the body louse: *South American spotted fever*, found in Brazil and transmitted by the dog tick; *murine typhus*, present worldwide, transmitted by the rat flea; *Q fever*, found worldwide, transmitted by the wood and cattle tick; *rickettsialpox*, found in North America and Europe, transmitted by mites from house mice; and still others found in particular areas of the world outside North America.

After the bite of an infected insect, a 3- to 10-day incubation period follows before major symptoms occur, although there may be loss of appetite and feelings of vague illness in the interim. Actual onset is marked by chills or chilly sensations, fever, headache, pain behind the eyes, joint and muscle pain, intolerance of light, nausea, vomiting, sore throat, and abdominal pain. Usually about three to five days after onset of symptoms, a rash appears on the wrists and ankles and spreads to the trunk and limbs, occasionally to the face. The appearance of small red spots that become larger sores distinguishes Rocky Mountain spotted fever from the other rickettsial diseases it resembles. In trench fever, the fever first may run for three to five days, disappear for 12 to 24 hours, then recur for another three to five days. In scrub typhus and rickettsialpox, a small oval or round ulcer with surrounding redness and covered by a black scab appears at the site of attachment of the insect. The rickettsial diseases respond well to antibiotics, particularly tetracycline and chloramphenical. If untreated, they can be serious, even fatal.

## ROSEOLA

An acute disease of infants and young children, believed caused by a virus, roseola is manifested by a fever of 103° to 104° for three to four days, often with convulsions, with the fever then falling and followed by a pink-reddish rash on the chest and abdomen, mildly on the face, arms, and legs. There is no specific drug for the disease, which is treated with aspirin and tepid water or alcohol sponge baths to bring the fever below 103°. When the temperature becomes normal and the rash appears, the child is usually so nearly well that no further treatment is needed.

## ROUNDWORM, GIANT INTESTINAL

Acquired through fecal contamination of the soil and contamination of vegetables, this parasite causes colicky pains and diarrhea, and can be treated effectively with piperazine, thiabendazole, or bephenium hydroxynaphthoate.

## SAINT VITUS' DANCE (see SYDENHAM'S CHOREA)

## SARCOIDOSIS

This chronic disease of unknown cause produces small, fleshy lumps or nodules in affected tissues, most often the lungs, skin, and lymph nodes. It is not communicable. Symptoms may be mild or absent; in more severe cases, there may be fever, weakness, lack of appetite and loss of weight, joint pain, sometimes cough, hoarseness, breathing difficulty. It appears most often in young adults and requires careful diagnosis to distinguish it from other problems such as tuberculosis. Often, sarcoidosis disappears spontaneously, although it may sometimes persist for years. Corticosteroids often provide relief for any severe symptoms. Colchicine may help joint pains, and hydroxychloroquine is useful for any skin lesions.

## SALMONELLA INFECTION (see GASTROENTERITIS, FOOD INFECTION)

## SCABIES ("THE ITCH")

Caused by a mite, which is readily transmitted from person to person and may affect a whole family, scabies is most likely to develop in the skin folds, webs of the hands, genital area, buttocks, underarms. It produces intense itching, usually worse at night, with slightly elevated grayish-white lines sometimes visible. For effective treatment, a hot bath with vigorous cleaning is used, followed by application of a cream or lotion containing a compound such as gamma benzene hexachloride, which is left on for 24 hours, then washed off. A second application sometimes may be needed.

## SCARLET FEVER

Also known as *scarlatina,* this acute contagious childhood disease is caused by streptococcal bacteria, occurs most commonly in late winter and spring, and may follow a strep infection of the throat, skin, ear, or other part of the body. After an incubation period of one to seven days, variable symptoms appear. They may include sore throat and swelling of neck lymph nodes. The tonsils may be covered by a patchy, pus-laden discharge. A bright red rash appears on the second day and may be mild or widespread. In mild cases, temperature may rise to 101°; in severe cases, to as high as 105°. Headache, chills, nausea, and fever may occur. The rash fades within a week. Antibiotic treatment is effective.

## SCHISTOSOMIASIS

A parasitic disease caused by blood flukes and also known as *bilharziasis,* schistosomiasis is endemic in Africa, the Middle East, Cyprus, some West Indies islands, the northern part of South America, Japan, central and south China, the Philippines, and occurs in some Puerto Ricans living in the United States. Infection develops from bathing or other contact with swimming parasites which penetrate the skin. A skin outbreak is followed by fever, hives, possibly bladder inflammation (cystitis) or chronic dysentery. Among the most effective treatment agents are tartar emetic and stibophen.

## SCIATICA

The sciatic nerve is one of the longest of the body, extending from the base of the spine down the thigh, with branches throughout the lower leg and foot. In sciatica, the nerve is inflamed, producing pain that may begin in the buttock and extend down the back of the thigh and leg to the ankle. In most cases, the cause is osteoarthritis in the lumbosacral area of the spine or rupture of an intervertebral disk. Occasionally a disease such as diabetes or gout or a vitamin deficiency may be the inciting factor. While surgery may sometimes be needed, most cases respond to conservative treatment, which may include use of a firm mattress, analgesic drugs, local heat, spraying with ethyl chloride, traction.

## SCLERODERMA

Also known as *progressive systemic sclerosis, dermatosclerosis,* and *hidebound skin,* this disease of unknown cause is more common in women than in men. It produces mottled reddening of the skin, followed after months or years by hardening and sometimes immobility of the skin, usually beginning in the hands and feet and spreading to other areas. It may sometimes involve the gastrointestinal tract, lungs, kidneys, and heart, producing heartburn, reflux of food from stomach to esophagus, and heart failure. No drug specific for scleroderma is available but helpful treatment may include use of a corticosteroid agent, small feedings, antacids, digitalis, and physiotherapy.

## SCURVY

Caused by vitamin C deficiency, scurvy in infants is usually due to lack of supplementary vitamin; in adults, to improper diet. In a child, symptoms may include irritability, appetite loss, failure to gain weight, anemia, fever. Adult symptoms may start with lassitude, weakness, irritability, weight loss, vague muscle and joint aches, and may go on to include swollen and bleeding gums, breakdown of old scars, failure of new wounds to heal, small black and blue spots on the skin. For treatment, vitamin C is given—in an infant, up to 150 milligrams a day for a month, less thereafter; in an adult, up to 500 milligrams a day until symptoms disappear, followed by lower maintenance doses.

## SEBACEOUS CYST (see CYST, SEBACEOUS)

## SEPTUM, DEVIATED (see DEVIATED SEPTUM)

## SERUM SICKNESS

This is an allergic reaction that may develop one to two weeks after administration of a drug or serum to which an individual is sensitive. Symptoms may include fever that is usually mild and lasts a day or two, hives or a skin rash, gland (lymph node) swelling, joint pains, and itching. The reaction is self-limiting. Treatment, which is directed at relieving symptoms, may include an antihistamine for itching, aspirin for joint pains, and, if these are not enough, a corticosteroid drug such as prednisone.

## SHIGELLOSIS (see BACILLARY DYSENTERY)

## SHAKING PALSY (see PARKINSON'S DISEASE)

## SHINGLES (see HERPES ZOSTER)

## SHOCK

A disruption of circulation, shock is a dangerous condition that occurs when blood pressure falls so low as to be inadequate for getting blood to vital tissues. It may follow a wide variety of disturbances such as severe injury, major surgery, hemorrhage, dehydration, heart attack, overwhelming infection, poisoning, drug reaction. Symptoms may include pallor, moist and cool skin, racing pulse, apathy or agitation, but can vary. When heart attack leads to shock, there may be weakness, nausea, sweating, chest pain, breathing difficulty. In a massive heart attack, the victim is pale, cold, has labored breathing, can breathe only in upright position, and experiences severe chest pain. In shock caused by severe infection, the skin may be warm, the patient somnolent.

Shock requires quick treatment even as the cause is sought. For first aid, the patient should be placed on his back with head low to ensure as much blood flow as possible to the brain. But if a severe head, neck, or back injury is present, the patient should not be moved without instructions from a physician. If foreign material is obstructing the airway, it should be removed. If the tongue is in the way, the tongue and jaw should be pulled forward. If the patient is not breathing, lungs should be inflated by mouth-to-mouth resuscitation (see under CARDIAC ARREST). Active bleeding should be controlled with pressure or a bandage directly over the bleeding site.

## SILICOSIS

A lung disease from inhalation of silica dust, silicosis is most likely to be contracted in such jobs as sandblasting in tunnels and hard-rock mining, but can occur with habitual exposure to dust of silica, one of the most common minerals, and almost any miner may be subject to it. The silica produces a reaction that scars the lungs, making them prone to further complications of bronchitis and emphysema. Symptoms include breathing difficulty, with respiration deeper and more rapid than normal, sometimes with dry cough. In advanced stages, there may be malaise, sleep disturbance, appetite loss, chest pains, hoarseness, blueness, coughing and spitting of blood. Regular chest x-rays are needed by all workers exposed to silica dust for early detection of the disease, which can usually be arrested by change of occupation. In advanced cases, improvement of symptoms may be obtained with drainage of bronchial secretions, bronchodilators, other measures.

## SILO-FILLER'S DISEASE

Caused by inhalation of oxides of nitrogen, most often nitrogen oxide, when working in a silo or burning nitrocellulose film, this serious disease (also known as *bronchiolitis obliterans*) produces labored breathing, blueness, cough, blood-flecked sputum. In treatment, oxygen and a corticosteroid such as prednisone may be used.

## SINOATRIAL EXIT BLOCK

This is a blocking of the electrical impulse in the heart (which is required for contraction of the heart chambers) and may lead to the omission of one or more heartbeats, producing dizziness, faintness, or convulsions. The block may develop in coronary heart disease and chronic rheumatic heart disease but most often occurs as a result of treatment with digitalis, quinidine, or potassium salts. Usually, if the block occurs infrequently and only a few beats are omitted, there are no symptoms. If overdosage of a drug is responsible for the block, that can be corrected. If necessary, symptoms may be relieved with atropine, ephedrine, or isoproterenol.

## SINUS BRADYCARDIA

This is a slowing of heartbeat to less than 60 per minute. Unless very severe, when it may lead to fainting and convulsions, sinus bradycardia produces no symptoms. It may sometimes be caused by meningitis, hemorrhage, gastrointestinal disturbances. In some people with a very sensitive carotid sinus (part of the carotid artery) in the neck area, pressure such as that produced by a tight collar may lead to severe sinus bradycardia. Often, no treatment is needed. The wearing of tight collars should be avoided by the sensitive. A drug such as atropine may sometimes be used.

## SINUS TACHYCARDIA

This fast, forceful beat of the heart, greater than 100 a minute, comes on gradually and slackens off when the cause is removed. Possible causes include emotion, exercise, infection, anemia, low blood pressure, hyperthyroidism. A sedative such as phenobarbital may sometimes be used until the cause can be eliminated.

## SINUSITIS

This inflammation of the sinuses, the hollow cavities in the skull that are connected with the nasal cavity, may be caused by anything that can irritate, infect, or obstruct the interior of the nose: colds and other upper respiratory infections, allergies, tooth infection. Symptoms may include headache, nasal and postnasal discharge, fever, dizziness, toothache, generalized aches, puffiness about the eyes. In most cases, sinusitis can be controlled by antibiotics, moist heat, and drugs that shrink the membrane lining of nose and sinuses to permit drainage. In some cases, surgery may be needed.

## SKIN CANCER (see CANCER OF THE SKIN)

## SLEEPING SICKNESS (see ENCEPHALITIS, VIRAL)

## SMALLPOX

This viral infection, one of the most contagious diseases known, is also called *variola*. It has become rare, almost nonexistent, throughout the world because of widespread vaccination. The first symptoms are severe headache, chills, and high fever. Children may suffer from vomiting and convulsions. Within three to four days, a rash of small, red pustules appears, first on the face, then on the arms, wrists, hands and legs. A small number of spots appear on the trunk. In a day or two blisters develop and fill with clear fluid. Over the next week, the fluid turns into a yellowish, puslike substance, and begins to dry up, leaving a crust or scab on the skin. The scabs fall off after three or four weeks, leaving disfiguring pits in the skin. There is no specific medication for smallpox. Treatment may consist of rest, nourishment, medication to lower fever and prevent or soothe itching, sedatives, antibiotics to counteract secondary infection. Vaccination to prevent the disease is highly effective.

## SPERMATOCELE (see under SCROTAL MASS in Symptoms Section)

## SPONDYLITIS, ANKYLOSING (see ANKYLOSING SPONDYLITIS)

## SPOROTRICHOSIS

An infectious disease caused by a fungus, sporotrichosis most often affects farmers, horticulturists, and laborers. It produces small, solid skin lesions, often on the finger, that slowly enlarge and ulcerate. There is usually no local pain. Diagnosis is made by recovering and identifying the fungus. The infection responds to potassium iodide taken orally in water.

## SPRUE, NONTROPICAL (see CELIAC DISEASE)

## SPRUE, TROPICAL

Occurring almost entirely in the Caribbean, India, and southeast Asia, tropical sprue involves abnormalities in the mucous membrane lining of the small intestine and malabsorption, including malabsorption of vitamins. The disease is of unknown cause, although there is some suspicion it may result from infection. It begins with diarrhea, appetite and weight loss, followed by anemia which can be severe, and appearance of fat in the stools. In treatment, a diet high in protein and normal in fat may be used, with folic acid supplements. In advanced stages, vitamin $B_{12}$ injections may be required, along with supplements of other vitamins and a tetracycline drug, to correct anemia, nutritional deficiencies, and produce weight gain.

## STOMACH INFLAMMATION (see GASTRITIS, ACUTE AND CHRONIC)

## STOMATITIS

This is an inflammation of the mucous membranes of the mouth. Both gingivitis (gum inflammation) and glossitis (tongue inflammation) are forms of it. Stomatitis may result from local irritants, vitamin deficiency, infection, injury to the inside of the mouth as from cheek-biting, irritating substances such as alcohol, tobacco smoke, very hot or spicy foods, or anemia. It may produce redness and swelling of tissues, which may become sore especially during eating, sometimes with unpleasant mouth odor, dryness of mouth, or excessive salivation. In some cases, stomatitis may be accompanied by chills, fever, and headache. Treatment may vary with cause. When anemia, vitamin deficiency, or a body infection is involved, both the underlying problem and the stomatitis are treated. Antibiotics are often helpful. A prescribed mouthwash may be used.

## STOMATITIS, RECURRENT APHTHOUS

Suspected but not proven to be of viral origin, recurrent aphthous stomatitis produces outbreaks of painful ulcers in the mouth from two or three times a year to as often as once a month. For treatment, a warm solution of 10 percent sodium bicarbonate used as a mouthwash may be soothing. Relief of symptoms may be aided by anesthetic troches, ointments, or solutions.

## STONES, URINARY (see URINARY CALCULI)

## STRABISMUS

A deviation of the eye which is also called *cross-eye, walleye* and *squint,* strabismus almost always appears at an early age. If not corrected, it may impair vision as well as mar appearance, as one eye, through less use or no use at all, suffers deterioration of vision. In treatment, a patch may be used over the stronger eye to force use of the weaker eye and restore its strength. Eyeglasses or special eye exercises may in some cases help correct the eye deviation. In others, a relatively simple surgical procedure on eye muscles may be required.

## STROKE

Involving destruction of a brain area because of loss of blood supply to the region, stroke may result from blood vessel spasm, rupture of a vessel and bleeding within the cranium, blockage of an artery by a locally formed clot or one traveling there from elsewhere in the body. Depending upon the part of the brain affected, stroke may produce paralysis of one side of the body, speech disturbance, defective vision, deep coma. In some cases, warning symptoms may precede a major stroke and may include moments of dizziness, nausea, vomiting, burning or tingling sensations, or weakness of one side of the body. In some cases, when the warning symptoms can be traced to a blockage in an artery outside the brain—in the neck area, for example—surgery to remove or bypass the blockage may be possible and preventive. When a major stroke occurs, skilled nursing care is essential and, during convalescence, physiotherapy to help overcome paralysis, and sometimes speech therapy.

## STY

An infection of one of the sebaceous glands of the eyelid, a sty may begin with a foreign body sensation in the eye, tearing, and then pain and redness of the lid margin and appearance of a pimplelike lesion. Often, a sty can be localized by application of hot compresses for 10 to 15 minutes every several hours. In some cases, an antibiotic may be prescribed to increase the likelihood of clearance without pus formation and discharge.

## SUBARACHNOID HEMORRHAGE

Involving bleeding into a space in the brain membranes, subarachnoid hemorrhage is most often due to head injury but may also occur as the result of rupture of a congenital aneurysm (a ballooning out) of a brain blood vessel. Symptoms include sudden, severe head pain, with neck stiffness, dizziness, nausea, vomiting, convulsions. Treatment entails bed rest until bleeding stops. Spinal puncture may be needed to relieve pressure within the brain. Surgery may be required to clip or otherwise correct an aneurysm to prevent recurrence.

## SUNSTROKE (see HEAT HYPERPYREXIA)

## SWEATING, EXCESSIVE (see HYPERHIDROSIS)

## SYDENHAM'S CHOREA

Also called *chorea minor, rheumatic chorea,* and *St. Vitus' dance,* this disorder is a central nervous system inflammatory complication of streptococcal infections and may occur sometimes as long as six months afterward, so it may seem to have nothing to do with an infection. It is more common in childhood and in girls, tending to occur in summer and early fall, and is characterized by purposeless, irregular movements. The spasmodic jerking movements often begin as awkwardness with facial grimacing. In mild cases, there may be clumsiness, slight difficulty in dressing and eating. In severe cases, heavy sedation may be needed to prevent self-injury from wildly flailing arms or legs. With medical treatment, which may include, as needed, use of a barbiturate or tranquilizer, or sometimes an aspirin-like compound or a corticosteroid agent, complete recovery is the rule.

## SYPHILIS

A contagious venereal disease caused by a spiral-shaped bacterium which enters the body through a break or abrasion of the skin or a mucous membrane, syphilis first produces a painless sore, called a *chancre,* about three weeks after infection, on or near the head of the penis in men, commonly on the labia but sometimes inside the vagina in women. In some cases, however, the chancre may develop elsewhere—on a lip, breast, finger, or in the anal area. The chancre marks primary syphilis, which can be cured readily by antibiotic treatment. If syphilis then is untreated, the sore disappears in 10 to 40 days, but 2 to 6 months later, secondary syphilis develops, with a rash that may cover any part of the body, white sores that appear on mucous membranes of mouth and throat and around genitalia and rectum, sometimes with hair falling out in patches and accompanied by pain in bones and joints. Secondary syphilis, like primary, can be cured by antibiotics. If untreated, it disappears usually within 3 to 12 weeks but may return later as tertiary syphilis, with the disease invading almost any cell of the body and damaging any organs it invades, including the heart, nervous system, eyes, and brain. Tertiary syphilis may be treated with antibiotics but therapy must be longer and is more difficult.

## TAPEWORM, DWARF

Transmitted through the mouth via tapeworm eggs contaminating the environment, dwarf tapeworm infestation produces abdominal discomfort, diarrhea, dizziness, and exhaustion similar to what would occur from lack of food in a child. It is treated with quinacrine hydrochloride.

# TAPEWORM, PORK OR BEEF

Acquired from poorly cooked or raw, infected beef or pork, this infestation may produce abdominal distress, sometimes severe enough to resemble an "acute appendix." Diagnosis can be made when segments of a worm are found in clothing or bedding or when eggs or segments are found in the stool. Treatment is with quinacrine hydrochloride.

# TELANGIECTASIA, HEREDITARY HEMORRHAGIC

In this disorder, involving a blood vessel anomaly, small red to violet spots appear on the skin and mucous membranes and tend to bleed spontaneously or after trivial injury. The spots consist of thin, dilated blood vessels and occur most often on lips, tongue, fingertips, and toes. No specific treatment is available. Bleeding spots may be treated with pressure, styptics, or other measures including electrocautery.

# TEMPORAL ARTERITIS

An inflammation of the temporal arteries, temporal arteritis produces headache, pain and tenderness of the arteries in the head, sometimes with vision loss. Diagnosis can be aided by microscopic examination of a small artery sample. The inflammation responds well to a corticosteroid such as prednisone.

# TEMPOROMANDIBULAR JOINT DISORDERS

The temporomandibular joint, connecting the upper and lower jaw on each side of the face, can be affected by arthritis, malocclusion, grinding of the teeth, poorly fitted dentures, and emotional disturbances. Symptoms may include pain in the face and in front of the ear, clicking or grating sounds on chewing, limited jaw motion due to pain and spasm. In treatment, muscle relaxants, analgesics, and tranquilizers along with a soft diet may be used for a short period. To overcome the cycle of muscle spasm and pain, heat applications, diathermy, injection of the joint with a corticosteroid, and bite adjustment may be needed. When arthritis is involved, aspirin may be continued.

**TENNIS ELBOW** (see BURSITIS)

**TESTICULAR CANCER** (see CANCER OF THE TESTIS)

## TETANUS

A serious infection, tetanus is caused by bacilli in soil and dust which enter the body through a break in the skin, especially a puncture wound such as caused by a nail, splinter, insect bite, or gunshot. Usually the first symptom is jaw stiffness. Other early symptoms may include stiff neck, stiff arms or legs, swallowing difficulty, fever, sore throat, chilliness, restlessness, irritability, constipation, convulsions. As the disease progresses, opening the jaws becomes difficult, and facial muscle spasm causes elevation of eyebrows and a fixed smile. Tetanus can and should be prevented by immunization. Mortality is greatest in children and the elderly. Treatment requires early use of antitoxin to neutralize the bacillary toxin. Sedation and almost constant nursing care may be required.

## TETANY

Caused by inadequate blood levels of calcium, leading to nerve and muscle irritation, tetany may occur in pregnancy or after childbirth if an excess amount of the mother's body calcium has been used up. In a newborn, tetany may result from temporarily underactive parathyroid glands, which ordinarily produce a secretion to keep blood calcium and phosphate content at normal levels. In children, tetany may occur because of inadequate calcium or vitamin D in the diet, the vitamin being needed if calcium is to be utilized by the body. Another cause of tetany in children is loss of calcium through prolonged diarrhea. In adults, tetany may occur with prolonged vomiting or excessive use of alkalis such as sodium bicarbonate and may also result from hyperventilation, or overbreathing. Symptoms may include abnormal flexion or bending of wrist and ankle joints, muscle twitching, cramps, convulsions. Treatment varies with cause and is usually successful. Measures may include administration of calcium, vitamin D, and parathyroid hormone.

## TETRALOGY OF FALLOT

Tetralogy of Fallot, a congenital heart condition, involves four structural anomalies: narrowing of the pulmonary artery, a ventricular septal defect (hole in the wall separating the two ventricles, or pumping chambers, of the heart), increase in size of the right ventricle, and mispositioning of the aorta so it receives blood from both ventricles instead of from the left ventricle alone. The condition causes blueness, clubbing of ends of fingers, coughing and spitting of blood, labored breathing on exertion, poor growth. Commonly a young child with the condition will squat after exertion. Once beyond treatment, tetralogy today can be overcome by surgery, with virtually complete reconstruction (sometimes partial in a very young child and completed later). Results are usually excellent.

## THREADWORM

Occurring in the southern part of the United States, threadworm infestation is acquired through the bare feet from soil contaminated with worm larvae. Symptoms are abdominal pain and diarrhea. Treatment is with thiabendazole.

## THROAT INFECTION (see PHARYNGITIS)

## THROMBOPHLEBITIS (see VENOUS THROMBOSIS)

## THRUSH (see CANDIDIASIS)

## THYROID CANCER (see CANCER OF THE THYROID)

## THYROID OVERACTIVITY (see HYPERTHYROIDISM)

## THYROID UNDERACTIVITY (see HYPOTHYROIDISM)

## THYROIDITIS, HASHIMOTO'S

A thyroid gland inflammation, Hashimoto's thyroiditis may be an autoimmune disease, in which the body, in effect, becomes allergic to and attacks thyroid tissue. The inflammation, which may occur at any age but most often does in the 30s and 40s, more often in women than in men, leads to swelling in front of the neck from thyroid gland enlargement, often with fullness in the throat, sometimes with symptoms of hypothyroidism. Treatment requires lifelong use of thyroid hormone and, in some cases, use of a corticosteroid such as prednisone for a few weeks.

## THYROIDITIS, SUBACUTE GRANULOMATOUS

A thyroid gland inflammation which may be caused by viral infection, this condition produces neck pain, which may radiate to jaws, arms or chest, sometimes with low-grade fever. It often subsides spontaneously within a few weeks. Aspirin or, in severe cases, prednisone may be used to alleviate discomfort. Almost always full recovery occurs.

## TIC DOULOUREUX (see NEURALGIA)

## TICS

Sometimes called *habit* or *mimic spasms,* tics are sudden, quick, repetitive, purposeless movements such as eye blinking, grimacing, head nodding or shaking, throat clearing, shoulder shrugging. Almost always without physical cause, they can occur at any time of life but most commonly affect 5- to 12-year-olds. They often are fleeting and disappear on their own. Psychotherapy may be helpful in some cases. A tranquilizer or mild sedative such as phenobarbital may sometimes be used.

## TONGUE INFLAMMATION (see GLOSSITIS)

## TONSILLITIS

The tonsils—two masses of lymph tissue in the sides of the throat, behind and above the tongue—and the adenoids, which are similar but smaller masses close to the openings of the eustachian tubes which drain the ears, serve useful purposes. They act as filters and remove impurities, especially bacteria from the air. Sometimes they become overloaded by a heavy germ invasion and, instead of destroying the invaders, themselves become overwhelmed and infected. The result, acute tonsillitis, leads to sore throat with pain in the tonsil area especially during swallowing, chills, fever to 105° or 106°, headache, malaise, sometimes stiff neck. Acute tonsillitis usually responds dramatically to antibiotic therapy. Chronic tonsillitis, which may result from repeated acute infections, may cause recurrent sore throat, chronic nasal discharge, neck gland swelling, sometimes low-grade fever, failure to gain weight, and lassitude. Surgical removal may be required. But surgery, once routine, no longer is and should be done only when clearly indicated.

## TOOTHACHE (see PERIAPICAL ABSCESS; PULPITIS)

## TORTICOLLIS, SPASMODIC (WRYNECK)

A contracted state of the neck muscles producing twisting of the neck, spasmodic torticollis may be a congenital deformity or may result from neck gland inflammation or muscle spasm. Sometimes, spasmodic torticollis may be temporarily overcome by slight pressure on the jaw on the side to which the head is being turned. Atropine or scopolamine sometimes may be helpful, as may be other drugs such as meprobamate and chlorpromazine.

## TOXIC AMBLYOPIA

Leading to reduced vision, usually in both eyes, toxic amblyopia is commonly the result of excessive use of alcohol or tobacco but may also follow long-term exposure to carbon monoxide, carbon tetrachloride, arsenic, lead, benzene, or quinine. Immediate elimination of the causative agent may bring improvement.

## TOXOPLASMOSIS

A worldwide disease, toxoplasmosis is caused by a protozoan parasite. Cysts of the parasite may be found in beef, pork, lamb, and poultry; and meat is believed to be the most common infectious source, although vegetarians are not immune. Cysts also have been found in the feces of infected animals, suggesting that the disease may be transmitted fecally. In the mild form of toxoplasmosis, symptoms may include swelling of neck and underarm glands (lymph nodes), malaise, muscle pain, irregular mild fever, mild anemia, and low blood pressure. An acute fulminating form often produces high fever, chills, skin rash, and prostration. A chronic form may produce muscular weakness, headache, diarrhea, weight loss, inflammation of the retina of the eye or of the uvea (iris, ciliary body, and choroid). A congenital toxoplasmosis, appearing soon after birth, apparently the result of infection of the mother, may produce many disturbances including those of the eye and central nervous system, with convulsions. Affected children may die in infancy or experience chronic destructive nervous system effects. For other than congenital toxoplasmosis, the outlook is good. Treatment may include use of sulfa drugs, pyrimethamine, and prednisone.

## TRACHOMA

Caused by a viruslike organism, trachoma is a chronic communicable disease of the eye, widespread in many parts of the world but rare in the United States. Symptoms include reddening of the eyes, swelling and sticking together of the lids, later with the lids becoming pocked and scarred and with granules forming on the lid interior surface. In treatment, tetracycline eye ointment applied several times a day for up to six weeks is often effective.

## TRANSPOSITION OF THE GREAT VESSELS

In this congenital heart defect, the pulmonary artery arises from the left instead of right ventricle, while the aorta arises from the right instead of left ventricle. As a result, most of the used blood returning from the body goes to the aorta without traveling to the lungs to be oxygenated. Symptoms are blueness at birth, becoming progressively more severe, with great breathing difficulty and growth failure. In emergency treatment a balloon catheter or tube is inserted into a blood vessel and maneuvered into the heart, to make an opening in the septum (or wall) between the two atria (or top chambers of the heart). This reroutes some of the blood and increases the flow of oxygenated blood to body tissues. Later, often at about the age of 3, a permanent reconstructive operation may be performed.

**TRENCH FEVER** (see ROCKY MOUNTAIN SPOTTED FEVER AND OTHER RICKETTSIAL DISEASES)

**TRENCH MOUTH** (see GINGIVOSTOMATITIS, NECROTIZING ULCERATIVE)

## TRICHINOSIS

This is an infection caused by a parasitic roundworm, usually acquired by eating poorly cooked pork. The larvae, or early forms of the worm, are embedded in tiny cysts in muscle tissue of infected pork and are killed by high cooking temperatures. If they survive in undercooked pork, the cysts dissolve during digestion, freeing the larvae, which grow to maturity in the intestines, produce new larvae, and then are carried via the bloodstream to one or many body tissues and organs. Even as the larvae develop into mature worms in the intestinal tract, there may sometimes be diarrhea, nausea, abdominal pain, and fever. But identifying symptoms come after a one- to two-week incubation period and include swelling of the eyelids, pain in the eyes, extreme sensitivity to light, muscle soreness and pain, thirst, chills, profuse sweating, hives, weakness, and prostration. Usually, by about the third month, most symptoms disappear, although vague muscular pains and fatigue may linger for several months more. Purgatives and worm-killers are of little use, since the worms are within the intestinal lining. Treatment is directed at relieving symptoms with analgesics, bed rest, and in some cases a corticosteroid such as prednisone, until the infection disappears.

## TRIGEMINAL NEURALGIA (see NEURALGIA)

## TUBERCULOSIS

This infectious, communicable disease commonly attacks the lungs although the organism responsible, the tubercle bacillus, can go on to invade virtually all parts of the body, including bone, kidneys, bladder, and genitalia. The source is often the sputum of an infected person which, even when dried, can harbor live organisms for months. The bacilli may be spread by droplets and can be carried in air, on eating utensils, and in unpasteurized milk and other dairy products from tuberculous cattle. In early stages of tuberculosis, some patients have no symptoms; others experience fever and weight loss. In children, early TB may appear as a flulike illness with fever, drowsiness, fatigue, loss of appetite and weight. In adults, listlessness and vague pains in the chest may go unnoticed because often they are not severe enough to call attention to themselves. The symptoms commonly thought of in connection with TB—cough, purulent sputum, night sweats, bleeding from the lungs—do not occur in the earliest stages of the disease. As TB progresses, severe cough develops, sputum becomes yellowish and often is streaked with blood, chest pain is present and aggravated by breathing effort. Tuberculosis of bones and joints in the legs leads to joint pain and swelling, and a limp. Disease in the arms causes joint swelling, limitation of movement, and tenderness. In the spine, the disease may produce painful muscle spasm, limitation of movement, followed by curvature of the spine and abscess formation. Among the drugs used effectively to treat tuberculosis are INH (isoniazid), PAS (para-aminosalicylic acid), ethambutol, and rifampin. Treatment often must continue for 18 to 24 months.

## TUBERCULOSIS OF THE ALIMENTARY TRACT

Infection of the digestive tract by tuberculosis may occur as the result of swallowing infected sputum or, uncommonly, as the result of drinking contaminated milk. Rarely the infection may produce masses that may partially fill the alimentary passageway. The usual result of infection is ulceration, which may develop in any area from mouth through to anus, producing symptoms such as appetite loss, abdominal discomfort and cramps, and diarrhea. For treatment the same drugs employed in tuberculosis of the lungs are used.

## TULAREMIA

Also known as *rabbit* or *deer-fly fever,* this acute infectious disease is transmitted by rodents and other animal hosts. Most frequently affected are hunters, farmers, butchers, fur handlers, and laboratory workers, most often through contact with wild rabbits. One to ten days after exposure, tularemia begins with sudden onset of chills and fever, headache, nausea, vomiting, and severe weakness. Within 24 to 48 hours, a small sore usually develops at the site of infection and ulcerates. A generalized red rash follows. Fever of 103° or 104° may last for three to four weeks. Treatment is with an antibiotic such as tetracycline, streptomycin, or chloramphenicol. Wet dressings may help the sore.

## TYPHOID FEVER

A bacterial infection, typhoid fever is transmitted by water, milk, or other food contaminated by people who are carriers of the bacteria. After a period of three days to several weeks, depending upon the number of organisms ingested, the disease produces chilly sensations, malaise, headache, appetite loss, nosebleeds, backache, and diarrhea or constipation. Sore throat and respiratory symptoms may occur. Temperature rises daily, reaching a peak of 105° after 7 to 10 days, remaining there for 7 to 10 days more, then falling. After a week or more, rose spots may appear on the chest and abdomen. Delirium and stupor are common. In some cases, there may be atypical symptoms of nausea, vomiting, rigidity, bronchitis, pneumonia. Where once death occurred in as many as 30 percent of patients, mortality with prompt use of suitable anitbiotics now is less than 1 percent.

## TYPHUS (see ROCKY MOUNTAIN SPOTTED FEVER AND OTHER RICKETTSIAL DISEASES)

## ULCERATIVE COLITIS (see COLITIS, CHRONIC ULCERATIVE)

## UNDULANT FEVER (see BRUCELLOSIS)

## UREMIA

Uremia is an accumulation in the blood of substances ordinarily eliminated in the urine. It develops when the kidneys lose much of their ability to filter out waste products from the blood. The loss of kidney function may result from temporary poisoning or obstruction or may occur in the final stages of severe kidney disease. In *acute uremia* the first symptom is a sudden drop in urine volume, followed by other symptoms such as fatigue, decreased mental acuity, muscular twitching, muscle cramps, nausea, vomiting, convulsions, appetite loss, yellow-brown discoloration of the skin, urine smell on breath and sweat, and itching; the cause of acute uremia may be injury or surgical shock, severe transfusion reaction, severe burn, severe infection, various kinds of poisoning, or drug reaction. *Chronic uremia*, without a sudden drop in the urine but with many of the other symptoms making their appearance gradually, may result from chronic nephritis or advanced pyelitis or hypertensive kidney disease. Diabetes, polycystic kidneys, untreated prostate enlargement, kidney stones and other obstructions may also cause uremia.

In acute uremia, the kidneys are rested by restriction of fluid intake while the cause of the kidney failure is sought and treated. Most patients with acute uremia respond well and the kidneys often recover in one to six weeks. If they do not, an artificial kidney may be used to give the damaged kidneys time to regain function. In chronic uremia, treatment is directed if possible at the cause. If correction is impossible, a low-protein diet may help decrease symptoms. Other measures may be employed. Patients who once would have died now can be kept in reasonable health for long periods with periodic kidney machine dialysis. Transplantation may be used and may allow return to virtually normal living.

## URETHRAL STRICTURE (see under SCROTAL MASS in Symptoms Section)

## URETHRITIS, NONGONOCOCCAL

A common inflammation of the urethra, the canal extending from the bladder to the outside, in men, nongonococcal urethritis (of venereal origin in most cases) is caused by an unknown organism. It produces a slight, watery, whitish secretion, sometimes with mild pain on urination and lower abdominal pain. Treatment with an antibiotic such as tetracycline, sometimes combined with a sulfa drug, is often effective. If not, other antibiotics may be used. Another form of urethral inflammation, occurring in women after menopause, may be associated with urethral atrophy. Local treatment measures such as urethral dilation and estrogen suppositories may be used.

## URINARY CALCULI (STONES)

Stones may form anywhere in the urinary tract and sometimes may produce excruciating, intermittent, colicky pain, usually starting in the kidney area and radiating across the abdomen into the genital area and inner aspects of the thigh, with nausea, vomiting, chills, fever, urinary frequency. Many people have one stone or a few without any obvious cause for the stone formation. Chronic stone-formers in some cases have predisposing infection or obstruction of the urinary tract. In some cases, there is an underlying disease such as gout. Many single stones without obstruction or infection require no treatment. Colic symptoms can be relieved by morphine or meperidine. Impacted stones usually must be removed by surgery. When stones are composed of uric acid, they may be dissolved by long-term use of alkalis to alkalinize the urine.

## URINARY TRACT INFECTIONS (see also GLOMERULONEPHRITIS; PYELONEPHRITIS)

Common symptoms of urinary tract infections include frequency, urgency, pain and burning, often with chills and fever, nausea and vomiting, general muscle aches, and lassitude. In cystitis, infection centers in the bladder. One form, *honeymoon cystitis*, occurs in young women early in marriage when frequent coitus may lead to fluid retention and swelling of the bladder neck and urethra, interfering with bladder emptying and favoring introduction of bacteria through the urethra. Honeymoon cystitis is often avoidable with high fluid intake and complete bladder emptying before and after intercourse. A hemorrhagic form of cystitis usually manifests itself first by blood in the urine followed by frequency, urgency, and pain. Cystitis also may occur with benign prostate enlargement. In acute prostatitis, urinary disturbances may be followed by severe fever and swelling and tenderness of the prostate. To treat urinary infections, antibiotics and sulfa drugs may be used. Other agents, such as belladonna, atropine, hyoscine, and hyoscyamine may be prescribed for relief of frequency and urgency of urination. If obstructive lesions are present, they may be corrected by surgery.

## URTICARIA (see HIVES)

## UTERINE CANCER (see CANCER OF THE UTERUS)

## UTERUS, MYOMA OF THE

Also called *fibroid tumor*, this is a benign tumor of smooth muscle fibers of the uterus, the most common of all tumors in women. It may occur in any part of the uterus. Although a single tumor may occur, usually there are several. Commonly, they are small but they may grow large and occupy most of the uterine wall. Growth usually stops after menopause. With growth, the tumors may exert pressure on nearby organs and cause painful menstruation, abnormal menstrual bleeding, vaginal discharge, or urinary frequency. When small, myomas may be checked frequently. Larger ones may be removed surgically. In some cases, hysterectomy may be performed.

## UTERUS, PROLAPSED (see PROLAPSE OF THE UTERUS)

## UVEITIS

Sometimes related to a specific allergy-causing agent but often of unknown cause, uveitis is an inflammation of the uvea, which is made up of the iris, ciliary body, and choroid of the eye. Symptoms include eye pain, sensitivity to light, inflammation around the cornea. In some cases, bacterial vaccines have been found helpful. Often, treatment is with a corticosteroid such as prednisone.

## VARICOCELE (see under SCROTAL MASS in Symptoms Section)

## VARICOSE VEINS

Varicose veins are swollen, distended, and knotted veins visible especially in the legs. They may result from sluggish blood flow in combination with defective valves and weakened vein walls. Prolonged standing or sitting without movement tends to favor their development, since return of blood from the legs is aided by leg muscle activity. Without leg muscle activity blood tends to back up, and its weight pressing down against the closed valves in the veins causes the veins to distend. When a number of valves no longer function effectively, blood pools or collects in the veins, which become distended further and swollen. During pregnancy, the uterus may press against veins coming from the legs, inhibiting free flow and setting up back pressure that may lead to varicosities. There is some evidence that constipation and straining at stool cause back pressure that may be an important factor in varicosity formation.

In mild cases of varicose veins, treatment may involve bathing the legs in warm water to help stimulate blood flow, several rest periods daily with the feet above the body to encourage return flow, and changes in daily routine to permit more movement. Stockings lightly reinforced with elastic add support for the veins. In more severe cases, when such measures are inadequate, a hardening or sclerosing solution may be injected into the veins, causing them to atrophy after a period of time, with blood channeled into other vessels. Alternatively, since recurrences may develop after injection, surgery in which a varicosed vein is tied off and removed may be performed.

## VENOUS THROMBOSIS

Variously referred to as thrombophlebitis, phlebitis, phlebothrombosis, and milk leg, venous thrombosis means a clot in a vein. *Phlebothrombosis* indicates that little or no inflammation is present with the clot, whereas *thrombophlebitis* and *phlebitis* indicate definite inflammation of the vein wall. The term *milk leg* is sometimes used to indicate a clot in the iliac or femoral vein, with massive leg swelling. Symptoms of venous thrombosis include leg swelling, pain or tenderness. Clot formation may occur because of accidental injury of the vein lining, the presence of microorganisms, or stasis (standstill) of blood in a vein with inactivity or bed rest. A clot, which may develop in a muscle vein of the calf or foot, gradually grows, developing a kind of "tail" that waves freely. As its diameter increases, it may obstruct a vein. Part or sometimes all of the clot may break loose and be carried by the blood to a vessel in the lung, becoming a pulmonary embolus. Alternatively, growth of the clot at its original site may stop, with the clot becoming firmly attached, and over a period of months a new channel for blood flow forms in the vein or new branches may form, allowing blood to be detoured around the clot obstruction.

In treatment, the patient is confined to bed, the leg elevated to encourage blood return to the heart, and moist warm packs are applied. An anticoagulant such as heparin helps prevent further clotting. Usually within five to ten days, tenderness and swelling are gone and the patient can walk with an elastic support, which may be worn for three months or longer. When the clot is in a superficial leg vein, bed rest may not be needed, and the patient may be allowed to walk with elastic support while taking time out for elevating the leg and moist heat applications several times a day for half an hour at a time. If improvement does not occur, the vein may be tied off to help prevent embolism.

## VENTRICULAR SEPTAL DEFECT

In this congenital heart abnormality, there is an opening in the septum (or wall) between the two ventricles (or lower chambers) of the heart. Symptoms include labored breathing, fatigue on exertion, sometimes impairment of growth. Permanent cure is obtained with surgery to close the opening.

## VIRAL ENCEPHALITIS (see ENCEPHALITIS, VIRAL)

## VITAMIN DEFICIENCIES (see also SCURVY; OSTEOMALACIA; and, in Missed Diagnoses Section, FOLIC ACID DEFICIENCY)

*Deficiency of vitamin A* may cause night blindness, sometimes with abnormal dryness of the surface of the conjunctiva and softening of the cornea. Therapeutic doses of vitamin are needed to correct the deficiency: thereafter, smaller maintenance doses are taken.

*Thiamine (vitamin B₁) deficiency* can cause a complex of symptoms of neurasthenia—appetite loss, lack of energy, aches and pains, irritability, poor memory, sleep disturbances—with chest pain, abdominal discomfort, constipation. The deficiency can arise not only from inadequate intake of the vitamin, but also from disorders increasing need for it, such as hyperthyroidism, fever, pregnancy, breast-feeding. Disorders such as severe liver disease, which impairs utilization of thiamine, and alcoholism, which interferes with both absorption and utilization, increase requirements as well. With continued deficiency, beriberi may develop, producing such symptoms as burning of the feet, calf muscle cramps, leg pains, mental confusion, congestive heart failure, pulmonary congestion. Treatment for neurasthenia symptoms may require 10 to 20 milligrams of thiamine daily in divided doses. In more advanced deficiency, injections of the vitamin may be required until improvement is obtained, after which oral supplements can be used.

*Riboflavin (vitamin B₂) deficiency* can produce dry scaling and fissuring of the lips and angles of the mouth, sometimes with red, scaly greasy areas on the ears, eyelids, scrotum, and labia majora, sometimes also with eye disturbances including light sensitivity and tearing. The deficiency may result from inadequate intake of milk or other animal proteins or may be associated with chronic diarrhea, liver disease, or chronic alcoholism. Dietary changes may be needed along with supplementary riboflavin of as much as 10 to 30 milligrams daily in divided doses until improvement begins, after which 2 to 4 milligrams per day may be used to full recovery.

*Niacin (nicotinic acid, vitamin B₃) deficiency* can cause fatigue, appetite loss, lack of energy, aches and pains, memory impairment, confusion, sore mouth, scarlet tongue and oral membranes, skin and gastrointestinal disturbances. The deficiency is common in some areas of the world where corn is a prime part of diet; niacin is present in corn in a form that makes it unavailable for proper absorption. The deficiency also may occur elsewhere with inappropriate diet, diarrheal disease, cirrhosis of the liver, and chronic alcoholism. In treatment, upward of 300 milligrams a day of the vitamin by mouth in divided doses are required.

*Pyridoxine (vitamin B₆) deficiency* can produce yellowish greasy scaling of the scalp, tongue inflammation, fissuring of the lips and angles of the mouth, anemia and, in infants, convulsions. Deficiency may result not only from lack of adequate intake of the vitamin but also from malabsorption or other disturbances. Symptoms respond to treatment with pyridoxine supplements, which in an adult may range from 50 to 100 milligrams per day.

*Vitamin K deficiency* can lead to bleeding into the skin and mucous membranes and vomiting of blood and darkening of feces with blood pigments. While some of the vitamin comes from the diet, much of it is produced in the gut by bacteria. Deficiency may result from impaired absorption, which may be due to varied causes including excessive use of mineral oil. The vitamin can be given by mouth or injection to control bleeding.


**VITAMIN POISONING** (see HYPERVITAMINOSIS A and D)


**VITILIGO (PIEBALD SKIN)**

Of unknown cause, vitiligo involves patchy losses of skin pigmentation and may occur anywhere on the body. The patches are milky white, sharply demarcated. They sometimes may be covered successfully with carefully matched cosmetic lotions or pastes. In some cases, repigmentation may occur with treatment combining a drug, methoxsalen, and carefully prescribed exposure to sunlight.


**VOCAL CORD POLYPS** (see POLYPOSIS OF THE VOCAL CORDS)


**von WILLEBRAND'S DISEASE**

This is a hereditary disease which may produce mild or severe bleeding into the skin and mucous membranes, bleeding in the gastrointestinal and genitourinary tracts, and often excessive menstruation in women. The disease is due to deficiency of a blood component, Factor VIII, and benefits from replacement of the component.

## VULVITIS

An inflammation of the vulva, vulvitis has many possible causes: injury; mechanical or chemical irritation; allergic reaction to clothing, detergents, or drugs; various infections; and venereal disease. Uncontrolled diabetes may also produce vulvitis.

Symptoms may include reddening, with edema and swelling, burning, itching, and sometimes pain severe enough to interfere with sitting and walking.

Vulvitis should be treated by a physician. The cause must be determined and combated. Antibacterial drugs may be used for bacterial or fungus infections. An oral antihistamine and either an oral or topically applied corticosteroid drug may be used for the inflammation and itching. Cold compresses of aluminum acetate solution may be prescribed for immediate relief in some cases; in others, hot compresses or warm sitz baths may be used.

## WARTS (see in Symptoms Section)

## WEN (see CYST, SEBACEOUS)

## WHIPPLE'S DISEASE

Occurring mostly in men, this is a disease, not very common, that produces symptoms similar to those of celiac disease and other malabsorption disorders—appetite and weight loss, anemia, weakness, fatigability—but in addition is characterized by fever of 100° to 103°, joint pains and arthritis of knees, wrists and back, nonproductive cough, abdominal and chest pain. Intensive antibiotic treatment, starting with up to two weeks of injections of penicillin and followed by another antibiotic such as tetracycline taken by mouth for up to a year, often is effective.

## WHIPWORM

This parasite, transmitted by fecal contamination of soil, is common in the Gulf Coast region and in warm moist climates. It produces diarrhea, nausea, anemia, retarded growth. Treatment is with thiabendazole or hexylresorcinol enemas.

## WHOOPING COUGH (PERTUSSIS)

A highly communicable bacterial disease, whooping cough can develop at any age but about half of all cases occur before the age of 2 years. Transmission is usually through air from an infected individual. After a 7- to 14-day incubation period, whooping cough often starts with running nose, sneezing, tearing of the eyes, appetite loss, listlessness, only rarely fever. There is also a hacking cough at night which gradually begins to appear by day. After 10 to 14 days, the cough becomes paroxysmal, taking place 8 to 10 times in one breath. The face may turn blue or purple. Finally, the breath is caught in a long noisy "whoop"-like intake. The coughing lasts for about four to six weeks, and the patient can transmit the disease for about four weeks after first symptoms appear. No specific treatment is available once whooping cough develops; a vaccine to prevent it is available. In a seriously ill infant, hospitalization and expert nursing care may be needed.

## WILMS' TUMOR (see CANCER OF THE KIDNEY)

## WILSON'S DISEASE

A rare hereditary disease in which a pair of abnormal genes lead to retention of abnormal amounts of the metal copper, Wilson's disease can produce tremor at rest and with movement, drooling, speaking difficulty, open-mouthedness, incoordination, rigidity, sometimes behavioral changes and anemia. In treatment a drug, penicillamine, by mouth is used to increase copper excretion. Lifelong treatment is required and a low-copper diet is prescribed. The vitamin pyridoxine also may be helpful.

## WRYNECK (see TORTICOLLIS, SPASMODIC)

## YELLOW FEVER

An acute viral disease transmitted by mosquito, yellow fever has an incubation period of three to six days. It manifests itself suddenly, intensely, with fever, headache, muscle aches, prostration. A few days later, the temperature suddenly falls only to rise again. Yellowing of the skin occurs, the urine becomes dark, frequent vomiting may occur with blood sometimes noticeable in the vomitus. The disease runs its course in a little more than a week, and those who recover—and most do—suffer no permanent damage.

# SECTION THREE  Missed Diagnoses

Diagnosis—the determination of what is causing a health problem—sometimes can be relatively simple for an experienced physician, sometimes complex but nonetheless achievable.

Some diagnoses, however, are missed.

There are those that are never sought: for nuisance ailments, bothersome but not acutely disturbing, that people get accustomed to living with even if not happily, seeking no medical help, sometimes mistakenly believing none is available.

But when help is sought, a diagnosis may be missed. That may be because a history is incomplete, the patient reporting a most bothersome symptom or set of symptoms but failing to recognize the significance of others and tell of them, which, if known to a physician, could provide clues to proper assessment of cause.

Diagnoses also may be missed for other reasons: the lack of experience of a physician, or even of many physicians, with a particular disorder; even a general opinion within the medical community that a particular disorder is rare, or limited to a certain group of people, or to one sex, or to certain specific symptoms and no others.

Here are more than three dozen conditions that, for such reasons, and although they may be treated successfully and in some cases even quite simply, often have gone and continue to go undiagnosed or are mistakenly diagnosed. According to some recent authoritative estimates, between them they affect millions in this country to some degree. For some of these missed-diagnosis conditions, it should be added, only recently have new insights been obtained that significantly aid diagnosis.

## AKITHISIA

A condition marked by an inability to sit still, a restless need to keep moving about, shifting the legs, tapping the feet, or rocking the body, akithisia may be triggered by drugs, especially tranquilizers. It can be readily eliminated, once recognized for what it is, by a change in drug dosage or a change to a different drug. The problem is that diagnosis may be missed, and often is, because patients mistake their restlessness for the anxiety for which they are taking a drug.

## ALLERGY, BLEACH-CHANGE

It's an old story that people allergic to the rubber elastic in undergarments suffer from itching rashes unless the elastic is avoided. A puzzling phenomenon has been the appearance of the same kind of rash in some people found by tests *not* to have the sensitivity. Recently, investigators have established the reason: When bleach is used in laundering underwear, the bleach action may cause a chemical change in the elastic that leads to a sensitivity that would not be shown by usual tests. The solution: use of underwear without elastic or rinsing without bleach.

## ANKYLOSING SPONDYLITIS

A disorder affecting the small joints of the spine, producing stiffening and painful, difficult movement, ankylosing spondylitis most often affects young adults. It has long been thought to be almost exclusively a male problem, affecting men at least ten times as often as women.

Recent investigations, however, indicate that women may be afflicted fully as often; that in some cases in women ankylosing spondylitis may be mistaken for rheumatoid arthritis; that in other cases women may suffer along for years with what they consider to be back trouble related to menstruation.

Ankylosing spondylitis is a chronic, progressive disorder. Its early recognition is important. If, with early recognition, pain can be relieved so as to permit good posture to be maintained, crippling may be prevented, a close-to-normal life made possible.

For this disorder, the corticosteroid drugs and gold salt injections often helpful in rheumatoid arthritis are not particularly effective.

Aspirin, however, is sometimes useful and, when it is not adequate, either of two drugs—indomethacin or phenylbutazone—can help 90 percent of patients.

## ARTERITIS, GIANT CELL

An artery inflammation, almost always limited to people over 50, and mostly over 65, giant cell arteritis is now believed to affect half a million or more of the elderly, often going unrecognized despite the potential for dramatic improvement with specific treatment.

When the temporal artery in the head is affected, there are severe headache and swelling and tenderness of the artery, often with intermittent jaw pain. When other arteries, alone or in addition to the temporal, are involved, there may be aching pain and stiffness in muscles of the neck, back, shoulder, upper arm, hip and thigh, often with mental depression, and low-grade fever.

Because patients often also complain of appetite loss and lassitude and because, too, of the diffuseness of the muscle aches and the fact that muscles and joints appear to be normal, it is easy for the problem to be dismissed as a matter of either senile depression or psychogenic aches and pains.

The cause of giant cell arteritis—called that because of the presence, with inflammation, of abnormally large cells—is unknown.

An aid to diagnosis is a simple blood test, called the *sedimentation rate,* which checks the rapidity with which red blood cells settle out of blood in an hour. The rate in arteritis is high.

Once diagnosed, giant cell arteritis responds remarkably to treatment with a corticosteroid drug such as prednisone in a daily dose of 40 to 60 milligrams. Pain disappears, usually in 48 hours or less, along with fever, apathy, and other symptoms.

## ATHLETE'S FOOT

A nuisance affliction with its between-the-toes itching, athlete's foot, at its height, can produce distracting, whitish, soggy, malodorous, itching lesions. Although it has long been supposed to result from infection with a fungus picked up in locker rooms, public showers, and swimming pool walkways, that, it now turns out, is just half the problem.

At its start, when it produces no symptoms, only dry scaling, athlete's foot is a fungal infection. When, however, the symptoms appear, they result from bacteria rather than fungi, and the latter, in fact, may no longer be present.

At some point after the original fungal infection, bacteria multiply because of the presence between the toes of excessive moisture, which may be there as the result of exercise, hot weather, tight shoes, or even emotionally triggered excessive sweating. Ideal for bacteria, the moisture allows them to multiply and displace the fungi.

With these facts uncovered by very recent studies, other research, making use of Philadelphia prison volunteers, has led to the finding of effective treatment which, at once, has a necessary drying effect along with antibacterial action. It's a solution of 30 percent aluminum chloride ($AlCl_3 \cdot 6H_2O$) which a druggist can prepare at moderate cost (approximately two to three dollars for four ounces). Applied twice daily with a cotton-tipped applicator, it has abolished itching and malodor within 72 hours and produced marked relief of all symptoms within a week. After complete clearance, it may be used once a day in very hot, humid weather. It should *not* be used because of the possibility of irritation when a fissure—a narrow, deep slit—is present and can allow penetration of the solution to living skin below the scaling and horny layers.

## CAFFEINISM

Among the symptoms of a psychiatric disorder, chronic anxiety, are dizziness, agitation, restlessness, recurrent headache, sleeping trouble, irritability, muscle twitching and, occasionally, vomiting and diarrhea.

Yet exactly such symptoms can be produced by unsuspected caffeinism, and recognition of the problem can avoid needless psychiatric treatment.

In pioneering research carried out at the Walter Reed Army Medical Center, Washington, D.C., where he was then director of psychiatric research, Dr. John F. Greden, now at the University of Michigan School of Medicine, uncovered the ability of caffeinism to mimic anxiety neurosis in a series of patients already diagnosed as being chronically anxious.

In each case, intake of caffeine—in coffee, tea, cola drinks, cocoa, and in caffeine-containing headache remedies—was high. In each case, symptoms disappeared when caffeine intake was cut, with improvement often occurring within 36 hours.

Greden's studies indicate that individual sensitivity to caffeine varies and in some people symptoms may be induced by an intake of as little as 250 milligrams, an amount exceeded by many people every day since, for example, the caffeine in three cups of coffee, a cola drink, and two caffeine-containing headache tablets amounts to about 500 milligrams.

## CHILDREN'S HEADACHES AND DEPRESSION

Children may get the same types of headaches as adults: migraine, tension or muscular contraction headaches, and inflammatory headaches associated with sinusitis or allergy.

They may also, along with adults, suffer from headaches induced by mental depression, although such headaches may escape proper diagnosis.

Recent research among children with severe headaches provides guidelines for diagnosis of childhood depression headaches.

In the research, each child was checked for certain specific factors: significant mood change, social withdrawal, progressively deteriorating performance in school, sleep disturbance, newly developed aggressive behavior, self-deprecation, beliefs of persecution, loss of energy, weight or appetite.

Children showing four or more of the factors and not suffering from other apparent psychiatric illness (the most common factors: mood change, social withdrawal, self-deprecation) were taken to be depressed. With treatment using an antidepressant agent such as amitriptyline or imipramine, their headaches as well as low mood improved markedly.

## CHILDREN WITH RAP (RECURRENT ABDOMINAL PAIN)

RAP, it is now estimated, occurs in 10 percent of school-age children. The possible causes are many.

Among those that sometimes may be missed are abdominal migraine and abdominal epilepsy. In such cases, the abdominal pain may be an initial indication of a migraine or convulsive disorder.

According to recent studies, the most frequently missed cause of RAP in young girls is urinary tract infection which may or may not produce any urinary symptoms but can be revealed by urine testing. RAP also may be caused by upper respiratory tract infection and tonsillitis, but the child may not have a sore throat. Another possible cause is PINWORMS.

## CHILDREN'S "SEIZURES" AND HEARTBURN

Reflux of acid from the stomach back up into the esophagus is well known for the heartburn it can produce. But can reflux sometimes be responsible in children for what seem like epileptic seizures and for other unusual effects? So it appears from a recent study at the University of Utah College of Medicine, Salt Lake City, with 12 children, aged 3 months to 5 years. Six suffered from seizures and, in addition, like the other six, from one or more such problems as difficulty in swallowing, wryneck, extreme irritability, abdominal pain, developmental retardation, or episodes of temporary breathing cessation. In 11 of the 12, x-ray studies revealed reflux. In most cases, treatment for the reflux eliminated symptoms.

## CHILDREN'S URINARY TRACT INFECTION AND COLIC

Colic, a common problem of infancy, may sometimes be the sole symptom of urinary tract infection. This, a new finding, comes from studies by Dr. Joseph N. H. Du of the University of Manitoba (Winnipeg) Health Sciences Center.

Among babies with persistent, severe colic, he found some who, like a 2-month-old girl, had to be hospitalized for study. Despite a physical examination that revealed nothing obviously abnormal, she had paroxysms of acute abdominal pain presumably of intestinal origin, associated with almost continuous crying and irritability. When urine examination revealed the presence of pus and disease organisms and she was treated with an antibiotic, ampicillin, the urinary infection—and the colic—disappeared. That was the case, too, in several other infants with colic associated with urinary infection.

## COUGH, ALLERGIC

A nonproductive, barking, foghorn cough in a child for which no physical cause can be found may be labeled "nervous" or "psychogenic." But at least in some cases, the problem may lie with allergy.

As an example, one medical report cites the case of a 10-year-old girl who coughed every 15 to 30 seconds, had undergone tonsil and adenoid removal, and had received varied medications without benefit. The cough clearly become worse when she was tense or excited, making it seem all the more likely that it was psychogenic.

Allergy tests, however, indicated hypersensitivity to molds and house dust. With allergy treatment that included injections of gradually increasing doses of the offending substances to build up tolerance, the cough finally subsided. At the time of the medical report, it had not recurred in four years.

## COUGH FROM A HAIR IN THE EAR

It may seem like the last place to look for a cause, but a chronic cough can result from a hair in the ear if the hair touches the eardrum. And physicians at Washington University School of Medicine have reported cures for several patients.

Actually, the phenomenon is easily explained. Upon receiving a message of irritation in the breathing passages, the cough center in the brain sends out impulses to produce the coughing response. Because a hair touching an eardrum is irritating, the cough center may receive an irritation message and respond chronically with cough-producing impulses until the irritating hair is removed.

## DEMENTIA, SENILE

Too often, senile dementia has been, and remains, a wastebasket diagnosis—or, more accurately, no diagnosis at all. Let an elderly person show behavioral changes and some evidence of intellectual decline and the tendency has been to equate these with irreversible brain atrophy and brain artery hardening, making any effort at treatment virtually useless.

Yet, even before the recent appearance of brain scanning machines, pioneering research has demonstrated that senility symptoms are not invariably linked with irreversible brain changes and that even when they are the problem may not be hopeless.

Many changes, not in the brain itself, often subtle changes, individually or collectively can conspire to produce the appearance or actuality of senility. The possible factors are many, ranging from thyroid or other hormone disturbances to low blood sugar, from anemia, smoldering infections, and injuries to intoxications from self-administered drugs such as bromides and sometimes from prescribed agents. Nor are these merely theoretical factors, for numerous reports recently have indicated that with their proper treatment, seemingly hopeless senility often can be reversed.

Some reversals are particularly dramatic. On admission to Mount Sinai Hosptial, New York, a 66-year-old judge was confused, disoriented, had memory deficits, paranoid suspiciousness, impaired gait, and was incontinent of urine and feces. His seeming senility had begun with an episode, two years before, of confusion and disorientation, and had become progressively worse. Within 48 hours after he was found to have a form of hydrocephalus—increased fluids in the brain exerting pressure on brain structures—and an operation was performed to eliminate the fluid accumulation, he was alert, cheerful, oriented, free of incontinence and paranoia.

Relatively few of the aged have that particular problem to account for their senility symptoms. But others may respond to other measures used individually or in combination as needed and including withdrawal of trouble-producing drugs, correction of anemia and congestive heart failure, treatment for mental depression or gland malfunctioning.

At Rush-Presbyterian–St. Luke's Medical Center, Chicago, physicians carried out one of the first studies with the new x-ray brain scanning machine as an aid to the diagnosis of patients with senility. With the new technique, some demented patients in whom conventional x-ray films had suggested cerebral atrophy were found to have moderate or questionable atrophy. Among them were patients with low thyroid functioning and pernicious anemia who were almost completely relieved of all indications of dementia after getting vigorous treatment for the thyroid condition and the anemia.

## DEPRESSION, MENTAL, IN PHYSICAL GUISES

The most common of all psychologic ills, mental depression is commonly regarded as involving only, although often devastatingly, a morbid sadness or melancholy. But depression can wear physical guises which can cloak the basic problem. And some studies indicate that elapsed time from onset of symptoms to accurate diagnosis can range up to three years, during which patients may be treated, if treated at all, for other illnesses.

Depression can produce such symptoms as these, and commonly does: easy tiring, sleeping difficulty (particularly a tendency to wake up early, feeling exhausted), remorse, guilt feelings, concentration difficulty, indecision, irritability, impatience, indifference, and suicidal thoughts.

But often there are physical symptoms which overshadow the "blues" to such an extent that patients, if they seek medical help, seek it for the physical symptoms which worry and bother them most, without revealing the depression.

Headaches are common, loss of appetite frequent, and gastrointestinal troubles can be diverse: digestive upsets, nausea, vomiting, constipation, diarrhea, gas, abdominal pain. Not uncommonly, the depressed may experience chest pains, ear noises, skin blotches, palpitation, numbness, tingling sensations.

Provided only that the depression is recognized, its treatment—which often may be with antidepressant drugs alone, or antidepressants combined with brief psychotherapy—can eliminate the physical as well as mental and behavioral symptoms.

A particularly astute physician may sometimes suspect depression under the physical cloak even without help from the patient. What's needed, however, is recognition on the part of patient, or family, of the importance of any mood disturbance that accompanies physical symptoms and its inclusion in presenting complaints to the physician.

## DEPRESSION, SHOULDER PAIN AND

Shoulder pain has numerous physical causes. But evidence that mysterious, often-unyielding shoulder pain may stem from mental depression comes from a study of 56 patients with such pain who were also found to be mentally depressed. When treated solely with antidepressant agents, 44 of the 56 experienced marked improvement in the shoulder pain. Noteworthy, too: x-ray studies after the antidepressant treatment showed clearing of calcification in the shoulder area.

## DOUCHING DISTURBANCES

Evidence to suggest that excessive douching may play a role in inflammation of the fallopian tubes (salpingitis) and pelvic inflammatory disease, producing such symptoms as lower abdominal pain and vaginal discharge, comes from a study in New Haven, Connecticut, of 101 consecutive women with those diseases and 743 in good health. Of the afflicted, almost 90 percent proved to be vigorous douchers, compared with half that many among the healthy women. The differences in douching frequency were even more marked, with three times as many of the diseased women in the habit of douching more than once a week. Considering the data, the investigators look with strong suspicion on douching as contributing to ascending infections by whatever disease organisms happen to be present in the vagina.

## DRINKING (MODERATE), MYSTERIOUS SYMPTOMS AND

Alcoholism is a well enough known problem. But drinking far short of the kind done by alcoholics may, in some people, be the unsuspected reason for headache, diarrhea, insomnia, and irritability. And in some cases, relatively low alcohol intake—as little as two drinks a day—may even cause more serious problems, including high blood pressure and heartbeat irregularities, a University of Wisconsin study indicates. The problems are often difficult to overcome, reports the chief investigator, not because they are incurable but because moderate drinkers find it difficult to believe their modest intake can cause any disturbances. And the problems may be compounded for people bothered by irritability and insomnia who request prescriptions for tranquilizers which may interact with the alcohol, adding to the effects.

## EPILEPSY, DISGUISED

Brief and mysterious episodes of delirium and other psychotic behavior may be caused by epilepsy, and although observable seizures do not accompany the episodes, treatment with anticonvulsant medication is effective. This was the finding of a Vanderbilt University study with a series of patients ranging in age from 10 to 75 years and previously mistakenly diagnosed as having various psychiatric disorders. According to the study, the epilepsy-related problem should be suspected when one or more of the following conditions are present: abrupt onset of psychotic episodes in a previously healthy person; unexplained delirium; a history of similar episodes with sudden accentuations and improvements; a history of fainting or falling spells.

## FAMILIAL MEDITERRANEAN FEVER

Two major new developments promise to help both knowing and unknowing victims of this strange disorder. It produces recurrent attacks of fever and severe abdominal pain, usually at monthly intervals. Common consequences have been depression, drug addiction, and underachievement. Some victims have been subjected to exploratory abdominal surgery which has revealed nothing. Many have gone through a wide variety of treatments—low-fat diets, hormone therapy, corticosteroid and other drug therapy, psychotherapy—without benefit.

What causes the disorder is unknown. And one of the two important developments is the recent research finding that the term *familial Mediterranean fever* is a misnomer; the disorder is *not* necessarily familial, it can occur sporadically rather than in families, and it can appear in people of non-Mediterranean as well as Mediterranean extraction.

The second major development is the finding that, after the failures experienced with all other treatment, an ancient drug, colchicine, long used for gout, is effective. Its mechanism of action is not yet understood, but in a series of patients treated at Massachusetts General Hospital, Boston, colchicine has produced striking reduction and in some cases elimination of attacks. In every case, there has been dramatic improvement in life-style, with some previously unable to hold jobs now at work again.

Trials elsewhere have confirmed colchicine's value, and because of its striking effectiveness, it can be used in all patients with recurrent unexplained abdominal pain and fever as a means of diagnosis as well as treatment, avoiding misdiagnosis, needless surgery, and useless medical therapy trials.

## FOLIC ACID DEFICIENCY

Many recent studies have been establishing that deficiency of folic acid, an essential vitamin, may long go unsuspected and be responsible for a wide variety of problems—and that such deficiency is common.

In one of the latest studies, at the Clinical Research Institute of Montreal, half a dozen women, aged 31 to 70, with long histories of mild depression, fatigability, burning feet, constipation, and diffuse muscular pain were found to be folic acid–deficient. All responded to treatment with the vitamin.

In other studies, some patients with numbness, burning and tingling sensations, malabsorption, redness, soreness and swelling of the tongue, fissuring and scaling of the lips and angles of the mouth have been found folic acid–deficient and have responded to treatment with the vitamin.

Folic acid deficiency can be easily induced. Body stores are small and may not be adequately replenished for any of several reasons. Although the vitamin is present in a wide variety of plant and animal tissue—richest sources include yeast, liver, and green vegetables, with moderate amounts in dairy foods, meat, and fish—only about 10 percent of the folic acid in these foods is nutritionally available. And losses in cooking and processing can be enormous. The vitamin is rapidly destroyed by heat. Cooking, especially boiling, or heat preservation in canning can destroy 50 to 90 percent of the available vitamin. The vitamin is unstable when exposed to air and tends to decline steadily in storage. Thus, a deficiency may occur when leafy vegetables, flesh foods, and liver are lacking in the diet or when they are stored too long under poor conditions or cooked too long or overly processed. Deficiency also may occur under conditions calling for greater amounts of folic acid—notably pregnancy, which at least triples the amount needed, and fever states and wound healing, which also greatly increase needs.

Although the deficiency can cause anemia—and, in fact, is one of the most common causes of anemia—it need not do so in order to produce neurologic and gastrointestinal symptoms.

Once suspected as the underlying problem behind such symptoms, folic acid deficiency can be readily diagnosed by a blood test and readily treated with oral doses.

## GIARDIASIS

One major and often unrecognized cause of gastrointestinal upsets among travelers—cramps, nausea, mucous diarrhea, with appetite and weight loss and fatigue, which may persist long after return home—is *Giardia lamblia,* a parasite transmitted in the form of a cyst. Infestation is unresponsive unless a particular drug is prescribed. The drug, quinacrine hydrochloride, an antimalarial, eliminates the parasite along with the symptoms. Typically, in one study at the Palo Alto (California) Medical Clinic, in which 70 returnees from vacations abroad were found to be afflicted with giardiasis, all responded to 100-milligram doses of quinacrine hydrochloride taken three or four times a day.

## HEADACHES AND BEDCOVERS

Among the many possible causes of headaches, one that can go unsuspected—and, in fact, has only been recently reported—is sleeping with bedcovers pulled up over the head. Called "turtle headaches" by the investigating physician who, quite literally, uncovered them, the headaches may be characterized by pain all over the head, but the pain is usually greatest in the front of the head. In some cases, victims may be awakened by the pain during the night; in others, the headaches are present on awakening in the morning. Cure for the problem, which may be the result of oxygen shortage, is to keep the covers down.

## HEARTBURN, CHRONIC, AND THE LES FACTOR

A bout of heartburn now and then after a dietary indiscretion is common, but chronic heartburn is a different problem. Unfortunately, it is also not uncommon, as witness the widespread advertising and sale of antacids, plain and otherwise.

If antacids are helpful insofar as they provide fleeting relief—neutralizing acid at best for about 45 minutes—they do nothing for the cause.

And the cause, it appears from recent research, is not so much, as commonly supposed, excess acid but rather a factor known as LES (lower esophageal sphincter) pressure.

The LES is an area at the lower end of the esophagus, in the region where the esophagus joins the stomach, that acts like a valve, opening to allow the passage of food into the stomach, then closing to prevent reflux of food (and acid) from the stomach back up into the esophagus.

Over the past decade, studies have been demonstrating that in people with chronic heartburn, LES pressure is low compared with the pressure in nonsufferers. More recently, studies have been directed at finding agents that might raise the pressure, and a valuable one has been found in a drug, bethanechol, which has previously been used to combat urinary retention and abdominal distention after surgery.

In trials with chronic heartburn volunteers, special measuring instrumentation has shown tripling and even greater elevations of LES pressure after use of bethanechol. Tried in patients with chronic heartburn not well controlled by even large amounts of antacids, 25-

milligram tablets four times a day relieved the heartburn and reduced consumption of antacids.

## HYPERVENTILATION

To many people an unrealized source of worry and anxiety, hyperventilation (abnormally prolonged and deep breathing often done unconsciously) can be responsible for a wide range of symptoms.

In one recent study of 95 consecutive patients with chest pain resembling that of the angina pectoris accompanying heart disease, 15 turned out to have the pain only because of hyperventilation.

Symptoms produced by the excessive breathing—which leads to respiratory alkalosis through the excessive exhalation of carbon dioxide—include faintness or impaired consciousness without actual unconsciousness, tightness of the chest, sensations of smothering, and apprehension. Other symptoms may be related to the heart and digestive tract—among them, palpitation or pounding of the heart, fullness in the throat, pain over the stomach region. In a prolonged attack, there may be muscle twitchings and cramps.

Itself a source of anxiety, hyperventilation may be provoked by acute anxiety or by emotional tension. A simple remedy that can be used to control the effects of hyperventilation is rebreathing in a paper bag so that "blown-off" carbon dioxide is replaced. But many people, unable to conceive that simple overbreathing could cause so many problems and worried that something serious may be wrong, have to be convinced by a thorough medical checkup that there is nothing organically at fault and that they can control attacks using bag rebreathing.

## HYPOTHYROIDISM

In extreme form, hypothyroidism (low thyroid gland activity) can produce symptoms unmistakable to physicians and even to many nonprofessionals: slowing of mental activity, physical weakness, listlessness that may approach apathy, extreme sensitivity to cold, coarse hair, brittle nails, thickening and rigidity of skin.

But in mild form, hypothyroidism can be far from obvious, even to physicians. More than 40 years ago, medical reports were noting that "In the practice of medicine today no more important condition is encountered or so often unrecognized as hypothyroidism"—largely because of an idea common among physicians that hypothyroidism could not exist unless there were drastic and obvious changes. Some present-day medical reports are still emphasizing that mild hypothyroidism may commonly remain undetected, often because patients with the problem come to live with it, even if not live well, sometimes because physicians ascribe the symptoms to other causes without checking on thyroid function.

These are among the symptoms that may stem from mild to moderate hypothyroidism, sometimes occurring singly, sometimes in various combinations: cold skin, abnormal sensations of coldness at temperatures considered comfortable by others, skin pallor, hair loss, breathing disturbances, hoarseness, swelling of feet and eyelids, constipation, palpitations, muscle aches and weakness, poor equilibrium, hearing disturbance, burning and prickling sensations, irritability, nervousness, emotional explosiveness, menstrual disturbances, infertility, proneness to infections, skin outbreaks, fatigue, depression.

When hypothyroidism is considered, it can be tested for and, when found, responds readily to thyroid medication in the right amount to make up for the existing deficiency.

## LEG CRAMPS AT NIGHT AND RESTLESS LEGS

The two complaints are far from uncommon. In one, restless legs, there is an acutely uncomfortable feeling in the legs, a need to move them continuously and, often, when an episode occurs at night, a need to get up and walk about. The episode may last several hours.

In the other, night leg cramps, which may occur independently or in association with the first, there are attacks of leg and foot muscle cramps that may occur one or more times a night, requiring use of heat and interfering with sleep.

Causes are obscure and treatments, which have included muscle relaxants, calcium, and quinine, have been less than satisfactory.

Recently, one study has suggested that excessive caffeine intake may play a major role in restless legs. All of 55 patients benefited from avoidance of caffeine-containing beverages and medications.

Another study was undertaken by a physician, himself and wife victims of leg cramps, after a patient being treated with vitamin E for an entirely different problem remarked that ever since he had begun to use the vitamin the nocturnal leg cramps which had bothered him for years had disappeared. Both physician and wife had the same experience. The study covered 125 patients with leg cramps, 9 with restless legs. Each received vitamin E—in the form of d-alpha-tocopheryl acetate or succinate—in doses of 400 units one to four times a day (except those with hypertension, heart disease, or diabetes who were started on lower doses). Of the 125 with cramps, 103 experienced complete or almost complete relief. Of the 9 with restless legs, 7 were completely relieved, the other 2 partially.

## MILK INTOLERANCE

Milk intolerance can cause abdominal cramps, bloating or diarrhea, and many victims are unaware of the source of their symptoms or, if they suspect milk, may find it difficult to believe it can be the cause—for, commonly, people with the intolerance are otherwise healthy, drank milk without ill effects as children, and are still able to drink it sometimes without penalty.

Nonallergic, the intolerance stems from a deficiency of an intestinal enzyme that is needed for digesting the lactose constituent of milk.

Recent research at Johns Hopkins University provides useful insights into some of the peculiarities of the intolerance. It shows that many with the enzyme deficiency, while unable to handle large amounts of milk, can take smaller amounts in cereals and coffee, and have less trouble when they drink milk with meals rather than alone and when they avoid ice-cold milk. They also tolerate well the milk in yogurt and cheese because in the preparation of these foods some of the lactose is converted to another substance.

## NARCOLEPSY

According to the best recent estimates from sleep disorder clinics, as many as 250,000 Americans may have undiagnosed narcolepsy, which can be the cause of difficulties in learning, trouble on the job, and marital difficulties.

The disorder, which often appears at puberty, is characterized by irresistible sleep attacks of short duration, usually less than 15 minutes, which occur at inappropriate times, such as when studying, working, driving, even dining. This bizarre symptom may be accompanied by one or more others: cataplectic attacks during which there is an abrupt brief loss of muscle control leading to partial weakness or, sometimes, body collapse; sleep paralysis, a brief period of inability to move while dozing or awakening; hypnagogic hallucinations, vivid auditory or visual sensations at the onset of sleep. In a mild case, a narcolepsy victim may feel persistently drowsy but seldom drops off to sleep.

According to an official of the American Narcolepsy Association, newly formed in Stanford, California, to serve as a clearinghouse of information on narcolepsy, so few doctors as well as patients are aware of narcolepsy that an average of more than ten years pass between the first appearance of symptoms and the initial correct diagnosis. Sufferers are often incorrectly treated for a variety of other illnesses or more commonly believed to be just lazy by their friends and even their doctors, and the average person with narcolepsy sees four or five doctors before one finally identifies the illness.

Not untypical, one patient finally seen at the Sleep Disorders Clinic at Stanford University at the age of 16 had her first attacks at the age of 9, was eventually labeled retarded, and over the years received psychiatric treatment and was subjected to many sophisticated and expensive tests. The inappropriate treatment and tests over the seven years cost her family $50,000.

Ironically, although it is rarely diagnosed, narcolepsy is simple to recognize. Usually, if there is an awareness of the existence of the disorder, a physician—and, sometimes, a patient—can suspect the disorder on the basis of the history of symptoms.

And although the cause is unknown and there is no cure, narcolepsy can be controlled effectively with stimulant drugs such as methylphenidate and dextroamphetamine. Imipramine is effective for the other narcolepsy symptoms but not for the sleep attacks.

## PAGET'S DISEASE

Affecting an estimated 2,500,000 people in the United States, Paget's disease is a bone disorder which leads to abnormal bone structure, weakness, pain, and deformity.

In some cases, the disease can be obvious through enlargement of the head, bowing of the legs, and hunching of the back as weakened bones in the spine collapse.

But often Paget's is not obvious, producing such nonspecific symptoms as headache, pain, hearing loss, ear ringing, or muscle or sensory disturbances if the diseased bone presses on nerves.

Yet, if only there is some suspicion that Paget's may be involved in producing such symptoms, the disease can be diagnosed with the help of x-rays that show characteristic changes and a blood test that reveals increased levels of an enzyme, alkaline phosphatase.

Diagnosis is all the more important now with the recent development of a new treatment using a thyroid gland hormone, calcitonin. Calcitonin has been found to help most patients, producing marked improvement or complete relief of pain and other symptoms, often within a two-week period.

## PARKINSONISM, FALLING EPISODES AND

The common manifestations of parkinsonism, or shaking palsy, are tremor and stooped, shuffling gait. Only recently have physicians at two major Chicago medical centers, Michael Reese and Rush-Presbyterian–St. Luke's, been able to trace to parkinsonism a previously mysterious problem: episodes of falling, forward or backward, while walking or standing, in a series of patients seen at both centers.

Although the patients had none of the usual manifestations of parkinsonism, the falling episodes were suspected to be related to the disorder. Most responded to amantadine, a drug often used for parkinsonism. Those who did not benefit from amantadine responded well to another antiparkinsonism agent, levo-dopa.

## PICA (BIZARRE APPETITES), IRON DEFICIENCY AND

Pica is the compulsive eating of anything. One well-known form is the eating of flaked old paint by children. Another is the eating of clay by black women in the South, which practice has spread to the cities where clay sometimes can be bought in supermarkets. To some extent, the eating of laundry starch has been substituted for clay eating.

There are other forms of pica: the compulsive eating of one kind of food and the compulsive eating of ice, whole trayfuls a day.

Like other compulsive behavior, pica is humiliating for its victims, a source of either shame or amusement for families and friends. Victims commonly try to hide the senseless eating.

Yet, where once pica was thought to be an indication of neurosis, superstition or mental aberration, pica is now known to be the result of iron deficiency in a high proportion of cases. And iron can cure the pica within a week or two.

## POISON IVY DERMATITIS WITHOUT POISON IVY

Organic food stores sell many items. One of them, raw cashew nuts, it turns out, is the answer to a mystery: why some people who are sensitive to poison ivy, poison oak, or poison sumac develop outbreaks when not exposed to the poison plants.

When roasted, cashews are harmless. But in the raw state they have on their surface a shell oil that closely resembles the oleoresin allergy-producing material of the poison plants and can produce a poison ivy-like outbreak when handled.

## SHOULDER PAIN AND THE DROOPY-SHOULDER SYNDROME

Shoulder pain, a common problem, has many possible causes. But one that may be overlooked, according to a recent study at the University of Saskatchewan, Canada, is the "droopy-shoulder syndrome." The typical patient is a young woman with a graceful, swanlike neck and drooping shoulders who has pain in one or both shoulders without any evidence of spine or nervous system abnormality. She is, however, mildly or moderately depressed mentally and, as a consequence, lets her shoulders droop, and the drooping causes a pull on nerves, resulting in pain. Where x-rays of the spine in the neck area normally show up only six or seven vertebrae, eight or nine appear in the droopy-shoulder condition, which improves with treatment for depression and measures to improve posture and shoulder girdle muscle tone.

## THE SPINE, ONE-SIDED WEAKNESS AND

Although weakness of an arm and leg on the same side of the body (hemiparesis) is usually due to brain or spinal cord disease, physicians at Duke University Medical Center and the University of North Carolina recently have found that there may be another cause in some cases: cervical spondylosis, or narrowing of between-the-disk spaces in the neck region of the spine. Surgery to laminate or fuse the affected disks can be effective.

In one case, for example, the patient had experienced increasing weakness of the right hand, dragging of the right foot, and burning and tingling sensations in both hand and foot. In another, the symptoms were right hand weakness, right arm numbness, and headaches. In both, substantial improvement followed laminectomy.

## TASTE AND SMELL DISTURBANCES

Disorders of taste and smell can be much more than mere esthetic problems. They include partial or complete loss of one or both senses, and distortions that make ordinary foods and odors taste and smell revolting. One serious consequence can be undernutrition. Others may include anxiety and severe depression.

Often in the past, victims of the disorders have had trouble convincing physicians that they actually experienced the disturbances, and many were sent to psychiatrists.

Recently, investigators at the National Institutes of Health and elsewhere have determined that a very common and easily corrected cause of the disturbances is zinc deficiency. In one of several studies, for example, 103 patients with the disturbances, ranging in age from 25 to 81, were found to have abnormally low blood zinc levels. Upon receiving zinc sulfate in doses of 25, 50, or 100 milligrams four times a day, all experienced rises in zinc blood levels, two thirds regained normal taste and smell, the remainder experienced marked improvement.

Recent research also has shown that for others with disturbances not associated with zinc deficiency, the problem may lie with thyroid deficiency. A study at Barnes Hospital, St. Louis, found half of hypothyroid patients experiencing, along with other symptoms of low thyroid functioning, disturbances in taste and smell, which in 80 percent of cases responded to thyroid treatment within a matter of weeks.

## TMJ/MPD

TMJ and MPD are finally beginning—but only beginning—to receive the recognition they deserve. One or the other affects more than 20 percent of the population to some degree—yet commonly escapes diagnosis.

TMJ stands for *temporomandibular joint,* the hinge at the side of the face connecting jaw to head, which moves every time the mouth is opened and closed. The joint may be affected by arthritis or poor "bite." MPD stands for *myofascial pain-dysfunction* syndrome and is one form of TMJ dysfunction; it results from muscle tension.

The TMJ-MPD problem is commonly undiagnosed or misdiagnosed because it can produce symptoms common to many diseases: severe headache and facial pain, jaw clicking and limited jaw motion, dizziness, ringing of the ears, ear pain, hearing loss. Its victims, as one recent medical report acknowledges, "belong to that segment of society who wander from specialist to specialist seeking relief."

Treatment, once diagnosis is made, can be effective.

At the University of Pennsylvania, Dr. Arnold Gessel has been able to obtain relief for 80 of 100 patients suffering severe MPD-caused headaches, using biofeedback to teach muscle relaxation.

At the University of Illinois, Dr. Richard Dohmann, a dentist, has used biofeedback with similar results for patients with facial pain, jaw clicking, and limited jaw motion.

Elsewhere, several hundred patients referred from headache clinics because of lack of response have been treated successfully for TMJ-MPD with muscle relaxants and other measures. Along with headaches, many suffered from dizziness and ear symptoms, which commonly improved.

At the White Memorial Medical Center, Los Angeles, Dr. Douglas H. Morgan says: "Many people I've treated had gone to doctor after doctor without success. TMJ is in a medical twilight area. Physicians think the jaw is for the dentist to work on and dentists send TMJ patients to the doctor because of the symptoms of headache and earache."

But Morgan adds: "There is gradually developing a group of dentists and physicians interested and knowledgeable in this area. More TMJ clinics will be developed in dental schools and hospitals. The future holds more hope for the large number of people afflicted with this most severe and perplexing problem."

## A note on biofeedback

The possible value of biofeedback is being explored in many areas other than TMJ, too.

Biofeedback is based on the discovery that many ordinarily involuntary activities of the body such as heart rate, rise and fall of blood pressure, and fluctuations in the state of muscles are not, as long believed, beyond voluntary control. Instead, if sensitive electronic equipment is used to give an individual indications of tiny internal fluctuations, the individual can, in effect, "will" the fluctuations to go one way or the other.

Various types of sensors can be applied to the skin over an area to detect muscle activity, temperature, blood pressure, etc. The signals picked up by the sensors are amplified and displayed on a meter or other instrument so the patient can see them.

By various methods—such as repeating a calming phrase like "I feel quiet" or thinking of a pleasant scene—a patient can make the needle on the meter, for example, move in a desired direction. The movement in that direction will indicate that a muscle is being relaxed or blood pressure is declining.

Once the patient, with some practice, can readily move the needle as desired, he or she is often able to accomplish the same result—such as muscle relaxation or blood pressure reduction—without need of the equipment, thus aborting or preventing difficulties.

## URETHRITIS, PUZZLING

Increased urination with pain and burning and urgency can stem from urethritis, an inflammation of the urethral canal which carries urine from bladder to outside the body. The inflammation often results from gonorrhea or other infection and responds to antibiotic treatment.

But in some men, urethritis is present without any evidence of infection. The cause in at least some of these mysterious cases, recent research indicates, may be an alkaline, irritative urine. When urine is strongly alkaline, it is unable to carry in solution, as it normally does, crystals of phosphate, which, on dropping out of solution, irritate the urethra and lead to inflammation.

When this is the problem, treatment is simple enough: massive doses, 3 grams a day for four days, of ascorbic acid (vitamin C), which acidifies the urine, allowing it to dissolve and carry out the phosphate crystals.

## URINARY INFECTIONS (RECURRENT), BATHING AND

That tub bathing may be a significant factor in some women with recurrent bladder infections is suggested by a study by Dr. Robert S. Gould of Wellesley, Massachusetts, with 50 women who had experienced as many as 10 infections each. Each woman was asked to replace tub bathing with showers. As long as they avoided the baths, 34 remained free of infection. Of the 16 who developed recurrent infections, 12 did so only after resuming tub baths.

## URINARY INFECTIONS (RECURRENT), SEX AND

Some women have repeated urinary tract infections, getting over one with the aid of antibacterial treatment only to have another appear not long afterward. Evidence that the recurrent infections are linked to sexual intercourse and that they may often be prevented by a single prophylactic oral dose of an antibacterial drug after intercourse comes from a study at Stanford University. Fourteen women followed that procedure—using either penicillin G, nitrofurantoin, cephalexin, nalidixic acid, or sulfonamide—for periods of up to 111 months, for a total of 761 patient-months. During that time, only 19 infections occurred in contrast to 90 during a previous period of 715 patient-months.

SECTION FOUR Symptoms
From Drugs

## AN IMPORTANT NOTE
## ABOUT DRUG SIDE-EFFECT SYMPTOMS

Without some background, a glance at the following pages may make it seem that drugs are poisons, calculated to produce harm rather than good. That, of course, is not the fact.

Most modern drugs are potent. Few, if any, are 100 percent specific, hitting only the target at which they are directed and nothing else. In combating a problem for which it is prescribed, a drug may produce unwanted effects.

For example, the gastrointestinal upsets—cramps, diarrhea, sore mouth, anal itch—that may occur with use of an antibiotic do so because even as the drug acts against the infection-causing organisms it acts against others also, sometimes to the extent of upsetting the natural microorganism balance in the body.

Many harmless, even useful bacteria are present in the gut. Some, in fact, are needed for digestion; some produce vitamins. If these should be decimated by the antibiotic, there is less competition for other, potentially harmful, organisms, which are always present in small numbers, and they may multiply and cause side-effect symptoms.

In some cases, side effects of drugs may develop because of inappropriate dosage. Drug dosages often are averages—to a large extent calculated for an "average" person who may have a body weight of about 150 pounds. You may weigh more or less, and an average dose, which may not be right for you, may cause trouble.

Moreover, even people of the same weight may not require the same dosage of a drug. You may know, from experience, that your body is very sensitive, that a relatively small dose of medication is all you need—and that is something to be discussed with your physician when he prescribes.

It is also a fact that there can be allergic sensitivity responses to medicine just as there are to foods. These vary considerably. One person may tolerate half a dozen eggs at a sitting; another cannot eat even one egg without developing an upset stomach. So with other foods; so, too, with drugs. Because of individual sensitivity, a drug beneficial for 95 percent or more of the population may cause trouble for the remainder. A good example is penicillin, which has saved millions of lives but has also caused severe sensitivity reactions in scores of thousands and has taken some lives.

Side effects can be peculiar. Some may appear at the beginning of use of a drug and may be mild and, before long, may disappear even as the drug is continued. Others may be mild or severe and not disappear.

When side effects develop, many people accept them as a price to be paid for treatment when, in fact, a change of dosage or a switch to another medication, equally good for the purpose, may eliminate them.

In many cases, too, people suffering symptoms from drugs are unaware of their origin, believing they may be added symptoms of their original problem.

A knowledge of what symptoms particular drugs may produce can be useful. It should not be scary. As you consider the listings in the following pages, remember that many of the symptoms or side effects indicated are extremely rare, some occurring possibly only in one person in a million. Some are more frequent but disappear with continued use of a drug. Some can be eliminated by change in dosage, others by a switch to another drug. Some can be countered by other measures your physician can suggest. Some may have to be borne in order to get well.

If, knowledgeably, you can discover that disturbing symptoms you are experiencing may be from a drug, you can and should discuss the problem with your physician, without delay. If you bring the problem to his attention—and you have every right to do so—almost certainly he can help in one way or another, either ameliorating it or providing reassurance that the disturbance will be only fleeting or, if not, and a price to be paid, not too high a price.

In the following pages the information for each drug is presented in this order: First, each heading gives the trade name of the drug, then in parenthesis the generic name or names. The initial paragraph after the drug name(s) lists the conditions for which the drug is used, and the second paragraph lists the symptoms (side effects) the drug may cause.

In the second part of this section, a symptom (side effect) is given in a heading, and the drugs that may cause it are then listed.

# *Individual drugs, their trade and generic names, uses, and the symptoms each may sometimes produce*

**Achromycin V** (tetracycline). See *Tetracycline.*

**Actifed** (tripolidine, pseudonephrine). For swollen nasal passage linings, as in the common cold or hay fever.
Sedation or stimulation.

**Actifed C Expectorant** (Actifed plus codeine). For cough relief.
Sedation or stimulation.

**Afrin** (oxymetazoline). For nasal congestion.
Burning, stinging, dryness of nasal passages, sneezing, headache, insomnia, light-headedness, palpitation, rebound nasal congestion.

**Aldactazide** (spironolactone, hydrochlorothiazide). For edema, high blood pressure.
Anemia, appetite loss, burning or tingling, blood disturbances, confusion, cramps, diarrhea, dizziness, drowsiness, fever, gynecomastia (breast enlargement in a male), headache, hives, itching, impotence, incoordination, jaundice, lethargy, abnormal hair growth, muscle spasm, menstrual irregularity, photosensitivity, rash, restlessness, nausea, vomiting, skin bruising, weakness.

**Aldactone** (spironolactone). For edema, high blood pressure.
Confusion, cramps, diarrhea, drowsiness, gynecomastia (breast enlargement in a male), fever, hives, impotence, incoordination, abnormal hair growth, headache, lethargy, irregular menses, rash, voice deepening.

**Aldomet** (methyldopa). For high blood pressure.

Angina aggravation, Bell's palsy, blood disturbances, breast enlargement, burning or tingling, constipation, depression, diarrhea, dizziness, eczema, edema, fever, flatulence, libido decrease, lightheadedness, headache, heart slowing, impotence, joint pain, gynecomastia (breast enlargement in a male), muscle pain, mental acuity decrease, nasal stuffiness, mouth dryness, sore or "black" tongue, nausea, vomiting, tremor, nightmares, weight gain.

**Aldoril** (methyldopa and hydrochlorothiazide). For high blood pressure.

Side effects may stem from either ingredient. See *Aldomet* and *Hydrodiuril*.

**Ambenyl Expectorant** (codeine, bromodiphenhydramine, diphenhydramine, ammonium chloride, potassium guaiacolsulfonate, menthol). For cough.

Confusion, constipation, anemia, dizziness, drowsiness, dryness of mouth, nose and throat, hives, insomnia, chest tightness and wheezing, thickening of bronchial secretions, nasal stuffiness, nausea, vomiting, palpitation, photosensitivity, rash, upper abdominal distress, nervousness, restlessness, tingling, heaviness and weakness of hands, difficulty in urination, vision blurring, double vision.

**Amcill** (ampicillin). Semisynthetic penicillin for infections.

See *Ampicillin*.

**Ampicillin.** Semisynthetic penicillin for infections.

Anemia, anaphylaxis, blood disturbances, diarrhea, hives, nausea, vomiting, rash, mouth inflammation, tongue inflammation, hairy tongue.

**Antivert** (meclizine). For motion sickness, vertigo from ear disturbances.

Drowsiness, dry mouth, vision blurring.

**Apresoline** (hydralazine). For high blood pressure.

Anxiety, appetite loss, blood disturbances, breathing difficulty, chills, constipation, chest pain, diarrhea, disorientation, conjunctivitis, depression, edema, fever, headache, hives, flushing, joint pain, itching, muscle cramps, nausea, vomiting, palpitation, fast heartbeat, nasal congestion, numbness, tearing of eye, tingling, tremor, rash, difficult urination, low blood pressure.

**Aristocort** (triamcinolone). For allergies, arthritic conditions, some skin disorders.

Abdominal distention, cataracts, Cushing-like state, convulsions, exophthalmos, fractures, fluid retention, glaucoma, facial redness, growth suppression, congestive heart failure, high blood pressure, osteoporosis, headache, pancreatitis, peptic ulcer, dizziness, increased insulin requirements, ulcerative esophagitis, increased sweating, muscle weakness, thin fragile skin, menstrual irregularities, impaired wound healing.

**Artane** (trihexyphenidyl). For Parkinson's disease and control of some nervous system side effects of reserpine and other tranquilizers.

Constipation, dizziness, drowsiness, headache, nervousness, mouth dryness, nausea, vomiting, urinary hesitancy, vision blurring.

**Atarax** (hydroxyzine). For anxiety, tension.

Convulsions, drowsiness, mouth dryness, tremor.

**Atromid-S** (clofibrate). For reducing elevated blood-fat levels.

Anemia, abdominal distress, diarrhea, dizziness, drowsiness, dyspepsia, flatulence, fatigue, impotence, itching, hives, dry and brittle hair, excessive eating, headache, muscle cramping, aching or weakness, joint pain, decreased libido, weight gain.

**Azo Gantrisin** (sulfamethoxazole, phenazopyridine). For painful urinary infections.

Abdominal pain, anemia, appetite loss, blood disturbances, convulsions, depression, diarrhea, dizziness, headache, hives, hepatitis, hallucinations, insomnia, itching, edema about the eyes, joint pain, fever, chills, nausea, vomiting, photosensitivity, mouth inflammation, pancreatitis, ringing of ears, skin eruption, diminished urination.

**Bellergal** (phenobarbital, belladonna, ergotamine tartrate). For menopausal symptoms, premenstrual tension, recurrent throbbing headache, nervous stomach, uterine cramps, some heart conditions.

Drowsiness, flushing, dry mouth, blurred vision.

**Benadryl** (diphenhydramine). For allergy, motion sickness, insomnia.

Anemia, abdominal distress, chest tightness and wheezing, confusion, constipation, diarrhea, dizziness, drowsiness, headache, hives, insomnia, light sensitivity, low blood pressure, nausea, vomiting, palpitation, restlessness, rash, nasal stuffiness, tingling, heaviness and weakness of hands, urinary difficulty, vision blurring, double vision.

**Bendectin** (dicyclomine, doxylamine, pyridoxine). For nausea and vomiting of pregnancy.

Appetite loss, constipation, diarrhea, dizziness, drowsiness, dry mouth, fatigue, headache, irritability, palpitation, rash, sedation, nausea, vomiting, stomach pain, painful urination, vision blurring.

**Bentyl** (dicyclomine). For irritable bowel, intestinal inflammation.

Constipation, bloated feeling, dizziness, drowsiness, headache, hives, insomnia, impotence, mouth dryness, loss of taste, nausea, vomiting, palpitation, fast pulse, nervousness, pupil dilation, suppression of lactation, decreased sweating, vision blurring, urinary hesitance, urinary retention.

**Bentyl/Phenobarbital** (dicyclomine, phenobarbital). For irritable bowel, intestinal inflammation.

Side effects similar to *Bentyl* (above) plus excitement.

**Benylin Cough Syrup** (diphenhydramine, alcohol, chloroform). For cough.

Drowsiness.

**Butazolidin and Butazolidin Alka** (phenylbutazone). For arthritic conditions, gout, painful shoulder.

Anemia, blood disturbances, agitation, confusion, diarrhea, dizziness, dyspepsia, abdominal distention, fluid retention, gastritis, gastrointestinal bleeding, stomach pain, hepatitis, hearing loss, high blood sugar, lethargy, joint pain, fever, heart disturbance, kidney disturbance, hearing loss, insomnia, nausea, vomiting of blood, ulceration (colon, duodenum, esophagus, mouth, or stomach), thyroid disorder, rash, skin disturbance, headache, respiratory alkalosis, metabolic alkalosis, retinal hemorrhage, retinal detachment, vision blurring, skin disturbances.

**Butisol Sodium** (butabarbital). For sedation, sleep.

Drowsiness, headache, hangover, lethargy, nausea, vomiting, skin eruption.

**Chlor-Trimeton** (chlorpheniramine maleate). For allergy.

Appetite loss, dizziness, drowsiness, dry mouth, headache, heartburn, nervousness, nausea, skin disturbance, painful or excessive urination, weakness.

**Cleocin** (clindamycin). For infection.

Abdominal pain, blood disturbances, diarrhea, hives, jaundice, nausea, vomiting, rash.

**Combid** (prochlorperazine, isopropamide). For peptic ulcer, irritable bowel, diarrhea.

Allergic reaction, asthma, bloated feeling, blood disturbances, constipation, convulsions, dizziness, drowsiness, inhibition of ejaculation, fever, headache, itching, jaundice, leg swelling, involuntary movement, movement difficulty, dry mouth, menstrual irregularities, nasal congestion, nausea, skin disturbances, swallowing difficulty, urinary hesitancy, urinary retention, vision blurring.

**Compazine** (prochlorperazine). For severe nausea, excessive anxiety, tension, agitation.

Agitation, blood disturbances, dizziness, drowsiness, drooling, shuffling gait, insomnia, jaundice, jitteriness, involuntary movements, neck muscle spasm, skin disturbances, swallowing difficulty, vision blurring, tremor, tongue protrusion.

**Cordran** (flurandrenolide). For inflammatory skin conditions.

Acnelike eruption, burning, dryness of skin, folliculitis, hairiness, infection, irritation, itching, skin maceration, miliaria, skin pigmentation loss, striae (skin streaks or lines).

**Cortisporin** (polymyxin, neomycin, gramicidin, hydrocortisone). For skin infections and inflammatory skin conditions.

Possible deleterious effects on ears, kidneys, striae (skin streaks or lines).

**Coumadin** (warfarin). For venous thrombosis, pulmonary embolism, atrial fibrillation, coronary occlusion.

Abdominal cramping, diarrhea, fever, hair loss, hemorrhage, hives, nausea, "purple toes," skin eruption.

**Cyclospasmol** (cyclandelate). For intermittent claudication, thrombophlebitis, Raynaud's disease, nocturnal leg cramps, and some other blood vessel disorders.

Abdominal pain, flushing, heartburn, headache, rapid heartbeat, weakness.

**Dalmane** (flurazepam). For insomnia.

Appetite loss, shortness of breath, constipation, coma, chest pain, confusion, diarrhea, disorientation, dizziness, drowsiness, eye burning, falling, joint pains, faintness, flushes, light-headedness, lethargy, headache, hallucinations, heartburn, irritability, itching, mouth dryness, nausea, vomiting, nervousness, palpitation, rash, restlessness, staggering, stomach upset, sweating, talkativeness, speech slurring, vision blurring, weakness.

**Darvon** (propoxyphene); **Darvon Compound 65** (with aspirin, phenacetin, caffeine); **Darvon-N/ASA** (with aspirin); **Darvocet-N** (with acetaminophen). For mild to moderate pain.

Abdominal pain, constipation, dizziness, euphoria, headache, light-headedness, nausea/vomiting, rash, restlessness, sedation, visual disturbances, weakness.

**DBI-TD** (phenformin). For adult-onset diabetes.

Appetite loss, diarrhea, nausea/vomiting, metallic taste.

**Decadron** (dexamethasone). For endocrine disorders, arthritis, bursitis, some severe allergic, skin, eye, intestinal, respiratory, blood, and malignant diseases.

Abdominal distention, bone fractures, cushingoid state, convulsions, cataracts, diabetes, dizziness, eye protrusion, facial redness, fluid retention, growth suppression, headache, hypertension, glaucoma, menstrual irregularities, muscle weakness, osteoporosis, peptic ulcer, pancreatitis, thin and fragile skin, sweating, impairment of wound healing.

**Declomycin** (demeclocycline). For infection.

Angioneurotic edema (giant hives), appetite loss, anaphylaxis, anemia, blood disturbances, diarrhea, hives, intestinal inflammation, nausea/vomiting, rash, swallowing difficulty, tongue inflammation.

**Demerol** (meperidine). Narcotic analgesic for pain.

Agitation, breathing depression, breathing arrest, constipation, dry mouth, disorientation, dizziness, euphoria, faintness, headache, heart arrest, hives, hallucinations, itching, light-headedness, nausea/vomiting, palpitation, slow or racing heartbeat, restlessness, rash, sedation, sweating, tremor, urinary retention, visual disturbances.

**Demulen** (ethynodiol, ethinyl). Oral contraceptive.

Abdominal bloating, abdominal cramps, breast changes, cerebral thromobosis, edema, blood pressure rise, gallbladder disease, heart attack, jaundice, mental depression, menstrual flow change, migraine, nausea/vomiting, pulmonary embolism, rash, spotting, thrombophlebitis, weight change.

**Dilantin** (phenytoin). Anticonvulsant.

Blood disturbances, constipation, dizziness, headache, hepatitis, hirsutism, incoordination, insomnia, joint disease, liver damage, lymph gland (node) enlargement, nausea/vomiting, mental confusion, nervousness, rash, speech slurring, twitching.

**Dimetane** (brompheniramine). For allergy.

Hemolytic anemia, appetite loss, anaphylaxis, blood disturbances, chest tightness and wheezing, confusion, constipation, diarrhea, dizziness, euphoria, excitement, fatigue, fast heartbeat, headache, hives, incoordination, insomnia, dryness of mouth, nose, throat, nasal stuffiness, nervousness, palpitation, photosensitivity, rash, restlessness, ringing of ears, sedation, sleepiness, stomach distress, urinary frequency, difficulty, retention, vision blurring, double vision.

**Dimetapp** (brompheniramine, phenylephrine, phenylpropanolamine). Decongestant for allergy.

Abdominal distress, appetite loss, blood disturbances, chest tightness, constipation, diarrhea, dizziness, drowsiness, ear ringing, faintness, giddiness, hives, headache, incoordination, lassitude, nausea/vomiting, palpitation, pupil dilation, rash, urinary frequency, painful urination, visual disturbances.

**Diabinese** (chlorpropamide). For diabetes.

Anemia, appetite loss, blood disturbances, diarrhea, edema, fever, jaundice, nausea/vomiting, skin eruption, weakness.

**Diupres** (chlorothiazide, reserpine). For high blood pressure.

Anaphylaxis, aplastic anemia, appetite loss, breathing difficulty, chest pain, constipation, cramping, depression, diarrhea, dizziness, fainting, flushing, fluid retention, headache, hearing loss, itching, impotence, jaundice, mouth dryness, muscle aches, muscle spasm, nausea/vomiting, nightmares, nasal congestion, nervousness, rash, restlessness, salivary gland inflammation, sedation, stomach irritation, vision blurring, weakness, weight gain.

**Diuril** (chlorothiazide). For edema, hypertension, toxemia of pregnancy.

Aplastic anemia, appetite loss, blood disturbances, constipation, cramping, diarrhea, dizziness, fever, headache, hives, jaundice, muscle spasm, nausea/vomiting, pancreatitis, photosensitivity, rash, restlessness, salivary gland inflammation, stomach irritation, vision blurring, weakness.

**Donnagel-PG** (kaolin, pectin, hyoscyamine, atropine, hyoscine). For diarrhea.
Flushing, mouth dryness, skin dryness, urinary difficulty, vision blurring.

**Donnatal** (hyoscyamine, atropine, hyoscine, phenobarbital). For digestive disorders, gallbladder inflammation, urinary frequency, painful menstruation, premenstrual tension, motion sickness.
Flushing, mouth dryness, skin dryness, urinary difficulty, vision blurring.

**DORIDEN** (glutethimide). Nonbarbiturate sleeping medication.
Blood disturbances, excitement, hangover, nausea, rash, vision blurring.

**DRAMAMINE** (dimenhydrinate). For motion sickness.
Drowsiness.

**Drixoral** (dexbrompheniramine, *d*-isoephedrine). For nasal congestion.
Abdominal cramps, appetite loss, anxiety, chest pain, confusion, dizziness, drowsiness, headache, hypertension, insomnia, nausea/vomiting, palpitation, rash, restlessness, sweating, tension, stomach distress, painful urination, weakness.

**Dyazide** (triamterene, hydrochlorothiazide). For edema, hypertension.
Anaphylaxis, constipation, diarrhea, dizziness, headache, hives, mouth dryness, muscle cramps, nausea/vomiting, pancreatitis, photosensitivity, rash.

**Elavil** (amitriptyline). Antidepressant.
Appetite loss, anxiety, blood disturbances, breast enlargement, diminished concentration, constipation, diarrhea, disorientation, drowsiness, dry mouth, excitement, facial puffiness, fatigue, hallucinations, abnormal heart rhythms, heart attack, heart block, hives, hy-

pertension, hypotension, incoordination, insomnia, jaundice, nausea/ vomiting, nightmares, numbness, palpitation, fast pulse, rash, restlessness, ringing of ears, seizures, stroke, black tongue, tingling of extremities, tongue edema, tremor, urinary retention, urinary frequency, vision blurring, weakness.

**Empirin Compound/Codeine** (aspirin, phenacetin, caffeine, codeine). For pain.
  Mild stimulation.

**E-Mycin** (erythromycin). For infection.
  See *Erythromycin.*

**Equanil** (meprobamate). For anxiety, tension.
  Agranulocytosis, anaphylaxis, aplastic anemia, angioneurotic edema (giant hives), blood disturbances, bronchospasm, chills, diarrhea, dizziness, drowsiness, euphoria, excitement, faintness, fever, headache, abnormal heart rhythms, incoordination, nausea/vomiting, overstimulation, palpitation, proctitis, fast pulse, rash, speech slurring, tingling, vision disturbances, diminished urination, weakness.

**Erythyrocin** (erythromycin). For infections.
  See *Erythromycin.*

**Erythromycin.** For infections.
  Abdominal cramping, anaphylaxis, diarrhea, hives, nausea/vomiting, rash.

**Esidrix** (hydrochlorothiazide). For hypertension, edema, toxemia of pregnancy.
  Abdominal cramping, aplastic anemia, appetite loss, blood disturbances, constipation, diarrhea, dizziness, headache, hives, jaundice, muscle spasm, nausea/vomiting, pancreatitis, rash, restlessness, stomach irritation, tingling, color vision disturbance, weakness.

**Etrafon** (perphenazine, amitriptyline). For anxiety, agitation, depressed mood.
  Anaphylaxis, asthma, angioneurotic edema (giant hives), appetite loss, anxiety, confusion, constipation, edema of face and tongue, eczema, delusions, dizziness, excitement, headache, heartburn, abnormal heart rhythms, hypertension, hypotension, heart attack, heart block, hives, incoordination, insomnia, itching, laryngeal edema,

drowsiness, breast enlargement, fatigue, jaundice, menstrual disturbances, muscle tone impairment, movement difficulty, involuntary movement of face, tongue, mouth or jaw, mouth dryness, nausea/vomiting, nasal congestion, nervousness, palpitation, rash, seizures, salivation, spasm of head and feet, stroke, testicular swelling, tingling, tremor, urinary frequency, urinary incontinence, urinary retention, vision blurring, black tongue, weakness.

**Feosol** (ferrous sulfate). For iron deficiency and iron-deficiency anemia.
Constipation, diarrhea, nausea.

**Fiorinal** (butalbitol, caffeine, aspirin, phenacetin). For headache, other pain.
Constipation, dizziness, drowsiness, nausea, rash.

**Fiorinal/Codeine** (*Fiorinal* plus codeine). For pain, cough.
Constipation, dizziness, drowsiness, nausea, pupil contraction, rash.

**Gantanol** (sulfamethoxazole). For urinary and other infections.
Abdominal pain, aplastic anemia, hemolytic anemia, appetite loss, blood disturbances, bruising, chills, convulsions, depression, diarrhea, dizziness, fever, hallucinations, headache, hives, incoordination, insomnia, itching, joint pains, nausea/vomiting, eye puffiness, pancreatitis, ringing in ears, skin eruption, diminished urination.

**Gantrisin** (sulfisoxazole). For urinary and other infections.
Side effects similar to those of *Gantanol* (above).

**Garamycin** (gentamicin). For infections.
Anemia, appetite loss, convulsions, dizziness, fever, headache, hives, itching, muscle twitching, numbness, nausea/vomiting, rash, ringing in ears, skin reddening, tingling, diminished urination.

**Hydergine** (dihydroergocornine, dihydroergocristine, dihydroergokryptine). For mood depression, confusion, unsociability, dizziness in the elderly.
Nausea, stomach disturbances.

**Hydrodiuril** (hydrochlorothiazide). For edema.
Appetite loss, constipation, cramping, burning or tingling, blood disturbances, bruising, breathing distress, diarrhea, dizziness, head-

ache, fever, hives, jaundice, pancreatitis, nausea/vomiting, photosensitivity, rash, muscle spasm, restlessness, vision blurring, weakness.

**Hydropres** (hydrochlorothiazide, reserpine). For hypertension.

Side effects may include those of *Hydrodiuril* (above), and those of reserpine that follow: appetite loss, anxiety, breathing difficulty, breast engorgement, chest pain, dizziness, diarrhea, depression, drowsiness, gynecomastia (breast enlargement in a male), fainting, glaucoma, headache, heart rhythm disturbances, hearing impairment, impotence, muscle aches, nasal congestion, nausea/vomiting, nervousness, nightmares, mouth dryness, nosebleeds, tremor, uveitis, weight gain.

**Hygroton** (chlorthalidone). For hypertension, edema.

Aplastic anemia, appetite loss, blood disturbances, burning sensations, constipation, cramping, diarrhea, dizziness, gout, headache, hives, impotence, jaundice, muscle spasm, nausea/vomiting, pancreatitis, rash, restlessness, stomach irritation, tingling, color vision disturbance, weakness.

**Inderal** (propranolol). For angina pectoris, heart rhythm abnormality, pheochromocytoma, hypertension.

Abdominal cramping, blood disturbances, breathing difficulty, congestive heart failure, constipation, depression, diarrhea, fatigue, fever, temporary hair loss, hallucinations, hypotension, nausea/vomiting, rash, sore throat, tingling of hands, vision disturbances, weakness.

**Indocin** (indomethacin). For arthritic conditions.

Abdominal pain, aplastic or hemolytic anemia, appetite loss, blood disturbances, breathing difficulty, confusion, depression, diarrhea, dizziness, eye disturbances, fainting, gastritis, gastrointestinal bleeding, headache, hearing disturbance, hair loss, hives, itching, jaundice, light-headedness, mouth inflammation, nausea/vomiting, nosebleed, rash, ulcer, vaginal bleeding, vision blurring.

**Ionamin** (phentermine resin). For weight reduction.

Constipation, diarrhea, dizziness, euphoria, headache, hives, hypertension, insomnia, impotence, mouth dryness, overstimulation, palpitation, fast pulse, restlessness, tremor.

**Isordil** (isosorbide dinitrate). For angina pectoris.

Dizziness, flushing, headache, nausea/vomiting, pallor, perspiration, rash, restlessness, weakness.

**Kaon** (potassium gluconate). For correcting low blood-potassium levels.

Abdominal discomfort, confusion, diarrhea, heart rhythm disturbances, hypotension, listlessness, leg weakness and heaviness, nausea/vomiting, tingling.

**Keflex** (cephalexin). For infections.

Abdominal pain, diarrhea, dizziness, dyspepsia, fatigue, hives, headache, itching, nausea/vomiting, rash, vaginitis, vaginal discharge.

**Kenalog** (triamcinolone). For inflammatory skin conditions.

Acnelike eruption, burning, dryness, folliculitis, excessive hairiness, hyperpigmentation, infection, itching, irritation, miliaria, skin maceration.

**Lanoxin** (digoxin). For congestive heart failure, other heart conditions.

Appetite loss, apathy, diarrhea, gynecomastia (breast enlargement in a male), headache, heart rhythm abnormalities, nausea/vomiting, vision blurring, weakness.

**Lasix** (furosemide). For edema.

Anemia, aplastic anemia, blood disturbances, diarrhea, dizziness, fatigue, headache, hearing loss, hives, light-headedness, itching, jaundice, mouth burning, muscle cramps, nausea/vomiting, perspiration, ringing of ears, skin outbreaks, stomach burning, tingling, thrombophlebitis, thirst, urinary frequency, vision blurring, weakness.

**Librax** (chlordiazepoxide, clidinium bromide). For symptomatic relief of gastrointestinal disturbances.

In addition to symptoms of *Librium* (below), Librax may produce these others: mouth dryness, vision blurring, urinary hesitancy.

**Librium** (chlordiazepoxide). For anxiety, tension.

Blood disturbances, confusion, constipation, drowsiness, edema, faintness, incoordination, menstrual irregularities, nausea, skin eruptions.

**Lomotil** (diphenoxylate, atropine). For diarrhea.

Abdominal discomfort, angioneurotic edema (giant hives), appetite loss, breathing depression, coma, dizziness, depression, drowsiness, euphoria, gum swelling, headache, hives, itching, lethargy, malaise, nausea/vomiting, numbness of extremities, restlessness, sedation.

**Macrodantin** (nitrofurantoin). For urinary tract infections.

Abdominal pain, anaphylaxis, angioneurotic edema (giant hives), hemolytic anemia, appetite loss, blood disturbances, breathing difficulty, chills, chest pain, cough, diarrhea, dizziness, drowsiness, fever, temporary hair loss, headache, hepatitis, hives, itching, jaundice, joint pain, malaise, nausea/vomiting, skin eruption.

**Marax** (ephedrine sulfate, theophylline, hydroxyzine). For asthma.

Abdominal discomfort, chest pain, dizziness, drowsiness, excitement, gait unsteadiness, headache, heart rhythm disturbances, insomnia, muscle weakness, nausea/vomiting, nervousness, nose and throat dryness, palpitation, sweating, tremulousness, urinary hesitation, urinary retention.

**Medrol** (methylprednisolone). For endocrine and rheumatic disorders, serious skin diseases, allergic states, other conditions.

Abdominal distention, bruising, cataract, congestive heart failure, convulsions, Cushing-like state, dizziness, exophthalmos, esophagitis, facial redness, fluid retention, glaucoma, growth suppression, headache, hypertension, muscle weakness, menstrual irregularities, osteoporosis, peptic ulcer, pancreatitis, thin fragile skin, sweating.

**Mellaril** (thioridazine). For psychiatric disorders.

Agranulocytosis, agitation, angioneurotic edema (giant hives), anemia, aplastic anemia, appetite loss, asthma, blood disturbances, breast engorgement, confusion, constipation, drowsiness, diarrhea, excitement, ejaculation inhibition, fever, gynecomastia (breast enlargement in a male), headache, laryngeal edema, leg edema, lethargy, jaundice, libido alteration, menstrual irregularities, mouth dryness, movement difficulty, muscular rigidity, nausea/vomiting, nasal stuffiness, pallor, restlessness, skin eruption, tremor, urinary retention, urinary incontinence, vision blurring, weight gain.

**Meprobamate.** See *Equanil.*

**Minocin** (minocycline). For infections.

Anaphylaxis, anemia, angioneurotic edema (giant hives), anogenital inflammation, appetite loss, blood disturbances, diarrhea, hives, intestinal inflammation, nausea/vomiting, rash, swallowing difficulty, tongue inflammation.

**Mycolog** (nystatin, neomycin, triamcinolone, gramicidin). For some skin conditions.

Acnelike eruption, burning, dryness, folliculitis, excess hairiness, irritation, itching, secondary infection, miliaria, pigmentation loss, skin maceration.

**Mycostatin** (nystatin). For fungal infections of mouth, throat.

Diarrhea, gastrointestinal distress, nausea/vomiting.

**Mylanta** (aluminum and magnesium hydroxides, simethicone). For relief of gas and stomach hyperacidity symptoms.

If used with tetracycline, makes the antibiotic unavailable for absorption.

**Mysteclin-F** (tetracycline, amphotericin B). For infections.

Anaphylaxis, anemia, angioneurotic edema (giant hives), appetite loss, blood disturbances, diarrhea, fever, hives, hoarseness, intestinal inflammation, itching, joint pain, mouth inflammation, nausea/vomiting, nail discoloration, proctitis, rash, sunburn reaction, sore throat, swallowing difficulty, tongue inflammation, black hairy tongue.

**Naldecor** (phenylpropanolamine, phenylephrine, phenyltoloxamine, chlorpheniramine). For symptoms of colds, sinusitis, hay fever, other pollen allergies.

Drowsiness, sedation.

**Nembutal** (pentobarbital). For sedation, insomnia.

Allergy, breathing depression, temporary breathing cessation, drowsiness, excitement, hangover, lethargy, nausea/vomiting, rash.

**Neosporin** (polymixin B, neomycin, gramicidin). For skin infections, infected eczema, herpes and seborrheic dermatitis.

Allergy, possible deleterious effects on ears, kidneys.

**Nicotinic Acid.** For reducing high blood-fat levels.

Flushing, gastrointestinal upset, headache, hypotension, itching, jaundice, peptic ulcer activation, skin dryness, toxic amblyopia.

**Nitroglycerin.** For prevention or treatment of anginal attacks.

Dizziness, faintness, headache, palpitation, fast pulse, weakness.

**Noludar** (methyprylon). For insomnia.

Diarrhea, dizziness, drowsiness (morning), esophagitis, excitement, headache, nausea/vomiting, rash.

**Norgesic** (orphenadrine, methylbenzhydryl, aspirin, phenacetin, caffeine). For pain.

Confusion, constipation, dizziness, drowsiness, headache, hives, mouth dryness, nausea/vomiting, palpitation, fast pulse, skin outbreak, urinary hesitancy or retention, vision blurring, weakness.

**Norlestrin** (norethindrone, ethinyl estradiol). Oral contraception.

Abdominal bloating, abdominal cramps, backache, breast tenderness, breast enlargement, breast secretion, blood pressure rise, cystitislike symptoms, edema, eye neuritis, depression, dizziness, fatigue, hirsutism, itching, jaundice, libido change, migraine, nausea/vomiting, nervousness, pulmonary embolism, rash, retinal thrombosis, scalp hair loss, stroke, thrombophlebitis, skin pigmentation, weight change.

**Norlestrin FE 28.** See *Norlestrin.*

**Novahistine-DH** (codeine, phenylephrine, chlorpheniramine, chloroform, alcohol). For cough, nasal congestion.

Drowsiness.

**Novahistine Expectorant** (*Novahistine-DH* plus glycerylguiaiacolate).

See *Novahistine-DH.*

**Omnipren** (ampicillin). For infections.

See *Ampicillin.*

**Oracon-21** (ethinyl estradiol, dimethistine). Oral contraceptive.

Possible side effects similar to *Norlestrin.*

**Orinase** (tolbutamide). Oral antidiabetic agent.

Aplastic anemia, hemolytic anemia, blood disturbances, headache, heartburn, hypoglycemia, hives, itching, jaundice, nausea, photosensitivity, porphyria cutanea tarda, skin redness, skin eruption.

**Ornade** (chlorpheniramine, phenylpropanolamine, isopropamide). For nasal congestion.

Abdominal distress, angina pain, appetite loss, blood disturbances, chest tightness, constipation, convulsions, diarrhea, dizziness, drowsiness, dryness of nose, mouth, throat, hypertension, hypotension, headache, incoordination, insomnia, irritability, nausea/vomiting, nervousness, palpitation, rash, tremor, urinary difficulty, painful urination, vision disturbances, weakness.

**Ortho-Novum, Ortho-Novum 1/50-21, Ortho-Novum 1/80-21** (norethindrone, mestranol, in varying dosages). Oral contraception.
Possible side effects similar to *Norlestrin.*

**Ovral** (norgestrel, ethinyl estradiol). Oral contraception.
Possible side effects similar to *Norlestrin.*

**Ovulen** (ethynodiol, mestranol). Oral contraception.
Possible side effects similar to *Norlestrin.*

**Parafon Forte** (chlorzoxazone, acetaminophen). For acute, painful musculoskeletal conditions.
Anaphylaxis, angioneurotic edema (giant hives), dizziness, drowsiness, gastrointestinal bleeding or upset, light-headedness, jaundice, rash, stimulation, urine discoloration.

**Paregoric** (powdered opium, anise oil, benzoic acid, camphor, glycerin, in diluted alcohol). For diarrhea.
May be habit-forming.

**Pavabid** (papaverine). For reduced blood flow conditions of heart, brain.
Abdominal distress, appetite loss, constipation, dizziness, diarrhea, drowsiness, headache, malaise, nausea, rash, sweating.

**Pediamycin** (erythromycin). For infection.
See *Erythromycin.*

**Penbritin** (ampicillin). For infection.
See *Ampicillin.*

**Penicillin G Potassium.** For infection.
Anaphylaxis, abdominal distress, hemolytic anemia, blood disturbances, chills, diarrhea, edema, fever, hives, joint pain, laryngeal edema, nausea/vomiting, rash, black hairy tongue.

**Penicillin VK** (phenoxymethyl penicillin). For infection.
Similar to *Penicillin G Potassium.*

**Pentids** (penicillin G potassium). For infection.
See *Penicillin G Potassium.*

**Pen-Vee K** (penicillin V potassium). For infection.
Similar to *Penicillin G Potassium.*

**Percodan** (oxycodone, aspirin, phenacetin, caffeine). For pain.
Constipation, dizziness, euphoria, itching, light-headedness, malaise, nausea/vomiting, restlessness, sedation.

**Periactin** (cyproheptadine). For allergies.
Abdominal distress, anaphylaxis, hemolytic anemia, appetite loss, blood disturbances, chest tightness, confusion, dryness of mouth, nose, throat, dizziness, ear ringing, excitation, euphoria, fatigue, faintness, hallucinations, headache, hives, hypotension, incoordination, insomnia, nausea/vomiting, nervousness, palpitation, photosensitivity, rash, restlessness, sedation, vision blurring, double vision, urinary difficulty, frequency, retention, wheezing.

**Peritrate** (pentaerythritol). For prevention and treatment of angina pectoris.
Collapse, dizziness, flushing, headache, nausea/vomiting, pallor, perspiration, rash, restlessness, weakness.

**Phenaphen/Codeine** (phenacetin, aspirin, phenobarbital, codeine). For pain and anxiety.
Constipation, drowsiness, nausea.

**Phenergan** (promethazine). For allergies, motion sickness, nausea/vomiting.
Blood disturbances, dizziness, mouth dryness, photosensitivity, vision blurring.

**Phenobarbital.** For sedation.
Allergy, excitement, musculoskeletal pain, rash.

**Placidyl** (ethchlorvynol). For insomnia.
Blood disturbances, dizziness, facial numbness, hangover, hypotension, hives, jaundice, nausea/vomiting, stomach upset, vision blurring.

**Polaramine** (dexchlorpheniramine). For allergies.

Appetite loss, dizziness, headache, heartburn, mouth dryness, nausea, nervousness, rash, restlessness, sweating, excessive or painful urination, vision doubling, weakness.

**Polycillin** (ampicillin). For infection.

See *Ampicillin*.

**Prednisone**. For severe skin and other diseases, hypersensitivity, malignancy.

Abdominal distention, bone fracture, cataract, convulsions, cushingoid state, diabetes, dizziness, esophagitis, exophthalmos, facial redness, fluid retention, glaucoma, growth suppression, headache, congestive heart failure, hypertension, menstrual irregularities, muscle weakness, osteoporosis, peptic ulcer, pancreatitis, thin fragile skin, sweating.

**Premarin** (conjugated estrogens). For amenorrhea, estrogen deficiency states, some abnormal uterine bleeding conditions, prostate cancer.

Abdominal bloating and cramps, appetite loss, bleeding breakthrough, breast tenderness and enlargement, endometriosis reactivation, edema, gynecomastia (breast enlargement in a man), headache, libido loss in a man, migraine aggravation, nausea/vomiting, rash.

**Principen** (ampicillin). For infection.

See *Ampicillin*.

**Pro-Banthine** (propantheline). For peptic ulcer.

Constipation, dizziness, drowsiness, headache, insomnia, impotence, nausea/vomiting, mouth dryness, nervousness, pupil dilation, rash, taste loss, vision blurring.

**Proloid** (thyroglobulin). For low thyroid function.

From overdosage: abnormal heart rhythms, angina pectoris, menstrual irregularities, nervousness.

**Pyridium** (phenazopyridine). For urinary pain, burning, urgency, frequency.

Gastrointestinal disturbances.

**Quinidine Sulfate**. For heart rhythm abnormalities.

Apprehension, blueness, breathing distress, confusion, coma, dizziness, edema, gastrointestinal upset, excitement, fever, headache, hearing disturbance, nausea/vomiting, rash, shock, cold sweat, vision disturbances.

**Rauzide** (rauwolfia, bendroflumethiazide). For hypertension.
Aplastic anemia, anxiety, appetite loss, blood disturbances, breathing difficulty, chest pain, constipation, cramping, diarrhea, dizziness, drowsiness, depression, heart rhythm abnormalities, headache, hives, hypotension, impotence, jaundice, mouth dryness, nasal congestion, muscle aches, muscle spasm, nausea/vomiting, nervousness, pancreatitis, burning or tingling sensations, photosensitivity, rash, stomach irritation, tremor, painful urination, color vision disturbance, weakness, weight gain.

**Regroton** (chlorthalidone, reserpine). For hypertension.
Aplastic anemia, appetite loss, blood disturbances, chest pain, constipation, deafness, diarrhea, dizziness, drowsiness, depression, flushing, gout, glaucoma, headache, hives, impotence, itching, jaundice, mouth dryness, myopia, muscle aches, muscle cramps, nightmares, nausea/vomiting, nasal congestion, pancreatitis, photosensitivity, rash, restlessness, stomach irritation, skin eruptions, tremor, uveitis, painful urination, color vision disturbance, vision blurring, weakness, weight gain.

**Reserpine.** For hypertension.
Anxiety, appetite loss, breathing difficulty, chest pain, increased susceptibility to colds, diarrhea, drowsiness, deafness, depression, dizziness, glaucoma, heart rhythm disturbances, headache, itching, impotence, libido decrease, muscle aches, mouth dryness, nasal stuffiness, nightmares, skin eruption, tremor, uveitis, vision blurring, weight gain.

**Ritalin** (methylphenidate). For mild depression, apathetic or withdrawn senile behavior, minimal brain dysfunction in children.
Abdominal pain, anemia, appetite loss, chest pain, dizziness, drowsiness, fever, hair loss, heart rhythm disturbances, headache, hives, insomnia, joint pains, movement difficulty, nervousness, palpitation, rash, skin eruption, weight loss.

**Salutensin** (hydroflumethiazide, reserpine). For hypertension.
Abdominal cramping, anxiety, aplastic anemia, appetite loss, breathing difficulty, blood disturbances, chest pain, constipation, increased susceptibility to colds, diarrhea, deafness, dizziness, depres-

sion, fainting, flushing of skin, fluid retention, glaucoma, headache, hives, impotence, itching, jaundice, libido decrease, mouth dryness, muscle ache, muscle spasm, nausea/vomiting, nightmares, nasal congestion, nervousness, pancreatitis, nosebleeds, rash, restlessness, sedation, stomach irritation, tremor, painful urination, uveitis, color vision disturbance, vision blurring, weakness, weight gain.

**Seconal** (secobarbital sodium). For insomnia.

Excitement, hangover, pain, sensitivity reactions in some people with asthma, hives, or angioneurotic edema.

**Ser-Ap-Es** (reserpine, hydralazine, hydrochlorothiazide). For hypertension.

Aplastic anemia, anxiety, appetite loss, blood disturbances, breast engorgement, breathing difficulty, chest pain, conjunctivitis, constipation, deafness, depression, diarrhea, disorientation, drowsiness, fainting, glaucoma, gynecomastia (breast enlargement in a male), headache, heart rhythm abnormalities, hepatitis, hives, itching, impotence, joint pains, jaundice, mouth dryness, muscle aches, muscle cramps, nasal congestion, nausea/vomiting, nervousness, nightmares, nosebleeds, numbness, palpitation, pancreatitis, rash, restlessness, stomach irritation, tremor, tingling, uveitis, painful urination, difficult urination, weakness, weight gain.

**Serax** (oxazepam). For anxiety, tension, agitation, irritability.

Blood disturbances, disorientation, dizziness, drowsiness, edema, euphoria, fainting, fever, hallucinations, headache, incoordination, incontinence, jaundice, lethargy, libido alteration, menstrual irregularities, nausea, rash, slurred speech, stupor, tremor, vision blurring, double vision.

**Sinequan** (doxepin). For anxiety, depression.

Appetite loss, blood disturbances, breast enlargement, burning, chills, confusion, constipation, diarrhea, disorientation, dizziness, drowsiness, facial edema, fatigue, flushing, gynecomastia (breast enlargement in a male), hair loss, hallucination, indigestion, incoordination, itching, jaundice, libido alteration, nausea/vomiting, photosensitivity, mouth dryness, ringing in ears, rash, taste disturbance, testicular swelling, tingling, tremor, urinary retention, vision blurring, weakness.

**Stelazine** (trifluoperazine). For anxiety, tension, agitation, psychotic disorders.

Agitation, amenorrhea, anaphylaxis, appetite loss, blood disturbances, cardiac arrest, constipation, dizziness, drowsiness, edema, fatigue, fever, headache, hives, insomnia, itching, jaundice, laryngeal edema, menstrual irregularities, mouth dryness, muscular weakness, muscle spasm, nasal congestion, nausea, rash, skin disorders, swallowing difficulty, tongue protrusion, tremor, vision blurring.

**Sterazolidin** (phenylbutazone, prednisone, aluminum hydroxide, magnesium trisilicate). For arthritis, bursitis, gout, acute fibrositis.

Side effects may be those of prednisone (see *Prednisone*) and phenylbutazone (see *Butazolidin*).

**Sudafed** (pseudoephedrine). For colds, ear infections, asthma, acute tracheobronchitis, other upper respiratory infections.
Stimulation.

**Sumycin** (tetracycline). For infections.
See *Tetracycline*.

**Synalar** (fluocinolone). For inflammatory skin conditions.
Burning, excessive hair, folliculitis, irritation, itching, miliaria, pigmentation loss, skin dryness, skin eruptions, skin maceration, striae (skin streaks or lines).

**Synthroid** (sodium levothyroxine). For thyroid deficiency.
Hyperthyroidism with overdose.

**Talwin** (pentazocine). For moderate to severe pain.
Abdominal distention, appetite loss, breathing depression, chills, constipation, diarrhea, dizziness, euphoria, excitement, fainting, flushing, headache, hallucinations, hives, insomnia, light-headedness, nausea/vomiting, numbness, rash, ringing in ears, sweating, sedation, tingling, tremor, urinary retention, vision blurring, weakness.

**Tandearil** (oxyphenbutazone). For arthritis, gout, painful shoulder, some other inflammatory conditions.
Side effects similar to those of phenylbutazone (see *Butazolidin*).

**Tedral** (theophylline, ephedrine, phenobarbital). For symptomatic relief of asthma, bronchitis.
Abdominal distress, insomnia, palpitation, stimulation, tremulousness, urinary difficulty.

**Teldrin** (chlorpheniramine maleate). For allergies.

Drowsiness, dizziness, gastrointestinal upset, fast heartbeat, mouth dryness.

**Tenuate** (diethylpropion). For short-term use in weight reduction.

Abdominal discomfort, anxiety, blood disturbances, blood pressure elevation, chest pain, constipation, depression, diarrhea, dizziness, drowsiness, euphoria, gynecomastia (breast enlargement in a male), headache, fast heartbeat, heart rhythm disturbances, hair loss, impotence, insomnia, jitteriness, menstrual upset, muscle pain, malaise, mouth dryness, nervousness, nausea/vomiting, palpitation, pupil dilation, rash, restlessness, stimulation, tremor, painful urination, excessive urination.

**Terramycin** (oxytetracycline). For infections.

See *Tetracycline*.

**Tetracycline**. For infections.

Anemia, hemolytic anemia, abdominal distress, anaphylaxis, angioneurotic edema (giant hives), anal itching, appetite loss, blood disturbances, diarrhea, dizziness, fever, headache, hives, hoarseness, intestinal inflammation, joint pains, mouth inflammation, nausea/vomiting, nail discoloration, proctitis, rash, swallowing difficulty, black hairy tongue.

**Tetrex** (tetracycline phosphate complex). For infections.

See *Tetracycline*.

**Thorazine** (chlorpromazine). For psychotic disorders, nausea and vomiting, tetanus, agitation, excessive anxiety, tension.

Agranulocytosis, blood disturbances, breast enlargement, convulsive seizures, constipation, dizziness, eye changes, fainting, fever, fast heartbeat, hives, jaundice, mouth dryness, nasal congestion, psychotic symptoms, pupil dilation, skin disturbances, skin pigmentation changes, sore throat, tremor, urinary retention, weight increase.

**Thyroid**. For thyroid deficiency.

With excessive doses: chest pain, diarrhea, fast heartbeat, fever, headache, hypertension, heat intolerance, insomnia, nausea, nervousness, sweating, tremor.

**Tigan** (trimethobenzamide). For nausea and vomiting.

Blood disturbances, coma, convulsions, depression, diarrhea, disorientation, drowsiness, hypotension, jaundice, muscle cramps, skin reaction, tremor, vision blurring.

**Tofranil** (imipramine). For depression, childhood enuresis.

Abdominal distress, agitation, anxiety, blood disturbances, breast enlargement, confusion, constipation, diarrhea, delusions, disorientation, dizziness, drowsiness, edema, fatigue, fever, flushing, heart rhythm disturbances, heart attack, gynecomastia (breast enlargement in a male), fast heartbeat, hypertension, hypotension, headache, hallucinations, hair loss, hives, insomnia, incoordination, impotence, jaundice, mouth dryness, mouth inflammation, nausea/vomiting, nightmares, numbness, parotid gland swelling, palpitation, photosensitivity, rash, restlessness, seizures, sweating, stroke, testicular swelling, tingling, black tongue, tremor, urinary retention, vision blurring, weakness.

**Tolinase** (tolazamide). For diabetes.

Anemia, blood disturbances, dizziness, fatigue, gas, headache, hypoglycemia, hives, jaundice, malaise, nausea/vomiting, photosensitivity, rash, weakness.

**Tranxene** (chlorazepate). For anxiety.

Confusion, depression, dizziness, drowsiness, fatigue, gastrointestinal upset, headache, incoordination, irritability, insomnia, mouth dryness, nervousness, rash, speech slurring, vision blurring.

**Triaminic** (phenylpropanolamine, pheniramine, pyrilamine). For nasal congestion, postnasal drip.

Dizziness, drowsiness, gastrointestinal upset, flushing, nervousness, palpitation, vision blurring.

**Triavil** (perphenazine, amitriptyline). For anxiety and/or depression.

Side effects may be those of phenothiazine agents (see *Compazine*) and amitriptyline (see *Elavil*).

**Tuinal** (secobarbital, amobarbital). For insomnia.

Angioneurotic edema (giant hives), excitement, hangover, hives, pain.

**Tuss-Ornade** (caramiphen, chlorpheniramine, phenylpropanolamine). For cough, upper respiratory congestion, excessive nasal secretion.

Abdominal distress or pain, appetite loss, blood disturbances, chest pain or tightness, convulsions, diarrhea, dizziness, drowsiness, dryness of nose, throat or mouth, headache, incoordination, insomnia, irritability, nausea/vomiting, nervousness, palpitation, rash, tremor, urinary difficulty, urinary pain, vision disturbances, weakness.

**Tylenol** (acetaminophen). For pain.
    Liver damage from overdose.

**Tylenol/Codeine** (acetaminophen and codeine).
    Liver damage from overdose.

**Valisone** (betamethasone). For inflammatory skin disorders.
    Burning, dryness, folliculitis, infection, irritation, itching, excessive hair growth, acnelike skin outbreak, miliaria, maceration, pigmentation loss.

**Valium** (diazepam). For tension, anxiety, muscle spasm.
    Anxiety, blood disturbances, confusion, constipation, depression, dizziness, drowsiness, fatigue, headache, hypotension, incoordination, insomnia, jaundice, joint pain, libido changes, nausea, rage, rash, slurred speech, tremor, double vision, vision blurring, urinary incontinence, urine retention.

**Vasodilan** (isoxsuprine). For blood vessel disorders, threatened abortion.
    Dizziness, palpitation, rash.

**V-Cillin K** (penicillin V potassium). For infections.
    Similar to *Penicillin G Potassium.*

**Vibramycin** (doxycycline). For infections.
    Anaphylaxis, angioneurotic edema (giant hives), anemia, anogenital inflammation, blood disturbances, diarrhea, hives, intestinal inflammation, mouth inflammation, nausea/vomiting, photosensitivity, rash, swallowing difficulty.

**Vioform-Hydrocortisone**    (iodochlorhydroxyquin,    hydrocortisone). For some skin disorders.
    Burning, irritation, itching, rash, striae (skin streaks or lines).

**Vistaril** (hydroxyzine). For anxiety, tension, agitation.
    Convulsions, drowsiness, mouth dryness, tremor.

Zyloprim (allopurinol). For gout.
Abdominal pain, blood disturbances, cataracts, chills, diarrhea, fever, hair loss, hives, itching, joint pain, nausea/vomiting, rash.

# Individual symptoms and the drugs that may produce them

**Abdominal bloating/distention.** Aristocort, Butazolidin, Butazolidin Alka, Decadron, Demulen, Medrol, Norlestrin preparations, Oracon preparations, Ortho-Novum preparations, Ovral, Ovulen 21, Sterazolidin, Tandearil.

**Abdominal cramps.** Aldactazide, Aldactone, Aldoril, Coumadin, Demulen, Diuril, Drixoril, E-Mycin, Erythrocin, Erythromycin, Esidrix, Hydrodiuril, Hygroton, Inderal, Norlestrin preparations, Oracon preparations, Ortho-Novum preparations, Ovral, Ovulen 21, Pediamycin, Premarin, Rauzide, Salutensin.

**Abdomimal discomfort.** Kaon, Lomotil, Marax, Tenuate.

**Abdominal distress.** Ambenyl Expectorant, Atromid-S, Benadryl, Dimetapp, Ornade, Pavabid, penicillin G potassium, Penicillin VK, Pentids, Pen-Vee K, Periactin, Sumycin, Talwin, Terramycin, tetracycline, Tetrex, Tofranil, Tuss-Ornade, V-Cillin K.

**Abdominal pain.** Azo Gantrisin, Cleocin, Cyclospasmol, Darvon preparations, Gantanol, Gantrisin, Indocin, Keflex, Macrodantin, Ritalin, Zyloprim.

**Agitation.** Butazolidin, Butazolidin Alka, Compazine, Demerol, Mellaril, Stelazine, Sterazolidin, Tandearil, Tofranil, Triavil.

**Agranulocytosis.** Equanil, Mellaril, Thorazine.

**Allergic reactions.** Combid, Nembutal, Neosporin, phenobarbital, Seconal.

**Amblyopia, toxic.** Nicotinic acid.

**Anaphylaxis.** Amcill, ampicillin, Declomycin, Dimetane, Diupres, Dyazide, E-Mycin, Equanil, erythromycin, Erythrocin, Etrafon, Macrodantin, Mellaril, Minocin, Omnipen, Parafon Forte, Pediamycin, penicillin G potassium, Pentids, Penicillin VK, Pen-Vee K, Penbritin, Periactin, Polycillin, Principen, Stelazine, Sumycin, Terramycin, tetracycline, Tetrex, V-Cillin K, Vibramycin.

**Anemia.** Achromycin V, Aldactazide, Ambenyl Expectorant, Amcill, ampicillin, Atromid-S, Azo Gantrisin, Benadryl, Butazolidin, Butazolidin Alka, Declomycin, Diabinese, Garamycin, Lasix, Mellaril, Mysteclin-F, Omnipen, Penbritin, Polycillin, Principen, Ritalin, Sterazolidin, Sumycin, Tandearil, tetracycline, Terramycin, Tetrex, Tolinase, Vibramycin.

**Anemia, aplastic.** Diupres, Diuril, Equanil, Esidrix, Gantanol, Gantrisin, Hygroton, Indocin, Lasix, Mellaril, Orinase, Periactin, Rauzide, Regroton, Salutensin, Ser-Ap-Es.

**Anemia, hemolytic.** Dimetane, Gantanol, Gantrisin, Indocin, Macrodantin, Minocin, Orinase, penicillin G potassium, Penicillin VK, Pentids, Pen-Vee K, Sumycin, Terramycin, tetracycline, Tetrex, V-Cillin K.

**Angina aggravation.** Aldomet, Aldoril.

**Angioneurotic edema (giant hives).** Declomycin, Equanil, Etrafon, Lomotil, Macrodantin, Mellaril, Minocin, Mysteclin-F, Parafon Forte, Sumycin, Terramycin, tetracycline, Tetrex, Tuinal, Vibramycin.

**Anogenital irritation/itching.** Minocin, Sumycin, Terramycin, tetracycline, Tetrex, Valium, Vibramycin.

**Anxiety.** Apresoline, Drixoril, Elavil, Etrafon, Hydropres, Rauzide, reserpine, Salutensin, Ser-Ap-Es, Tenuate, Tofranil, Triavil, Valium.

**Appetite loss.** Achromycin V, Aldactazide, Aldomet, Aldoril, Apresoline, Azo Gantrisin, Bendectin, Chlor-Trimeton, Dalmane, DBI-TD, Diabinese, Dimetane, Dimetapp, Diupres, Diuril, Drixoril, Esidrix, Etrafon, Gantanol, Gantrisin, Garamycin, Hydrodiuril, Hydropres, Hygroton, Indocin, Lanoxin, Lomotil, Macrodantin, Mellaril, Minocin, Mysteclin-F, Ornade, Pavabid, Periactin, Polaramine, Premarin, Rauzide, Regroton, reserpine, Ritalin, Salutensin, Ser-Ap-Es, Sinequan, Stelazine, Sumycin, Terramycin, tetracycline, Tetrex, Triavil, Tuss-Ornade, Vibramycin.

**Asthma.** Combid, Etrafon.

**Backache.** Norlestrin preparations, Oracon preparations, Ortho-Novum preparations, Ovral, Ovulen 20.

**Bleeding, breakthrough.** Premarin.

**Bleeding, gastrointestinal.** Butazolidin, Butazolidin Alka, Indocin, Parafon Forte, Sterazolidin, Tandearil.

**Bloated feeling.** Bentyl, Combid.

**Blood disturbances.** Aldactazide, Aldomet, Aldoril, Amcill, ampicillin, Apresoline, Azo Gantrisin, Butazolidin, Butazolidin Alka, Cleocin, Combid, Compazine, Declomycin, Diabinese, Dilantin, Dimetane, Dimetapp, Diuril, Doriden, Elavil, Equanil, Esidrix, Gantanol, Gantrisin, Hydrodiuril, Inderal, Indocin, Lasix, Librax, Librium, Macrodantin, Mellaril, Minocin, Mysteclin-F, Omnipen, Orinase, Ornade, Penbritin, penicillin G potassium, Penicillin VK, Pentids, Pen-Vee K, Periactin, Polycillin, Principen, Phenergan preparations, Placidyl, Rauzide, Regroton, Salutensin, Ser-Ap-Es, Serax, Sinequan, Stelazine, Sterazolidin, Sumycin, Tandearil, Tenuate, Terramycin, tetracycline, Tetrex, Thorazine, Tigan, Tofranil, Tolinase, Triavil, Tuss-Ornade, Valium, V-Cillin K, Vibramycin, Zyloprim.

**Bone fractures.** Aristocort, Decadron, prednisone, Sterazolidin.

**Breast engorgement.** Hydropres, Mellaril, Ser-Ap-Es, Thorazine.

**Breast enlargement.** Aldomet, Aldoril, Demulen, Elavil, Norlestrin preparations, Oracon preparations, Ortho-Novum preparations, Ovral, Ovulen 21, Premarin, Sinequan, Tofranil, Triavil.

**Breast secretion.** Norlestrin preparations, Oracon preparations, Ortho-Novum preparations, Ovral, Ovulen 21.

**Breast tenderness.** Norlestrin preparations, Oracon preparations, Ortho-Novum preparations, Ovral, Ovulen 21, Premarin.

**Breath, shortness of.** Dalmane.

**Breathing cessation, temporary.** Nembutal.

**Breathing depression.** Demerol, Lomotil, Nembutal, Talwin.

**Breathing difficulty.** Aldoril, Apresoline, Diupres, Hydrodiuril, Hydropres, Inderal, Indocin, Macrodantin, quinidine sulfate, Rauzide, reserpine, Salutensin, Ser-Ap-Es.

**Bronchial secretion thickening.** Ambenyl Expectorant.

**Bronchospasm.** Equanil, meprobamate.

**Bruising.** Aldactazide, Aldoril, Hydrodiuril, Medrol.

**Burning.** Afrin, Aldactazide, Aldomet, Aldoril, Cordran, Hydrodiuril, Hygroton, Kenalog, Mycolog, Sinequan, Synalar, Valisone, Vioform-Hydrocortisone.

**Cardiac arrest.** Stelazine.

**Cataracts.** Aristocort, Decadron, Medrol, prednisone, Sterazolidin, Zyloprim.

**Cerebral thrombosis.** Demulen.

**Chest pain.** Apresoline, Dalmane, Diupres, Drixoril, Hydropres, Macrodantin, Marex, Ornade, Proloid, Rauzide, Regroton, reserpine, Ritalin, Salutensin, Ser-Ap-Es, Tenuate, thyroid, Tuss-Ornade.

**Chest tightness.** Ambenyl Expectorant, Benadryl, Dimetane, Dimetapp, Ornade, Periactin, Tuss-Ornade

**Chills.** Apresoline, Azo Gantrisin, Equanil, Gantanol, Gantrisin, Macrodantin, meprobamate, penicillin G potassium, Penicillin VK, Pentids, Pen-Vee K, Sinequan, Talwin, V-Cillin K.

**Colds, increased susceptibility to.** Reserpine, Salutensin.

**Collapse.** Peritrate.

**Colon ulceration.** Butazolidin, Butazolidin Alka, Sterazolidin, Tandearil.

**Coma.** Dalmane, Lomotil, quinidine sulfate, Tigan.

**Concentration, disturbed.** Elavil, Triavil.

**Confusion.** Aldactazide, Aldactone, Ambenyl Expectorant, Benadryl, Butazolidin, Butazolidin Alka, Dalmane, Dilantin, Dimetane, Drixoril, Elavil, Etrafon, Indocin, Kaon, Librax, Librium, Mellaril, Norgesic, Periactin, quinidine sulfate, Sinequan, Sterazolidin, Tandearil, Tofranil, Tranxene, Triavil, Valium.

**Conjunctivitis.** Apresoline, Ser-Ap-Es.

**Constipation.** Aldomet, Aldoril, Ambenyl Expectorant, Apresoline, Artane, Benadryl, Bendectin, Bentyl, Bentyl/phenobarbital, Combid, Dalmane, Darvon preparations, Demerol, Dilantin, Dimetane, Dimetapp, Diupres, Diuril, Dyazide, Elavil, Esidrix, Etrafon, Feosol, Fiorinal, Fiorinal/codeine, Hydrodiuril, Hygroton, Inderal, Ionamin, Librax, Librium, Mellaril, Norgesic, Ornade, Pavabid, Percodan, Phenaphen/codeine, Pro-Banthine, Rauzide, Regroton, Salutensin, Ser-Ap-Es, Sinequan, Stelazine, Talwin, Tenuate, Thorazine, Tofranil, Triavil, Valium.

**Convulsions** (see also *Seizures*). Aristocort, Atarax, Azo Gantrisin, Combid, Decadron, Gantanol, Gantrisin, Garamycin, Medrol, Ornade, prednisone, Sterazolidin, Tandearil, Thorazine, Tigan, Tuss-Ornade, Vistaril.

**Cough.** Macrodantin.

**Cushing-like state.** Aristocort, Decadron, Medrol, prednisone, Sterazolidin.

**Cystitislike syndrome.** Norlestrin preparations, Oracon preparations, Ortho-Novum preparations, Ovral, Ovulen 21.

**Delusions.** Etrafon, Tofranil, Triavil.

**Depression.** Aldomet, Aldoril, Apresoline, Azo Gantrisin, Demulen, Diupres, Gantanol, Gantrisin, Hydropres, Inderal, Indocin, Lomotil, Norlestrin preparations, Oracon preparations, Ortho-Novum preparations, Ovral, Ovulen 21, Rauzide, Regroton, reserpine, Ser-Ap-Es, Tenuate, Valium.

**Diabetes.** Decadron, prednisone, Sterazolidin.

**Diarrhea.** Aldactazide, Aldactone, Aldomet, Aldoril, Ambenyl Expectorant, Amcill, ampicillin, Apresoline, Atromid-S, Azo Gantrisin, Benadryl, Bendectin, Butazolidin, Butazolidin Alka, Cleocin, Coumadin, Dalmane, DBI-TD, Declomycin, Diabinese, Dimetane, Dimetapp, Diupres, Diuril, Dyazide, Elavil, E-Mycin, Endrix, Equanil, Erythrocin, erythromycin, Feosol, Gantanol, Gantrisin, Hydrodiuril, Hydropres, Hygroton, Inderal, Indocin, Ionamin, Kaon, Keflex, Lanoxin, Lasix, Macrodantin, Mellaril, meprobamate, Minocin, Mycostatin, Mysteclin-F, Noludar, Omnipen, Ornade, Pavabid, Pediamycin, Penbritin, penicillin G potassium, Penicillin VK, Pentids, Pen-Vee K, Polycillin, Principen, Rauzide, Regroton, reserpine, Salutensin, Ser-Ap-Es, Sinequan, Sterazolidin, Talwin, Tandearil, Terramycin, tetracycline, Tetrex, Tigan, Tofranil, Triavil, Tuss-Ornade, Vibramycin, V-Cillin K, Zyloprim.

**Disorientation.** Apresoline, Dalmane, Demerol, Elavil, Ser-Ap-Es, Serax, Sinequan, Tigan, Tofranil, Triavil.

**Dizziness/vertigo.** Aldactazide, Aldomet, Aldoril, Ambenyl Expectorant, Apresoline, Aristocort, Artane, Atromid-S, Azo Gantrisin, Benadryl, Bendectin, Bentyl, Bentyl/phenobarbital, Butazolidin, Butazolidin Alka, Chlor-Trimeton, Combid, Compazine, Dalmane, Darvon preparations, Decadron, Demerol, Dilantin, Dimetane, Dimetapp, Diupres, Diuril, Drixoril, Dyazide, Elavil, Equanil, Esidrix, Etrafon, Fiorinal, Fiorinal/codeine, Gantanol, Gantrisin, Garamycin, Hydropres, Hygroton, Indocin, Ionamin, Isordil, Keflex, Lasix, Lomotil, Macrodantin, Marex, Medrol, meprobamate, nitroglycerin, Noludar, Norgesic, Norlestrin preparations, Oracon preparations, Ornade, Ortho-Novum preparations, Ovral, Ovulen 21, Parafon Forte, Pavabid, Percodan, Periactin, Peritrate, Phenergan preparations, Placidyl, Polaramine, prednisone, Pro-Banthine, quinidine sulfate, Rauzide, Regroton, reserpine, Ritalin, Salutensin, Ser-Ap-Es, Serax, Sinequan, Stelazine, Sterazolidin, Sumycin, Talwin, Teldrin, Tenuate, Terramycin, tetracycline, Tetrex, Thorazine, Tofranil, Tolinase, Tranxene, Triaminic, Triavil, Tuss-Ornade, Valium, Vasodilan.

**Drooling.** Aldactazide, Aldactone, Combid, Compazine, Triavil.

**Drowsiness.** Aldactazide, Aldactone, Ambenyl Expectorant, Antivert, Artane, Atarax, Atromid-S, Bellergal, Benadryl, Bendectin, Bentyl,

Bentyl/phenobarbital, Benylin Cough Syrup, Butisol Sodium, Chlor-Trimeton, Combid, Compazine, Dalmane, Dimetane, Dimetapp, Dramamine, Drixoril, Elavil, Equanil, Etrafon, Fiorinal, Fiorinal/codeine, Hydropres, Librax, Librium, Lomotil, Macrodantin, Marax, Mellaril, meprobamate, Naldecor, Nembutal, Noludar, Norgesic, Novahistine-DH, Novahistine Expectorant, Ornade, Parafon Forte, Pavabid, Phenergan/codeine, Pro-Banthine, Rauzide, Regroton, reserpine, Ritalin, Ser-Ap-Es, Serax, Sinequan, Stelazine, Teldrin, Tenuate, Tigan, Tranxene, Triaminic, Triavil, Tuss-Ornade, Valium, Vistaril.

**Dyspepsia.** Atromid-S, Butazolidin, Butazolidin Alka, Keflex, Sinequan, Sterazolidin, Tandearil.

**Ear Ringing.** Azo Gantrisin, Dimetane, Dimetapp, Elavil, Gantanol, Gantrisin, Garamycin, Lasix, Periactin, Sinequan, Talwin, Triavil.

**Ear toxicity.** Cortisporin, Neosporin.

**Eating, excessive.** Atromid-S.

**Edema** (fluid accumulation). Aldomet, Aldoril, Apresoline, Aristocort, Butazolidin, Butazolidin Alka, Combid, Decadron, Demulen, Diabinese, Diupres, Etrafon, Librax, Librium, Medrol, Norlestrin preparations, Oracon preparations, Ortho-Novum preparations, Ovral, Ovulen 21, penicillin G potassium, Penicillin VK, Pentids, Pen-Vee K, prednisone, Premarin, quinidine sulfate, Salutensin, Serax, Sinequan, Stelazine, Sterazolidin, Tandearil, Tofranil, Triavil, V-Cillin K.

**Ejaculation inhibition.** Combid, Mellaril.

**Endometriosis reactivation.** Premarin.

**Esophagitis.** Aristocort, Medrol, Noludar, prednisone, Sterazolidin.

**Euphoria.** Demerol, Dimetane, Equanil, Ionamin, Lomotil, meprobamate, Percodan, Periactin, Serax, Talwin, Tenuate.

**Excitement.** Dimetane, Doriden, Elavil, Equanil, Etrafon, Marax, Mellaril, meprobamate, Nembutal, Noludar, Periactin, phenobarbital, quinidine sulfate, Seconal, Triavil, Tuinal.

**Exophthalmos.** Aristocort, Decadron, Medrol, prednisone, Sterazolidin.

**Eye burning.** Dalmane.

**Eye disturbances.** Indocin, Thorazine.

**Eye edema.** Azo Gantrisin, Gantanol, Gantrisin.

**Eye neuritis.** Norlestrin preparations, Oracon preparations, Ortho-Novum preparations, Ovral, Ovulen 21.

**Eye protrusion.** See *Exophthalmos*.

**Eye tearing.** Apresoline.

**Facial paralysis.** Aldomet, Aldoril.

**Facial redness.** Aristocort, Decadron, Medrol, prednisone, Sterazolidin.

**Faintness.** Dalmane, Demerol, Dimetapp, Diupres, Equanil, Hydropres, Indocin, Librax, Librium, meprobamate, nitroglycerin, Periactin, Salutensin, Ser-Ap-Es, Serax, Talwin, Thorazine.

**Falling.** Dalmane.

**Fatigue.** Atromid-S, Bendectin, Dimetane, Elavil, Inderal, Keflex, Lasix, Norlestrin preparations, Oracon preparations, Ortho-Novum preparations, Ovral, Ovulen 21, Periactin, Sinequan, Stelazine, Tofranil, Tolinase, Tranxene, Triavil, Valium.

**Fever.** Aldactazide, Aldactone, Aldoril, Apresoline, Azo Gantrisin, Butazolidin, Butazolidin Alka, Combid, Coumadin, Diabinese, Diuril, Equanil, Gantanol, Gantrisin, Garamycin, Hydrodiuril, Inderal, Macrodantin, Mellaril, meprobamate, Mysteclin-F, penicillin G potassium, Penicillin VK, Pentids, Pen-Vee K, quinidine sulfate, Ritalin, Serax, Stelazine, Sterazolidin, Sumycin, Tandearil, Terramycin, tetracycline, Tetrex, Thorazine, thyroid, Tofranil, V-Cillin K, Zyloprim.

**Flatulence.** Aldomet, Aldoril, Atromid-S.

**Fluid accumulation.** See *Edema*.

**Flushing.** Apresoline, Bellergal, Cyclospasmol, Dalmane, Demerol, Donnagel-PG, Donnatal, Diupres, Isordil, nicotinic acid, Peritrate, Regroton, Salutensin, Ser-Ap-Es, Sinequan, Talwin, Tofranil, Triaminic.

**Folliculitis.** Cordran, Kenalog, Mycolog, Synalar, Valisone.

**Gait, shuffling or unsteady.** Compazine, Marax.

**Gallbladder disease.** Demulen.

**Gastrointestinal bleeding.** See *Bleeding, gastrointestinal*.

**Gastrointestinal upset.** Mycostatin, nicotinic acid, Pyridium, Parafon Forte, quinidine sulfate, Tranxene, Triaminic.

**Giddiness.** Dimetapp.

**Glaucoma.** Aristocort, Decadron, Hydropres, Medrol, prednisone, Regroton, reserpine, Salutensin, Ser-Ap-Es, Sterazolidin.

**Gout.** Hygroton, Regroton.

**Growth suppression.** Aristocort, Decadron, Medrol, prednisone, Sterazolidin.

**Gum swelling.** Lomotil.

**Gynecomastia** (breast enlargement in a male). Aldactazide, Aldactone, Aldomet, Aldoril, Hydropres, Lanoxin, Mellaril, Premarin, Ser-Ap-Es, Sinequan, Tenuate, Tofranil.

**Hair, abnormal growth of** (hirsutism). Aldactazide, Aldactone, Cordran, Kenalog, Mycolog, Norlestrin preparations, Oracon preparations, Ortho-Novum preparations, Ovral, Ovulen 21, Synalar, Valisone.

**Hair, dry, brittle.** Atromid-S.

**Hair loss.** Coumadin, Inderal, Indocin, Macrodantin, Norlestrin preparations, Oracon preparations, Ortho-Novum preparations, Ovral, Ovulen 21, Ritalin, Sinequan, Tenuate, Tofranil, Zyloprim.

**Hallucinations.** Azo Gantrisin, Dalmane, Demerol, Elavil, Gantanol, Gantrisin, Inderal, Periactin, Serax, Sinequan, Talwin, Triavil.

**Hands, heaviness of.** Ambenyl Expectorant, Benadryl.

**Hands, tingling.** Benadryl.

**Hands, weakness of.** Ambenyl Expectorant, Benadryl.

**Hangover.** Butisol Sodium, Doriden, Nembutal, Placidyl, Seconal, Tuinal.

**Headache.** Afrin, Aldactazide, Aldomet, Aldoril, Ambenyl Expectorant, Apresoline, Aristocort, Artane, Atromid-S, Azo Gantrisin, Benadryl, Bendectin, Bentyl, Bentyl/phenobarbital, Butazolidin, Butazolidin Alka, Butisol Sodium, Chlor-Trimeton, Combid, Cyclospasmol, Dalmane, Darvon preparations, Decadron, Demerol, Demulen, Dilantin, Dimetane, Dimetapp, Diupres, Diuril, Drixoril, Dyazide, Equanil, Esidrix, Etrafon, Gantanol, Gantrisin, Garamycin, Hydrodiuril, Hydropres, Hygroton, Indocin, Ionamin, Isordil, Keflex, Lanoxin, Lasix, Lomotil, Macrodantin, Marax, Medrol, Mellaril, meprobamate, nicotinic acid, nitroglycerin, Noludar, Norgesic, Orinase, Ornade, Pavabid, Periactin, Polaramine, prednisone, Premarin, Pro-Banthine, quinidine sulfate, Rauzide, Regroton, reserpine, Ritalin, Salutensin, Ser-Ap-Es, Serax, Stelazine, Sterazolidin, Sumycin, Talwin, Tandearil, Tenuate, Terramycin, tetracycline, Tetrex, thyroid, Tofranil, Tolinase, Tranxene, Tuss-Ornade, Valium.

**Healing, impaired.** Aristocort, Decadron.

**Hearing loss.** Butazolidin, Butazolidin Alka, Diupres, Hydropres, Indocin, Lasix, quinidine sulfate, Regroton, reserpine, Salutensin, Ser-Ap-Es, Sterazolidin, Tandearil.

**Heart attack.** Demulen, Elavil, Etrafon, Tofranil, Triavil.

**Heartbeat, fast** (see also *Pulse, fast*). Apresoline, Bentyl, Bentyl/phenobarbital, Cyclospasmol, Demerol, Dimetane, Teldrin, Tenuate, Thorazine, thyroid, Tofranil.

**Heartbeat, slow.** Aldomet, Aldoril, Demerol.

**Heartburn** (see also *Dyspepsia*). Chlor-Trimeton, Cyclospasmol, Dalmane, Etrafon, Orinase, Polaramine.

**Heart Disorders.** Butazolidin, Butazolidin Alka, Demerol, Elavil, Etrafon, Sterazolidin, Tandearil.

**Heart failure, congestive.** Aristocort, Inderal, Medrol, prednisone, Sterazolidin.

**Heart rhythm disturbances.** Elavil, Hydropres, Kaon, Lanoxin, Marax, Proloid, Rauzide, reserpine, Ritalin, Ser-Ap-Es, Tenuate, Tofranil, Triavil.

**Hemorrhage.** Coumadin.

**Hepatitis.** Azo Gantrisin, Butazolidin, Butazolidin Alka, Dilantin, Macrodantin, Ser-Ap-Es, Sterazolidin, Tandearil.

**Hives.** Achromycin V, Aldactazide, Aldactone, Aldoril, Ambenyl Expectorant, Amcill, ampicillin, Apresoline, Atromid-S, Azo Gantrisin, Benadryl, Bentyl, Bentyl/phenobarbital, Butazolidin, Butazolidin Alka, Cleocin, Coumadin, Declomycin, Demerol, Dimetane, Dimetapp, Diuril, Dyazide, Elavil, E-Mycin, Erythrocin, erythromycin, Esidrix, Etrafon, Gantanol, Gantrisin, Garamycin, Hydrodiuril, Hygroton, Indocin, Ionamin, Keflex, Lasix, Lomotil, Macrodantin, Minocin, Mysteclin-F, Norgesic, Omnipen, Omnipres, Orinase, Pediamycin, Penbritin, penicillin G potassium, Pentids, Penicillin VK, Pen-Vee K, Periactin, Placidyl, Polycillin, Principen, Rauzide, Regroton, Ritalin, Salutensin, Ser-Ap-Es, Stelazine, Sterazolidin, Sumycin, Tandearil, Talwin, Terramycin, tetracycline, Tetrex, Thorazine, Tofranil, Tolinase, Triavil, Tuinal, Vibramycin, Zyloprim.

**Hoarseness.** Sumycin, Tetrex, Terramycin, tetracycline.

**Hyperglycemia** (elevated blood sugar). Butazolidin, Butazolidin Alka, Sterazolidin, Tandearil.

**Hypertension.** Aristocort, Decadron, Demulen, Drixoril, Elavil, Etrafon, Ionamin, Medrol, Norlestrin preparations, Oracon preparations, Ornade, Ortho-Novum preparations, Ovral, Ovulen 21, prednisone, Sterazolidin, Thyroid, Tofranil, Triavil.

**Hyperthyroidism.** Synthroid, thyroid.

**Hypotension.** Ambenyl Expectorant, Apresoline, Benadryl, Elavil, Etrafon, Inderal, Kaon, nicotinic acid, Ornade, Periactin, Placidyl, Rauzide, Tigan, Tofranil, Triavil, Valium.

**Impotence.** Aldactazide, Aldactone, Aldomet, Aldoril, Atromid-S, Bentyl, Bentyl/phenobarbital, Diupres, Hydropres, Hygroton, Ionamin, Pro-Banthine, Rauzide, Regroton, reserpine, Salutensin, Ser-Ap-Es, Tenuate, Tofranil.

**Incoordination (ataxia).** Aldactazide, Aldactone, Dilantin, Dimetane, Dimetapp, Elavil, Equanil, Etrafon, Gantanol, Gantrisin, Librax, Librium, meprobamate, Ornade, Periactin, Serax, Sinequan, Tofranil, Tranxene, Triavil, Tuss-Ornade, Valium.

**Infection.** Cordran, Kenalog, Mycolog, Valisone.

**Insomnia.** Afrin, Ambenyl Expectorant, Azo Gantrisin, Benadryl, Bentyl, Bentyl/phenobarbital, Butazolidin, Butazolidin Alka, Compazine, Dilantin, Dimetane, Drixoril, Elavil, Etrafon, Gantanol, Gantrisin, Ionamin, Marax, Ornade, Periactin, Pro-Banthine, Ritalin, Stelazine, Talwin, Tedral, Tenuate, thyroid, Tofranil, Tranxene, Triavil, Tuss-Ornade, Valium.

**Intestinal inflammation.** Declomycin, Minocin, Mysteclin-F, Sumycin, Terramycin, tetracycline, Tetrex, Vibramycin.

**Irritability.** Bendectin, Dalmane, Ornade, Tranxene, Tuss-Ornade.

**Itching.** Aldactazide, Apresoline, Atromid-S, Azo Gantrisin, Combid, Cordran, Dalmane, Demerol, Diupres, Etrafon, Gantanol, Gantrisin, Garamycin, Indocin, Keflex, Kenalog, Lomotil, Lasix, Macrodantin, Mycolog, Mysteclin-F, nicotinic acid, Norlestrin preparations, Oracon preparations, Orinase, Ortho-Novum preparations, Ovral, Ovulen 21, Percodan, Regroton, reserpine, Salutensin, Ser-Ap-Es, Sinequan, Stelazine, Synalar, Valisone, Vioform-Hydrocortisone, Zyloprim.

**Jaundice.** Aldactazide, Aldoril, Cleocin, Combid, Compazine, Demulen, Diabinese, Diupres, Diuril, Elavil, Esidrix, Etrafon, Hydrodiuril, Hygroton, Indocin, Lasix, Macrodantin, Mellaril, nicotinic acid, Norlestrin preparations, Oracon preparations, Orinase, Ortho-Novum preparations, Ovral, Ovulen 21, Parafon Forte, Placidyl, Rauzide, Regroton, Salutensin, Ser-Ap-Es, Serax, Sinequan, Stelazine, Thorazine, Tigan, Tofranil, Tolinase, Triavil, Valium.

**Jitteriness.** Compazine, Tenuate, Triavil.

**Joint disease.** Dilantin.

**Joint pain.** Aldomet, Aldoril, Apresoline, Atromid-S, Azo Gantrisin, Butazolidin, Butazolidin Alka, Dalmane, Gantanol, Gantrisin, Macrodantin, Mysteclin-F, penicillin G potassium, Penicillin VK, Pentids, Pen-Vee K, Ritalin, Ser-Ap-Es, Sterazolidin, Sumycin, Tandearil, Terramycin, tetracycline, Tetrex, Valium, V-Cillin K, Zyloprim.

**Kidney disturbances.** Butazolidin, Butazolidin Alka, Sterazolidin, Tandearil.

**Kidney toxicity.** Cortisporin, Neosporin.

**Lactation suppression.** Bentyl, Bentyl/phenobarbital.

**Laryngeal edema.** Mellaril, penicillin G potassium, Penicillin VK, Pentids, Pen-Vee K, Stelazine, V-Cillin K.

**Lassitude.** Dimetapp.

**Leg swelling.** Combid, Mellaril.

**Leg Weakness.** Kaon.

**Lethargy.** Aldactazide, Aldactone, Butisol Sodium, Butazolidin, Butazolidin Alka, Dalmane, Lomotil, Mellaril, Nembutal, Serax, Sterazolidin, Tandearil.

**Libido alteration.** Aldomet, Aldoril, Atromid-S, Mellaril, Norlestrin preparations, Oracon preparations, Ortho-Novum preparations, Ovral, Ovulen 21, Premarin, reserpine, Salutensin, Serax, Sinequan, Valium.

**Light-headedness.** Afrin, Aldomet, Aldoril, Dalmane, Darvon preparations, Demerol, Indocin, Lasix, Parafon Forte, Percodan, Talwin.

**Light sensitivity** (photosensitivity). Achromycin V, Aldactazide, Aldoril, Ambenyl Expectorant, Azo Gantrisin, Benadryl, Diuril, Dyazide, Hydrodiuril, Orinase, Periactin, Phenergan preparations, Rauzide, Regroton, Sinequan, Tofranil, Tolinase, Vibramycin.

**Listlessness.** Kaon.

**Liver damage.** Dilantin, Tylenol and Tylenol/codeine (with overdosage).

**Lymph node enlargement.** Dilantin.

**Malaise.** Lomotil, Macrodantin, Pavabid, Percodan, Tenuate, To-linase.

**Menstrual irregularities.** Aldactazide, Aldactone, Aristocort, Combid, Decadron, Demulen, Etrafon, Librax, Librium, Medrol, Mellaril, prednisone, Proloid (overdose), Serax, Stelazine, Sterazolidin, Tenuate.

**Mental acuity, decreased.** Aldomet, Aldoril.

**Metabolic acidosis.** Butazolidin, Butazolidin Alka, Sterazolidin, Tandearil.

**Migraine.** Norlestrin preparations, Oracon preparations, Ortho-Novum preparations, Ovral, Ovulen 21, Premarin.

**Miliaria** (prickly heat). Cordran, Kenalog, Mycolog, Synalar, Valisone.

**Mouth burning.** Lasix.

**Mouth dryness.** Aldomet, Aldoril, Ambenyl Expectorant, Antivert, Artane, Atarax, Bellergal, Benadryl, Bendectin, Bentyl, Bentyl/phe-nobarbital, Chlor-Trimeton, Combid, Dalmane, Demerol, Dimetane, Donnagel-PG, Donnatal, Diupres, Dyazide, Etrafon, Hydropres, Ionamin, Librax, Librium, Mellaril, Norgesic, Ornade, Phenergan preparations, Pro-Banthine, Polaramine, Rauzide, Regroton, reserpine, Salutensin, Ser-Ap-Es, Sinequan, Stelazine, Teldrin, Tenuate, Thorazine, Tofranil, Tranxene, Tuss-Ornade, Vistaril.

**Mouth inflammation.** Amcill, ampicillin, Azo Gantrisin, Indocin, Mysteclin-F, Omnipen, Penbritin, Polycillin, Principen, Sumycin, Terramycin, tetracycline, Tetrex, Tofranil, Vibramycin.

**Mouth ulceration.** Butazolidin, Butazolidin Alka, Sterazolidin, Tandearil.

**Movement, difficult.** Combid, Etrafon, Mellaril, Ritalin.

**Movements, involuntary.** Aldomet, Aldoril, Combid, Compazine, Triavil.

**Muscle ache.** Atromid-S, Diupres, Hydropres, Rauzide, Regroton, reserpine, Salutensin, Ser-Ap-Es.

**Muscle cramps.** Apresoline, Atromid-S, Dyazide, Lasix, Regroton, Ser-Ap-Es, Tigan.

**Muscle pain.** Aldomet, Aldoril, phenobarbital, Tenuate.

**Muscle spasm.** Aldoril, Compazine, Diupres, Diuril, Esidrix, Hydrodiuril, Hygroton, Rauzide, Salutensin, Stelazine, Triavil.

**Muscle tone impairment.** Etrafon.

**Muscle weakness.** Aristocort, Atromid-S, Decadron, Medrol, Marax, prednisone, Stelazine, Sterazolidin.

**Muscular rigidity.** Mellaril.

**Myopia.** Regroton.

**Nail discoloration.** Mysteclin-F, Sumycin, Terramycin, tetracycline, Tetrex.

**Nasal congestion.** Afrin, Apresoline, Combid, Diupres, Etrafon, Hydropres, Regroton, reserpine, Ser-Ap-Es, Salutensin, Stelazine, Thorazine.

**Nasal dryness.** Afrin, Ambenyl Expectorant, Benadryl, Dimetane, Marax, Ornade, Tuss-Ornade.

**Nasal Stuffiness.** Aldomet, Aldoril, Ambenyl Expectorant, Benadryl, Dimetane, Mellaril.

**Nausea/vomiting.** Achromycin V, Aldactazide, Aldomet, Aldoril, Ambenyl Expectorant, Amcill, ampicillin, Apresoline, Artane, Atromid-S, Azo Gantrisin, Benadryl, Bendectin, Bentyl, Bentyl/phenobarbital, Butisol Sodium, Butazolidin, Butazolidin Alka, Cleocin, Coumadin, Dalmane, Darvon preparations, DBI-TD, Declomycin, Demerol, Demulen, Dilantin, Dimetapp, Diabinese, Diupres, Diuril, Doriden, Drixoril, Dyazide, Elavil, Equanil, Erythyrocin, erythyromycin, E-Mycin, Esidrix, Etrafon, Feosol, Fiorinal, Fiorinal/codeine, Gantanol, Gantrisin, Garamycin, Hydergine, Hydrodiuril, Hydropres, Hygroton, Inderal, Indocin, Isordil, Kaon, Keflex, Lanoxin, Lasix, Librax, Librium, Lomotil, Macrodantin, Marax, meprobamate, Mellaril, Minocin, Mycostatin, Mysteclin-F, Nembutal, Noludar, Norgesic, Norlestrin preparations, Omnipen, Oracon preparations, Orinase, Ornade, Ortho-Novum preparations, Ovral, Ovulen 21, Pavabid, Pediamycin, Penbritin, penicillin G potassium, Penicillin VK, Pentids, Pen-Vee K, Percodan, Periactin, Peritrate, Phenergan/codeine, Placidyl, Polaramine, Polycillin, Premarin, Pro-Banthine, quinidine sulfate, Rauzide, Regroton, Salutensin, Ser-Ap-Es, Serax, Sinequan, Stelazine, Sterazolidin, Sumycin, Talwin, Tandearil, Tenuate, Terramycin, tetracycline, Tetrex, thyroid, Tofranil, Tolinase, Triavil, Tuss-Ornade, Valium, V-Cillin K, Vibramycin, Zyloprim.

**Nervousness.** Ambenyl Expectorant, Artane, Bentyl, Bentyl/phenobarbital, Dalmane, Dilantin, Dimetane, Diupres, Hydropres, Marax, Norlestrin preparations, Oracon preparations, Ornade, Ortho-Novum preparations, Ovral, Ovulen 21, Periactin, Polaramine, Pro-Banthine, Proloid (overdose), Rauzide, Ritalin, Salutensin, Ser-Ap-Es, Tenuate, thyroid (overdose), Tranxene, Triaminic, Tuss-Ornade.

**Nightmares.** Aldomet, Aldoril, Diupres, Elavil, Hydropres, Regroton, reserpine, Salutensin, Ser-Ap-Es, Tofranil, Triavil.

**Nosebleed.** Indocin, Salutensin, Ser-Ap-Es.

**Numbness.** Apresoline, Elavil, Etrafon, Garamycin, Lomotil, Ser-Ap-Es, Talwin, Tofranil, Triavil.

**Osteoporosis.** Aristocort, Decadron, Medrol, prednisone, Sterazolidin.

**Pallor.** Isordil, Mellaril, Peritrate.

**Palpitation.** Afrin, Ambenyl Expectorant, Apresoline, Benadryl, Bendectin, Bentyl, Bentyl/phenobarbital, Dalmane, Demerol, Dimetane, Dimetapp, Drixoril, Elavil, Equanil, Etrafon, Ionamin, Marax, meprobamate, nitroglycerin, Norgesic, Ornade, Periactin, Ritalin, Ser-Ap-Es, Tedral, Tenuate, Tofranil, Triaminic, Triavil, Tuss-Ornade, Vasodilan.

**Pancreatitis.** Aristocort, Azo Gantrisin, Decadron, Diuril, Dyazide, Esidrix, Gantanol, Gantrisin, Hydrodiuril, Hygroton, Medrol, prednisone, Rauzide, Regroton, Salutensin, Ser-Ap-Es, Sterazolidin.

**Photosensitivity.** See *Light sensitivity*.

**Porphyria cutanea tarda.** Orinase.

**Proctitis.** Equanil, meprobamate, Mysteclin-F, Sumycin, Terramycin, tetracycline, Tetrex.

**Psychotic symptoms.** Thorazine.

**Pulmonary embolism.** Norlestrin preparations, Oracon preparations, Ortho-Novum preparations, Ovral, Ovulen 21.

**Pulse, fast.** Elavil, Equanil, Ionamin, meprobamate, nitroglycerin, Norgesic, Triavil.

**Pupil contraction.** Fiorinal/codeine.

**Pupil dilation.** Bentyl, Bentyl/phenobarbital, Dimetapp, Tenuate, Thorazine.

**Purple toes.** Coumadin.

**Rage.** Valium.

**Respiratory alkalosis.** Butazolidin, Butazolidin Alka, Sterazolidin, Tandearil.

**Restlessness.** Aldactazide, Aldoril, Ambenyl Expectorant, Benadryl, Chlor-Trimeton, Dalmane, Darvon preparations, Demerol, Dimetane, Diupres, Diuril, Drixoril, Elavil, Esidrix, Hydrodiuril, Hygroton, Ionamin, Isordil, Lomotil, Mellaril, Percodan, Periactin, Peritrate, Polaramine, Regroton, Salutensin, Ser-Ap-Es, Tenuate, Tofranil, Triavil.

**Retinal detachment.** Butazolidin, Butazolidin Alka, Sterazolidin, Tandearil.

**Retinal hemorrhage.** Butazolidin, Butazolidin Alka, Sterazolidin, Tandearil.

**Retinal thrombosis.** Norlestrin preparations, Oracon preparations, Ortho-Novum preparations, Ovral, Ovulen 21.

**Salivary gland inflammation.** Aldoril, Diupres, Diuril, Hydrodiuril, Tofranil.

**Salivation.** Etrafon.

**Sedation.** Actifed, Actifed-C Expectorant, Aldomet, Aldoril, Bendectin, Darvon preparations, Demerol, Dimetane, Diupres, Lomotil, Naldecor, Percodan, Periactin, Salutensin, Talwin.

**Seizures** (see also *Convulsions*). Elavil, Etrafon, Tofranil, Triavil.

**Shock.** Quinidine sulfate.

**Skin disturbances.** Butazolidin, Butazolidin Alka, Chlor-Trimeton, Combid, Compazine, Diabinese, Gantanol, Gantrisin, Stelazine, Sterazolidin, Tandearil, Triavil.

**Skin dryness.** Donnagel-PG, Donnatal, Kenalog, Mycolog, nicotinic acid, Synalar, Valisone.

**Skin irritation.** Cordran, Kenalog, Mycolog, Valisone, Vioform-Hydrocortisone.

**Skin maceration.** Cordran, Kenalog, Mycolog, Synalar, Valisone.

**Skin pigmentation alteration.** Cordran, Kenalog, Mycolog, Norlestrin preparations, Oracon preparations, Ortho-Novum preparations, Ovral, Ovulen 21, Synalar, Thorazine, Valisone.

**Skin rash or eruption.** Achromycin V, Aldactazide, Aldactone, Aldomet, Aldoril, Ambenyl Expectorant, Amcill, ampicillin, Apresoline, Atromid-S, Azo Gantrisin, Benadryl, Bendectin, Butisol Sodium, Butazolidin, Butazolidin Alka, Cleocin, Coumadin, Dalmane, Darvon preparations, Declomycin, Demerol, Demulen, Dilantin, Dimetane, Dimetapp, Diupres, Diuril, Doriden, Drixoril, Dyazide, Elavil, E-Mycin, Equanil, Erythrocin, erythromycin, Esidrix, Etrafon, Fiorinal, Fiorinal/codeine, Gantrisin, Garamycin, Hydrodiuril, Hygroton, Inderal, Indocin, Isordil, Keflex, Kenalog, Lasix, Librax, Librium, Macrodantin, Mellaril, meprobamate, Minocin, Mysteclin-F, Mycolog, Nembutal, Norgesic, Norlestrin preparations, Omnipen, Oracon preparations, Orinase, Ornade, Ortho-Novum preparations, Ovral, Ovulen 21, Parafon Forte, Pavabid, Pediamycin, Penbritin, penicillin G potassium, Pencillin VK, Pentids, Pen-Vee K, Periactin, Peritrate, phenobarbital, Polaramine, Polycillin, Premarin, Princi-pen, Pro-Banthine, quinidine sulfate, Rauzide, Regroton, reserpine, Ritalin, Salutensin, Ser-Ap-Es, Serax, Sinequan, Stelazine, Sterazoli-din, Sumycin, Synalar, Talwin, Tandearil, Tenuate, Terramycin, te-tracycline, Tetrex, Thorazine, Tigan, Tofranil, Tolinase, Tranxene, Triavil, Tuss-Ornade, Valisone, Valium, Vasodilan, V-Cillin K, Vibra-mycin, Vioform-Hydrocortisone, Zyloprim.

**Skin reddening.** Garamycin, Orinase.

**Skin, thin, fragile.** Aristocort, Decadron, Medrol, prednisone, Stera-zolidin.

**Sneezing.** Afrin.

**Speech, slurring.** Dalmane, Dilantin, Equanil, meprobamate, Serax, Tranxene, Valium.

**Staggering.** Dalmane.

**Stimulation.** Actifed, Actifed-C Expectorant, Empirin Compound/ codeine, Equanil, Ionamin, meprobamate, Parafon Forte, Sudafed, Tenuate, Tedral.

**Stinging.** Afrin.

**Stomach irritation, pain, or upset** (see also *Dyspepsia*). Aldoril, Ben-dectin, Butazolidin, Butazolidin Alka, Dalmane, Dimetane, Diupres, Diuril, Drixoril, Esidrix, Hydergine, Hydrodiuril, Hygroton, Indocin, Lasix, Placidyl, Rauzide, Regroton, Salutensin, Ser-Ap-Es, Sterazoli-din, Tandearil, Teldrin.

**Striae** (skin streaks or lines). Cordran, Cortisporin, Synalar, Vioform-Hydrocortisone.

**Stroke.** Elavil, Etrafon, Norlestrin preparations, Oracon preparations, Ortho-Novum preparations, Ovral, Ovulen 21, Tofranil, Triavil.

**Stupor.** Serax.

**Sunburn reaction** (see also *Light sensitivity*). Mysteclin-F.

**Swallowing difficulty.** Combid, Compazine, Declomycin, Minocin, Mysteclin-F, Stelazine, Sumycin, Terramycin, tetracycline, Tetrex, Triavil, Vibramycin.

**Sweat, cold.** Quinidine sulfate.

**Sweating.** Aristocort, Dalmane, Decadron, Demerol, Drixoril, Isordil, Lasix, Marax, Medrol, Pavabid, Peritrate, Polaramine, prednisone, Sterazolidin, Talwin, thyroid, Tofranil.

**Sweating, decreased.** Bentyl, Bentyl/phenobarbital.

**Talkativeness.** Dalmane.

**Taste disturbance.** Bentyl, Bentyl/phenobarbital, DBI-TD, Pro-Banthine, Sinequan.

**Tension.** Drixoril.

**Testicular swelling.** Sinequan, Tofranil.

**Thirst.** Bendectin, Lasix.

**Throat dryness.** Ambenyl Expectorant, Benadryl, Dimetane, Marax, Ornade, Tuss-Ornade.

**Throat, sore.** Inderal, Mysteclin-F, Tofranil.

**Thrombophlebitis.** Demulen, Lasix, Norlestrin preparations, Oracon preparations, Ortho-Novum preparations, Ovral, Ovulen 21.

**Thyroid disturbance.** Butazolidin, Butazolidin Alka, Sterazolidin, Tandearil.

**Tingling.** Aldactazide, Aldomet, Aldoril, Ambenyl Expectorant, Apresoline, Elavil, Equanil, Esidrix, Etrafon, Garamycin, Hydrodiuril, Hygroton, Inderal, Kaon, Lasix, meprobamate, Ser-Ap-Es, Sinequan, Talwin, Tofranil, Triavil.

**Tongue, black/hairy.** Amcill, ampicillin, Elavil, Mysteclin-F, Omnipen, Penbritin, penicillin G potassium, Penicillin VK, Pentids, Pen-Vee K, Polycillin, Principen, Sumycin, Terramycin, tetracycline, Tetrex, Tofranil, Triavil, V-Cillin K.

**Tongue inflammation.** Amcill, ampicillin, Declomycin, Mysteclin-F, Minocin, Omnipen, Penbritin, Polycillin, Principen.

**Tongue protrusion.** Compazine, Stelazine, Triavil.

**Tongue, sore.** Aldomet, Aldoril, Amcill, ampicillin, Omnipen, Polycillin.

**Tongue, swollen.** Elavil, Triavil.

**Tremor.** Aldomet, Aldoril, Apresoline, Atarax, Compazine, Demerol, Elavil, Etrafon, Hydropres, Ionamin, Mellaril, Ornade, Rauzide, Regroton, reserpine, Salutensin, Ser-Ap-Es, Serax, Sinequan, Stelazine, Talwin, Tenuate, Thorazine, Triavil, thyroid, Tigan, Tofranil, Tuss-Ornade, Valium, Vistaril.

**Tremulousness.** Marax, Tedral.

**Twitching.** Dilantin

**Ulcer, gastrointestinal** (Esophagus, Stomach, or Duodenum). Aristocort, Butazolidin, Butazolidin Alka, Decadron, Indocin, Medrol, nicotinic acid, prednisone, Sterazolidin, Tandearil.

**Urinary incontinence.** Etrafon, Mellaril, Valium.

**Urination, difficult.** Apresoline, Benadryl, Dimetane, Donnagel-PG, Donnatal, Ornade, Periactin, Ser-Ap-Es, Tedral, Tuss-Ornade.

**Urination, diminished.** Azo Gantrisin, Equanil, Gantanol, Gantrisin, Garamycin, meprobamate.

**Urination, excessive.** Chlor-Trimeton, Polaramine, Tenuate.

**Urination, frequent.** Dimetane, Dimetapp, Elavil, Etrafon, Periactin, Triavil.

**Urination hesitancy.** Bentyl, Bentyl/phenobarbital, Combid, Librax, Librium, Marax, Norgesic.

**Urination, painful.** Bendectin, Chlor-Trimeton, Dimetapp, Drixoril, Ornade, Polaramine, Rauzide, Regroton, Salutensin, Ser-Ap-Es, Tenuate, Tuss-Ornade.

**Urine, discoloration.** Parafon Forte.

**Urine retention.** Bentyl, Bentyl/phenobarbital, Combid, Demerol, Dimetane, Elavil, Etrafon, Marax, Mellaril, Norgesic, Periactin, Sinequan, Talwin, Thorazine, Tofranil, Triavil, Valium.

**Uveitis.** Hydropres, Regroton, reserpine, Salutensin, Ser-Ap-Es.

**Vaginal bleeding.** Indocin.

**Vaginal discharge.** Keflex.

**Vision blurring.** Aldoril, Ambenyl Expectorant, Antivert, Artane, Bellergal, Benadryl, Bendectin, Bentyl, Bentyl/phenobarbital, Butazolidin, Butazolidin Alka, Combid, Compazine, Dalmane, Dimetane, Donnagal-PG, Donnatal, Diupres, Diuril, Doriden, Elavil, Etrafon, Hydrodiuril, Indocin, Lanoxin, Lasix, Librax, Librium, Mellaril, Norgesic, Periactin, Phenergan preparations, Placidyl, Pro-Banthine, Regroton, reserpine, Salutensin, Serax, Sinequan, Stelazine, Sterazolidin, Talwin, Tandearil, Tigan, Tofranil, Tranxene, Triaminic, Triavil.

**Vision, color disturbance of.** Aldoril, Esidrix, Hydrodiuril, Hygroton, Rauzide, Regroton, Salutensin.

**Vision disturbance.** Darvon preparations, Demerol, Dimetapp, Equanil, Inderal, meprobamate, Ornade, quinidine sulfate, Tuss-Ornade.

**Vision, double.** Ambenyl Expectorant, Benadryl, Dimetane, Periactin, Polaramine, Serax.

**Voice deepening.** Aldactazide, Aldactone.

**Vomiting blood.** Butazolidin, Butazolidin Alka, Sterazolidin, Tandearil.

**Weakness.** Aldactazide, Aldomet, Aldoril, Artane, Bentyl, Bentyl/phenobarbital, Cyclospasmol, Dalmane, Darvon preparations, Diabinese, Diupres, Diuril, Drixoril, Dyazide, Elavil, Endrix, Equanil, Etrafon, Hydrodiuril, Hygroton, Inderal, Isordil, Lanoxin, Lasix, meprobamate, nitroglycerin, Norgesic, Ornade, Peritrate, Polaramine, Rauzide, Regroton, Salutensin, Ser-Ap-Es, Sinequan, Talwin, Tofranil, Tolinase, Triavil, Tuss-Ornade.

**Weight gain/loss.** Aldomet, Aldoril, Atromid-S, Demulen, Diupres, Hydropres, Mellaril, Norlestrin preparations, Oracon preparations, Ortho-Novum preparations, Ovral, Ovulen 21, Rauzide, Regroton, reserpine, Ritalin, Salutensin, Ser-Ap-Es, Thorazine.

**Wheezing.** Ambenyl Expectorant, Dimetane, Periactin.

# About the Author

LAWRENCE GALTON is a noted medical writer and editor and a former visiting professor at Purdue University. He is a columnist for the Washington Star Syndicate and *Family Circle,* and his articles frequently appear in *The New York Times Magazine, Reader's Digest, Parade,* and other national publications. He is the author of more than a dozen other books.